Multi–Agent Systems for Healthcare Simulation and Modeling:
Applications for System Improvement

Raman Paranjape
University of Regina, Canada

Asha Sadanand
University of Guelph, Canada

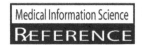

MEDICAL INFORMATION SCIENCE REFERENCE

Hershey · New York

Director of Editorial Content: Kristin Klinger
Senior Managing Editor: Jamie Snavely
Assistant Managing Editor: Michael Brehm
Publishing Assistant: Sean Woznicki
Typesetter: Jamie Snavely
Cover Design: Lisa Tosheff
Printed at: Yurchak Printing Inc.

Published in the United States of America by
        Medical Information Science Reference (an imprint of IGI Global)
        701 E. Chocolate Avenue
        Hershey PA 17033
        Tel: 717-533-8845
        Fax: 717-533-8661
        E-mail: cust@igi-global.com
        Web site: http://www.igi-global.com/reference

Library of Congress Cataloging-in-Publication Data

Multi-agent systems for healthcare simulation and modeling : applications for
system improvement / Raman Paranjape and Asha Sadanand, editors.
       p. ; cm.
 Includes bibliographical references and index.
 Summary: "This book provides theoretical frameworks and the latest empirical
research findings used by medical professionals in the implementation of
multi-agent systems"--Provided by publisher.
 ISBN 978-1-60566-772-0 (hardcover)
 1. Artificial intelligence--Medical applications. 2. Intelligent agents
(Computer software) I. Paranjape, Raman. II. Sadanand, Asha.
 [DNLM: 1. Delivery of Health Care--methods. 2. Models, Theoretical. 3.
Systems Theory. W 84.1 M961 2010]
 R859.7.A78M85 2010
 610.285'63--dc22
                         2009021413

British Cataloguing in Publication Data
A Cataloguing in Publication record for this book is available from the British Library.

Table of Contents

Section 3
Physician/Patient Support Systems

Section 4
Population Modeling Systems

Detailed Table of Contents

Section 1
Overview of Healthcare System Issues

Venkat Sadanand, University of Saskatchewan, Canada

This chapter reviews the current practices of healthcare delivery in three economically advanced countries namely Canada, U.S.A., and U.K. The review shows that medico-legal and technological prowess may not translate into a healthier life and better healthcare delivery. The chapter argues that poor allocation of ample resources is tantamount to resource insufficiency and cites anonymous but true cases of patients to illustrate the salient points.

Asha B. Sadanand, University of Guelph, Canada

This chapter examines the compatibility of the objectives of universality and public funding which are two important pillars of the Canadian health care system, with the objectives of cost effectiveness and more generally economic efficiency. Author recommends a market-based mechanism that utilizes mobile agents representing patients and their medical needs. The agents participates in virtual auctions using a needs based ranking as the currency for making bids in order to incorporate the basic goals of universality and public funding.

Simerjit Gill, University of Regina, Canada & TRLabs Regina, Canada
Raman Paranjape, University of Regina, Canada & TRLabs Regina, Canada

This chapter reviews and summarizes eight selected paper in the area of agent-based healthcare systems. The objective of the summaries is to provide an overview of recent research work in the area and to examine the characteristics of agent-based healthcare applications. The chapter also briefly discusses reasons for adopting agent-based simulation and modeling over traditional modeling techniques.

Section 2
Healthcare Modeling Systems

Chapter 4

Raman Paranjape, University of Regina, Canada & TRLabs Regina, Canada
Simerjit Gill, University of Regina, Canada & TRLabs Regina, Canada

This chapter examines the paradigm that a health care system's behavior may be examined using an agent simulation in order to illuminate its macroscopic characteristics and the effects of policy on its over all operation. Authors propose the development of a health care system model in which agents mimic the behavior of the key components of the system. These components interact and engage each other in a manor analogous to the operation of the health care system. This chapter present results from the development of a diabetic patient agent model, the development of an agent-based neurosurgery ward bed allocation system, and the development of an agent-based scheduling system that may be used to allocate resources within the health care system.

Chapter 5

Q. Peng, University of Manitoba, Canada
Q. Niu, University of Manitoba, Canada
Y. Xie, University of Manitoba, Canada
T. ElMekkawy, University of Manitoba, Canada

This chapter introduces the method of using simulation and agent-based technologies to enable a better understanding of the patient flow to improve the process performance in healthcare. The proposed method is used to identify the existing problem and to evaluate proposed solutions for the problem of the operating room (OR) at Winnipeg Health Sciences Centre. The chapter identifies issues including patient flows, operation schedules, demand and capacity of the system and the configuration of resources required. An optimum scheduling is proposed for the OR operation to shorten the patient waiting time.

Chapter 6

Xiaoqin Zhang, University of Massachusetts Dartmouth, USA
Haiping Xu, University of Massachusetts Dartmouth, USA
Bhavesh Shrestha, University of Massachusetts Dartmouth, USA

This chapter presents an integrated approach for modeling, designing and implementing a multi-agent health care simulation system using Role-based Agent Development Environment (RADE). The chapter describes the definition of role classes and agent classes, as well as the automatic agent generation process and also illustrate the coordination problem and present a rule-based coordination approach. In the end, the chapter presents present a runtime scenario of this health care simulation system, which demonstrates that dynamic task allocation can be achieved through the creation of role instances and the mapping from role instances to agents.

Section 3
Physician/Patient Support Systems

Chapter 7

David Isern, University Rovira i Virgili, Italy
Antonio Moreno, University Rovira i Virgili, Italy

This chapter focuses on the execution of Clinical guidelines (CGs) and describes the design and implementation of an agent-based platform in which the actors involved in health care coordinate their activities to perform the complex task of guideline enactment.

Chapter 8

Luigi Benedicenti, University of Regina, Canada
Chitsutha Soomlek, University of Regina, Canada

This chapter introduces an agent-based wellness visualization system. The visualization system integrates and analyzes health information collected from existing portable health monitoring devices, users, and other existing health information resources. Authors propose that using the visualization system the individual will have a better understanding in personal wellness and will be encouraged to be aware of both personal and public's health. The chapter shows initial results that indicate that the proof of concept of the research will provide direct benefits to the public, research communities, and enterprises.

Chapter 9

Vijay Kumar Mago, DAV College, India
M. Syamala Devi, Panjab University, India
Ajay Bhatia, CTIM&IT, India
Ravinder Mehta, Mehta Childcare Center, India

This chapter presents a novel approach of applying Probabilistic Neural Network (PNN) to classify the childhood disease and their respective medical specialist. The system presented in this chapter imitates the behavior of a pediatrician while selecting super specialist doctor. The aim of this chapter is to design the Multi-agent system, in which the software agents interact with each other to diagnose a disease and decide the treatment plan(s).

Section 4
Population Modeling Systems

Chapter 13

Georgiy Bobashev, RTI International, Russia
Andrei Borshchev, XJ Technologies, Russia

In this chapter, authors describe modeling approaches that consider human behaviour as it relates to health care using software agents. The chapter presents examples that demonstrate how accounting for the social network structure changes the dynamics of infectious disease, how social hierarchy affects the chances of getting HIV, how the use of low dead-space syringe reduces the risk of HIV transmission, and how emergency departments could function more efficiently when real-time activities are simulated. The chapter also discusses data needs and future applications for this method.

Foreword

AGENT SYSTEMS FOR HEALTH CARE SIMULATION AND MODELING

Agent systems is a major area of research in computer science and an extremely rewarding technology for the development of applications across a wide variety of domains. For example, agent research and development in medicine and healthcare has been the focus of a few volumes[1] and several international workshops: ECCAI (2002), CAEPIA-03 (2003), Agentcities ID-3 (2003), AgentLink Technical Forum (2004), ECCAI (2004), IJCAI (2005), ECCAI (2006), AAMAS (2008).

An agent is a computer system capable of flexible autonomous action in dynamic and unpredictable domains. Communities of agents, acting together in multi-agent systems, emerged in the 1990's as one of the most vibrant and important areas of research into how to handle the ever increasing complexity of computer systems. Indeed, agent technology is now well-established as an efficient and effective approach in many application domains relevant to medicine and healthcare. These include: ambient intelligence (electronic environments sensitive and responsive to the presence of people); electronic patient records; medical diagnosis; patient monitoring and treatment; resource and task coordination; Semantic Web (systems to share data, and to coordinate and provide services over the World Wide Web); and many others.

A particularly fruitful area of agent technology research and development is that of agent-based modeling and simulation, and in this book Raman Paranjape and Asha Sadanand have brought together an interesting set of papers that discuss the many practical issues that arise in building such applications in medicine and healthcare. However, the papers are not simply focused on medical and healthcare domains: they also succeed in raising a number of practical and theoretical issues of wide relevance to the general field of agent research.

One might ask, what is the relationship between *modeling* and *simulation*? More often than not the terms are used interchangeably but traditionally there is a difference. A model is a simplified representation or abstraction of a system at some particular point in time or space intended to promote understanding of the real system, whereas a simulation is the manipulation of a model in such a way that it operates on time or space to compress it, thus enabling one to perceive the interactions that would not otherwise be apparent because of their separation in time or space. So typically an abstract model of a particular system is developed and then a computer program or group of programs, usually on a network of computers, attempts to simulate the model. In fact, computer simulations have become a useful part of mathematical modeling of many natural systems to gain insight into the operation of those systems, or to observe their behavior. While computer simulations might use some algorithms from purely mathematical models, computers can combine simulations with reality or actual events, such as generating input responses, to simulate test subjects who are no longer present. As the missing test subjects are being simulated the system they use could be the actual equipment, revealing performance limits or defects in long-term use by the simulated users.

So why is agent technology an appropriate approach to modeling and simulation? There are several reasons. First, as mentioned above, many of the situations and scenarios that we wish to model have always been or are becoming too complex for traditional modeling approaches to be effective. In such cases the data and/or resources required to undertake a task are so varied and distributed in often non-standard forms that traditional methods would be too difficult or too time-consuming to be feasibly employed. Second, it has become possible to collect data at finer levels of granularity and organize that data into highly efficient databases, which can be used by simulated at a micro-level of detail not previously possible. And last, the computational power required is either already available or fast becoming so.

Many aspects of medicine and healthcare are modeled/simulated in the volume, which cover these broad areas:

- Physiological processes are simulated in order to diagnose disorders, such as diabetes, childhood diseases, kidney function, HIV and avian flu.
- Activities in health care are simulated in order to allocate scarce resources or determine states of physical or mental health, requiring the collection of data from diverse sources such as patient records, monitoring devices, and hospital resource databases.
- Roles and tasks in health care organizations are modeled and simulated in order to coordinate human resource allocation and enact clinical guidelines.

Thus, we see in this volume a valuable presentation of a range of projects and a persuasive demonstration of the types of applications and services that agent-based modeling and simulation can implement. Paranjape is to be congratulated for editing the papers into such a stimulating book, which is likely to be the forerunner of much more work in this field.

ENDNOTE

[1] Applications of Software Agent Technology in the Health Care Domain (Whitestein Series, 2003), e-Health: Application of Computing Sciences in Medicine and Health Care (Instituto Politécnico Nacional, Mexico, 2003), Agents Applied in Health Care (AI Communications, 2005).

Professor John Nealon
www.johnnealon.com

John Nealon is currently undertaking external examination and consultancy in higher education, and is a Visiting Professor. He was formerly Head of the School of Computing and Mathematical Sciences, Associate Dean of the School of Technology, and Chair of the Department of Computing at Oxford Brookes University. He studied pure mathematics at the University of Sussex and trained to become a teacher. He later gained a degree in Psychology (Open University) and a masters degree in Computer Science (Brunel University). He is a member of the British Computer Society (BCS) and the Association for Computing Machinery (ACM) and formerly an executive committee member of the Council of Professors and Head of Computing (CPHC), the Subject Body for University Computing in Great Britain. He was the founding head of the Intelligent Systems Research Group which developed into groups undertaking research in applied formal methods, natural computation, computer vision and web technology.

Preface

The challenges of improving healthcare systems through the use of information technology are many. However, the potential rewards of helping society and human condition are also great. Agent systems can have a real and significant impact in healthcare because healthcare systems are innately complex and a paradigm which is sufficiently sophisticated is needed when simulating these systems. The autonomy of agents, in a multi-agent system, naturally and logically maps into actors, components, and systems within healthcare. However, while the potential is great, the actual impact of agent simulation is currently still limited to primarily research focused endeavors. With this book we begin the process of moving the research closer to the practice. We do this because of the steady advances in agent simulations and the perspective that healthcare is moving more and more towards embracing technology and is part of the solution for effective and efficient services.

In this book, we present work from researchers around the world who describe their advances in agent-based systems in order to model and simulate components of the healthcare system. In order to put the collected works of these agent researchers in some type of context, we invited a physician to tell about the needs and challenges of healthcare environment. We also asked an economist to discuss the issues around resources and the mechanisms to value and rank factors within the healthcare system. Lastly, to enhance the understanding of the progress to date, a summary of a number of important research papers in the area of agents in healthcare is included.

We are truly fortunate to have such a competent and diverse list of contributing authors for this book. The works presented span the wide breadth of agent application in healthcare looking at both practical and theoretical issues. The contributions are sure to catch the interest of both researchers in the field of agent systems and also the practitioners of healthcare in terms of both active physicians and those involved in the administration of healthcare systems.

This book is organized into four sections. The first section is titled "An Overview of Healthcare Systems Issues" and includes a chapter by an active neuro-surgeon who is familiar with many aspects of healthcare delivery in Canada, the United States and the United Kingdom. This is followed by a chapter on the economics of resource allocation within healthcare. The final chapter in this section is a review of eight recent papers in agent-based systems in healthcare.

The second section is titled "Healthcare Modeling Systems" and includes a chapter on the development of a large multi-faceted healthcare model and its various components. This is followed by a chapter on an agent modeling system of an operating theatre. We follow with a more theoretical chapter of how to do modeling in healthcare using role-based systems.

The third section is titled "Physician/Patient Support Systems" and this section begins with a chapter on a multi-agent system that automates clinical guidelines. This is followed by a chapter that focuses on modeling wellness for both the patient as well as the physician. The next two chapters discuss agent systems to help pick specialists and to help medical personnel learn about the function of organs using an agent simulation.

The last section of the book is titled "Population Modeling Systems" and begins with a chapter focused on modeling mental health and the retrieval of appropriate information to manage and control this illness. The next chapter in this section looks at the use of agent systems to help understand the issues around healthcare service and delivery in developing countries, and the final chapter is focused on modeling social behaviors in populations using agents for illnesses such as HIV.

Chapters for this book were solicited by a public call on a number of web sites, list-servers and through direct email to active researchers. Authors were asked to submit a chapter proposal and the proposals were reviewed by the editors. We received 15 proposals and requested chapters from 14 researchers. The completed chapters were first reviewed by the editors and then double blind reviewed by other contributors. Of the 14 submitted chapters one was rejected and one was withdrawn by the authors. Thus 12 chapters were accepted for the final manuscript and enhanced by the authors based on the reviewers' comments. Ultimately, in consultation with the publisher, an additional review chapter was added in order to enhance the coverage of the subject matter. Thus, the final manuscript contains 13 chapters of original, new research contributions and one review chapter of recent research results.

Acknowledgment

The editors are grateful to Ms. Heather Probst and Mr. Tyler Heath of IGI Global for their advice and guidance throughout the entire book editing process. We are most grateful to Mr. Simerjit Gill for his detailed organization of all the chapters and for the final collation of the manuscript. We thank the University of Regina and TRLabs Regina for their support of this endeavor.

Raman Paranjape
University of Regina, Canada

Asha Sadanand
University of Guelph, Canada

Section 1
Overview of Healthcare System Issues

Chapter 1
Current Practices in Select Healthcare Systems

Venkat Sadanand
University of Saskatchewan, Canada

ABSTRACT

In this chapter, current practices of healthcare delivery in three economically advanced countries will be reviewed. Is healthcare delivery commensurate with economic prosperity? Countries with technological and economic advantages may be better poised to deliver healthcare efficiently. However, this is not the case in fact. The following review will show that medico-legal and technological prowess may not translate into a healthier life and better healthcare delivery. It will be argued that poor allocation of ample resources is tantamount to resource insufficiency. The chapter will cite anonymous but true cases of patients to illustrate the salient points.

INTRODUCTION

In this chapter, current practices of healthcare delivery in three G8 countries will be reviewed. Does economic prosperity lead to a better quality of delivered healthcare? Countries with technological and economic advantages may seem to be better poised to deliver healthcare efficiently. However, this may not be the case in fact. The following review will show that medico-legal and technological prowess may not translate into a healthier life and better healthcare delivery. Distribution of wealth does not necessarily correlate with the distribution of health. It will be argued that poor allocation of ample resources is tantamount to resource insufficiency.

In the attempt to provide improved healthcare for its citizens, many of the G8 countries have tried everything in the spectrum from a publicly funded healthcare system to a fully private system. Common to all these are the intimidating waiting lists for doctors' appointments or surgeries. Some may argue that a waiting list is an inevitable byproduct of an economically efficient healthcare system. Patients who are deemed to be surgical candidates are obviously quite ill and possibly in pain. If you ask such a patient if a waiting list is acceptable,

DOI: 10.4018/978-1-60566-772-0.ch001

the answer would be a resounding rejection of such a concept.

The issue at hand is more than an argument about what constitutes a welfare system. The concept of economic efficiency in healthcare is a red herring. To be efficient from an economic standpoint may not be the same as efficiency in the distribution of healthcare. One may argue that a competitive market resulting in economic efficiency may result in a distribution of wealth with people holding extremes of wealth or poverty. Inequities in health distribution may be a similar outcome of an economically efficient system. The United States of America is an example of this disparity in healthcare. There can be no such tradeoffs in healthcare. In an efficient healthcare system, one cannot accept a dichotomy with some people having ready access to healthcare and some having none. The existence of such a state of society is, admittedly, a failure of the healthcare system. Society must see to it that the last person who needs healthcare receives it.

Some may be quick to interpret this as an advocacy of socialism. In truth however, there is no such thing as socialism in healthcare. Socialism is an economic concept. Wealth distribution is an economic concept. But an equitable distribution of healthcare is as much a necessity as the distribution of oxygen. Everyone ages and every aging person is a potential healthcare consumer. Healthcare is a prime example of market failure. Therefore the allocation of healthcare by free markets is inherently inefficient. The reason a market for healthcare fails is due to (a) the existence of externalities discussed below and (b) the existence of transaction costs and asymmetric information. President Barrack Obama and Secretary of State Hillary Clinton have both strongly emphasized the philosophy that "every American has the right to affordable healthcare" during their 2008 presidential campaigns. Yet a waiting list is a denial of that essential service of healthcare.

In such a context what is a surgical or patient care waiting list? One may have a society where all its citizens have access to healthcare but are placed in a waiting list to see their doctor or to receive appropriate surgical intervention. How does this differ from a society where some have immediate treatment of their illnesses and some do not? The emergence and establishment of surgical waiting lists must therefore be considered a cost to society due to pain and suffering of those waiting patients. The impact on the patients' quality of life and society's productivity is obvious. In the written words of the Supreme Court of Canada Chief justice Beverly McLachlin in the 2005 *Chaoulli v. Quebec (Attorney General)* case, "Access to a waiting list is not access to healthcare."

Consider, for example, patient D.L. from Canada who has a brain tumor compressing on her optic nerve. She was virtually blind in one eye and was losing vision in the other. She was placed on a waiting list and it took several months for the surgery to decompress the tumor. On the day of the scheduled surgery, she was "bumped" and the surgery was cancelled due to unavailability of beds. One month later, her vision now worse, she was taken to surgery emergently. As another example, in the specialty of ophthalmology, the mean waiting time for cataract surgery in Canada was 17 weeks in 2005 (Conner-Spady, B.L., Sanmugasunderam, S., et al., 2005). Patients in the U.K. have had to endure long waiting lists for surgery, some as long as six to nine months (Martin, R., Sterne, J.A.C., Gunnel, D., et al., 2003). Even in the U.S. with a mostly private healthcare system, waiting lists are not uncommon (Hurst, J., & Siciliani, L., 2003).

How then do these waiting lists emerge? Can anything be done to improve such a system which tolerates the pain incurred by waiting patients in stark contradiction to its mission to care for the health and suffering of its citizens? In the Supreme Court of Canada judgment (Chaoulli v. Quebec, 2005) above, all justices of the Supreme Court agreed that such delays can affect the patient physically and psychologically and may cause irreparable harm.

This chapter will compare the healthcare systems of Canada, the United Kingdom and the United States of America. The purpose of this comparison is not only to understand the genesis of surgical waiting lists in economically advanced countries, but also to find solutions by increasing efficiencies in existing allocation of resources rather than additional capital investment. For example, it is seen in what follows that increasing capital expenditures or hospital capacity does not strongly correlate with improved healthcare status in the U.K. but it does in the U.S. This is possibly related to the way the healthcare system is financed.

CANADA

An attempt at universal healthcare was first legislated in Canada in the province of Saskatchewan in 1946. This eventually led to the Medical Care Act in 1966, which provided a framework for each province to offer a universal healthcare system. The success of this led to the Canada Health Act of 1984 and a commitment by the federal government to support the well-developed healthcare system predicated on the principles of universality, portability, comprehensiveness, public administration and accessibility (Lewis, S., Donaldson, C., et al., 2001). Thus, the government insures every Canadian and this insurance is portable anywhere in Canada. The Canada Health Act requires that every hospital and physician should be financed only by the government with no individual user charges. In addition, there cannot be any third party coverage for these services nor can a hospital or physician accept third party insurance for their services for Canadians. The fiduciary responsibility of healthcare delivery is relegated to individual provinces. However, there is a complex revenue sharing agreement between the federal government and the provinces that serves as a financial spigot, which can be turned off if individual provinces do not abide by the Act. This could

potentially threaten the transfer of funds from the federal to the provincial government should a province choose to accept third party insurance or charge extra billings to patients.

Year after year the federal government sits with the provinces to renegotiate the transfer payment agreements. The little band-aid changes to the transfer agreements negotiated during these meetings did not do much to fundamentally alter the efficacy of healthcare delivery. Population demographics was changing with time and the healthcare budgets were falling behind unable to respond to these changes. Eventually, there was a stagnation in the real amount of spending for healthcare in the provinces leading to nation-wide reviews of the healthcare system. This led to a series of reforms, most notably, a decentralization of healthcare budgetary decision to regional health boards (Province of Alberta, 1994).

The key requirement in the Canada Health Act is that physician and hospital services be 100% publicly financed. But the provision of these services can be private. Doctors need not be government employees. Hospitals are non-profit corporations. However, there have been some recent developments in several provinces that have to be considered in assessing their impact on patient waiting lists. (Figure 1)

The Canada Health Act governs the financial conduct of hospitals and physicians. With an aging population, there has been an increase in the relative financial outlay for prescription drugs and community care. The latter is not under the purview of the Act. For example, in 1971, the median age in Canada was 26 and in 2001 it was 37.2. In addition, the percentage of people over 65 years of age is expected to grow from 8% in 1971 to 26.5% in 2051 (Statistics Canada, n.d.)

Second, the federal and provincial governments seem to have done little to respond to changing demographics and increasing demands on the healthcare system. The regionalization system appears to have divided the accountability for patient care between the provincial governments

Figure 1. Canada: Financing of health care, 2004 (Source: Chart data from CIHI (2004) Improving the health of Canadians. Ottawa, Canadian Institute for Health Information. Chart in Marchildon GP. Health Systems in Transition: Canada. Copenhagen, WHO Regional Office for Europe on behalf of the European Observatory on Health Systems and Policies, 2005.)

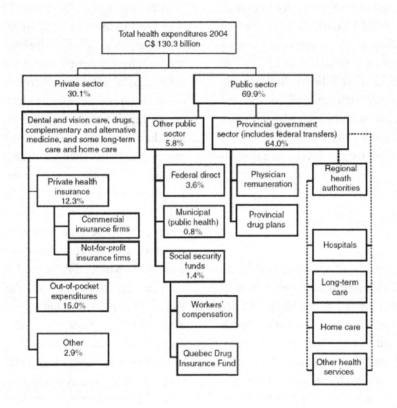

Notes:
* Percentages may not add up due to rounding.
* The distribution of expenditures between private insurance, out-of-pocket and other is based on figures from 2002.

and the regional boards. Thus, if a patient in Saskatoon needs urgent medical or surgical care of a certain kind, the regional boards seem to have no moral responsibility to provide that and, in fact, may be better off sending the patient to another province or to the U.S for that care. Patient care costs for medical care received in another province are borne by the province, not by the regional board. The way the incentives work, regional boards may as well have more services rendered to patients from outside the province and thereby use their limited resources for their immediate needs. In the economics literature this is a classic problem of what is known as 'externalities.' The best examples of these inefficiencies are derived from the polluting factory. Consider a factory that produces computer hardware. Supposing the firm installs a production process by which the chemicals used in the process of etching circuit boards and microprocessors are washed away and deposited in a nearby flowing river. Or, for that matter, pollutants may be released underground and thereby pollute the water table. In either case, the cost of polluting the river or the water table is not borne by the factory. It is indeed borne by downstream fisherman or those who consume that water. Since those costs do not enter the balance sheet of the polluting company, its production decisions, which are guided by its costs, are completely blind to the enormous costs imposed on others. Such myopic decision-making by firms are rectified by taxing the firm for it's output so that the costs of cleaning up the river or water table is seen by the firm as a tax. This will enter its balance sheet and thereby affect its production decision. Such a process is called "internalization of costs". The costs of certain decisions taken by the health boards are not borne by the health boards but accrue to the governments and the patients. Excess use of carbon-based fuels and resulting high pollution levels is another example of externalities and wrong production decisions. In the context of Canadian healthcare and the recent regionalization, these externalities must be internalized. One possible approach to achieve this is by imposing an actual or implicit tax on the regional health boards for patient pain and suffering from waiting lists. The problem, however, with this approach is that health boards are not for-profit organizations and such taxes will do little to internalize the externalities.

The next approach to rectifying the problem of waiting lists is to view the situation from another perspective. The literature on Game Theory has looked into the problem of incentives in complex contracts under asymmetric information. One of the most popular theory is the principal-agent model. In these situations, one individual (the principal) contracts with another individual (the agent) to undertake a task whose outcome will affect the welfare of the principal and when the principal lacks information about the efforts or production process known only to the agent. In the context of Canadian healthcare, the Federal government is the principal who hands over a sum of money to the agent who is the provincial government who has to undertake the task of providing healthcare to its citizens. The Ministry of Health

in the provincial government then pays its agent (the regional health boards) to deliver healthcare. So one has to examine the incentives to perform in a model where there is one principal-agent relationship (Federal Government – Provincial Government) and this, in turn, results in another principal-agent relationship (Provincial Government – Regional Health Board). The final output affects the welfare of the patients. The broader questions is: how can one structure incentives at all levels so that the healthcare is delivered with efficiency and patient welfare is maximized? This question and its solutions have been well-addressed by "Contract Theory". In their book on Economics, Organization and Management, Milgrom and Roberts (1992) develop the conditions for designing an efficient contract. One of the conditions is called the "informativeness principle". This states that any measure of performance that reveals information about the effort level chosen by the agent should be included in the compensation contract. Hence, waiting lists and underemployment of specialists are clearly monitored data. By including them in the Federal transfer of funds for healthcare, the two agents are given the proper incentives to reduce waiting times and hence patient suffering. Thus, if Federal transfer of funds are sensitive to patient waiting times and availability of specialists, then Provincial governments and regional health boards will find ways to reduce those waiting lists and provide an adequate supply of specialists for the patients. Short waiting lists should be rewarded with higher levels of funding while long waiting lists should trigger decreased funding. While this sounds counter-intuitive, the incentives it provides in a principal-agent setting will nevertheless achieve efficiency in healthcare delivery.

There is also the issue of strategic representation or misrepresentation by regional health boards with the current incentives. Larger waiting lists will provide sufficient rationale for the heath boards to request a budget increase. If the Provincial and Federal governments award such an increase, pursuit of higher budgets will result in increasing waiting lists and chronic shortage of specialists.

Finally, in some provinces, marginal privatization has developed. Day surgery clinics have sprouted that offer surgeries for which the patient does not require hospital admission.

How then do these factors affect healthcare delivery in Canada? First, in contrast to a market driven healthcare system, a public healthcare system ignores the realities of demand and supply. Supply decisions are made with little concern for current or future demand. This leads to rationing and wait lists. Patients have to wait for diagnostic imaging, surgery, hospital emergency room and even access to a primary care physician (Esmail N., Hazel, M., & Walker, M.A., 2008). From the time a specialist decided to undertake treatment to the time the patient actually receives treatment is a waiting time during which all parties agree treatment is needed, but treatment is however not given. In the specialty of neurosurgery, for example, the 2008 waiting time from decision to treat to treatment is 19.4 weeks, which is one of the highest in any OECD country (Milgrom, P., & Roberts, J., 1992). Mean 2008 waiting time for an MRI scan was 9.4 weeks. Second, the availability of modern medical technology is restricted. For example, neuroendovascular techniques have evolved into a subspecialty in neurosurgery several years ago and most countries have nation-wide centers of excellence for these modalities of treatment for cerebral aneurysms. However, the province of Saskatchewan has yet (at the time of writing this book) to have a neuroendovascular facility, which is already the standard of care throughout the world. Third, the recent trend of new private day-surgery centers have eased the burden on surgical waiting lists and the government has so far looked the other way as these centers have clearly improved patient access to critical surgeries and physicians.

In summary, the Canadian healthcare system is founded on principles that are now ignored.

Patients do not have timely access to healthcare and not having such access is, indeed, denial of healthcare. Suffering while on a surgical waiting list can only be appreciated by those who suffer, and least by those whose administrative decisions lead to waiting lists.

UNITED STATES OF AMERICA

In contrast to the Canadian healthcare system, the U.S. has adopted a market-based system. Private insurance companies cover a majority of individuals for their healthcare costs. Employers pay for the coverage. But employment is not a guarantee of health coverage. In 2005, nearly 15% of employees had no health insurance coverage from their employers (DeNavas-Walt, C.B.P., & Smith, J., 2007). In 2007, nearly 45 million Americans or about 16% of the population have no insurance coverage at all. Private insurance covered 68% of the population (DeNavas-Walt, C.B.P., & Smith, J., 2008). The insurance companies and the government depending upon the coverage held by the patients compensate physicians and hospitals. Most hospitals are private enterprises. Thus the purchase of medical equipment is viewed as an investment by the hospital, which reaps greater returns on the investment if more patients use the equipment. This is in contrast to Canada where new equipment is often viewed as a drain on a fixed budget. As a result of this availability of medical technology in the United States, it is currently one of the most advanced nations in the world in healthcare technologies. For example, in 1990, the number of MRI units per million population is 3.69 in the United States compared to 0.46 in Canada (DeNavas-Walt, C.B.P., & Smith, J., 2008). (Figure 2)

Despite market forces at work, patients in the United States do encounter waiting lists for surgeries, emergency medical care and physician appointments. Canada's rationing is supply based while the United States rations based on price.

Figure 2. United States: Financing of health care, 2003 (Source: OCED Secretariat, 2003)

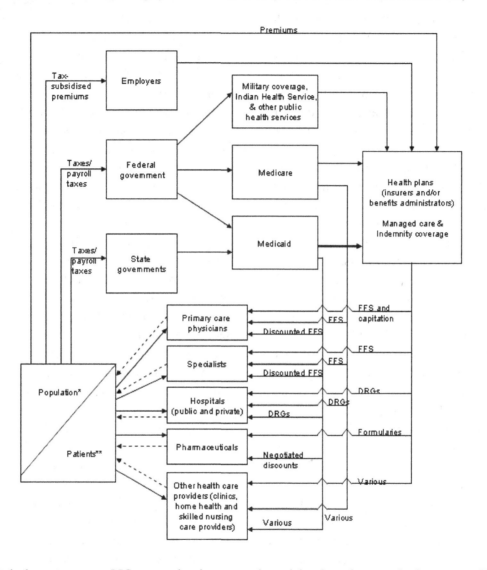

Note: FFS is fee-for-service payment DRGs are case-based payments to hospitals based on a diagnosis-related group system. *Health care for the 14% of the population lacking health insurance coverage is financed by publicly subsidized charity care and patients' out-of-pocket payments to health care providers.

**Patient cost-sharing arrangements vary widely by type of coverage. Indemnity coverage generally included deductibles and co-insurance. Managed care plans often require co-payments for certain services.

That is, those who cannot afford healthcare are doomed to a parallel inferior system where waiting lists and poor accessibility are the norm. In a market-based system, the allocation of resources is shifted in favor of those sectors where the marginal returns are higher. In 1986 the United States Congress passed an Act called EMTALA (Emergency Medical Treatment and Active Labor Act) requiring hospitals and ambulance services to provide care to anyone needing emergency treatment regardless of their ability to pay. Hence the uninsured patients crowd emergency rooms for routine ailments that are best managed in physician offices. This generates wait times for insured patients. The same price rationing consequences apply to surgical wait times. Although these times are much smaller than in Canada and the U.K. they nevertheless exist and represents a failure of a market based system.

A recent OECD study found that the major factors reducing waiting times for elective surgery are: higher number of acute care beds, higher surgical activity levels in hospitals, fee-for-service remuneration, a higher healthcare budget and a lack of fixed budgets for hospitals. Surprisingly, the study demonstrated that a younger population is not a factor in reducing waiting times. In a multivariate analysis in the same study it was found that the number of acute care beds and the number of physicians and specialists had the largest impact on waiting times (Fuchs, B.C., & Sokolovsky, J., 1990).

In summary, the United States does have waiting lists for elective surgeries, but the waiting times are an order of magnitude less than those in publicly funded systems. The humanitarian considerations for uninsured people, makes the system for insured people slightly inefficient. However, the principal (insurance company) – agent (doctors and hospitals) model in the United States is much closer to full efficiency than in Canada and the United Kingdom.

UNITED KINGDOM

Healthcare in the United Kingdom works under a blend of public and private systems. The National Health Service (NHS) refers to four publicly funded healthcare systems in the U.K. with its components in England, Scotland, Wales and Northern Ireland. In addition, citizens may choose to purchase private medical insurance for hospital and doctor services. In 2001, 11.5%

of the population held private medical insurance (Siciliani, L., & Hurst, J., 2003). Furthermore, 40% of adults with private medical insurance are in the top decile of income. As a percentage of total healthcare expenditure, public to private ratios were 83.3:16.7 (Laing, W., & Buisson, C., 2001). NHS does not cover all necessary medical treatment costs. The benefits are ill defined and its decisions are based on an analysis of costs and benefits of a particular medical technology, pharmaceutical or procedure. The National Institute for Clinical Excellence makes such recommendations. In some instances the health authorities may make rationing decisions. Drugs may be excluded because of poor therapeutic value or excessive costs. Employers mostly purchase private medical insurance provided by for-profit and non-profit organizations and most are group policies. NHS patients must have a referral from a GP to access secondary level care with specialists.

With poor hospital capacities and low per capita specialists figures, waiting times to see a specialist was on the average 13 weeks in 2001-2002 (Laing, W., & Buisson, C., 2001). NHS Trust hospitals had the longest waiting lists with between 52% and 83% of patients waiting longer than six months for elective surgery found in 25% of NHS hospitals (OECD Health Data, 2001). Interestingly, this study found that in contrast to the United States data, not much association was found between waiting times and hospital capacity and number of beds. Paradoxically increasing the number of specialists increased average waiting times suggesting that the supply of doctors induced demand. Individual level of employment, affluence and urgency of disease shortened waiting times. This mostly indicates the relative efficacy of the private medical insurance arm 40% of whose subscribers are in the top income decile as noted above. (Figure 3)

Figure 3. United Kingdom: Financing of health care, 1999 (Source: Health Care Systems in Transition: United Kingdom, 1999. European Observatory on Health Care Systems)

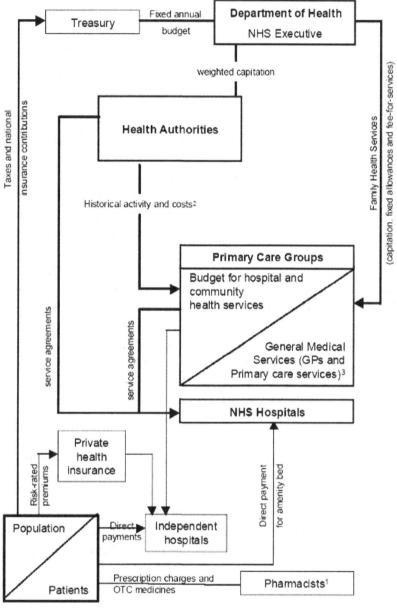

COMPARISONS

The three OECD countries discussed above have three different healthcare systems although many would argue that the U.K. and Canadian systems are closer in principle to each other than to the United States. Recent OECD health data revels some interesting differences among these three countries (Martin, R., Sterne, J.A.C., Gunnel, D., et al., 2003).

Table 1 below, gives an estimate of waiting times for surgery in the United States compared

Table 1.

Percentage of Patients Waiting > 4 months for Elective Surgery in 2001	
United States	5
Australia	23
Canada	27
New Zealand	26
United kingdom	38

to key OECD countries in 2001 (Mohan, R., Mirmirani, S., 2007).

The following comparisons of resource allocation in the three countries are from the OECD 2008 health data. (Table 2)

An Example

Given an understanding of the heathcare systems in the three countries, this section will consider as an example the generation of waiting lists in one of the provinces in Canada. We will specifically consider two kinds of surgical waiting lists: waiting lists by the specialist to see the patient after referral by a GP and patient waiting lists after a decision is made to undertake surgery.

Consider the first waiting list. Family physicians or GPs send a referral letter to the specialist. The specialist then places the patient on a clinic waiting list. This waiting list is generated due to the limited hospital and outpatient facility resources as well as the limited number of specialists that the health boards have decided to recruit. Thus, a

specialist can only run a fixed number of clinics per week. The number of clinics is independent of patient demand for referrals. There may be days when the specialist has time to see patients but the hospital and outpatient facilities do not have the resources to allow the specialist to see patients as the same resources are shared by several specialists. In one of the specialties, for example, the clinic waiting list is between 150-250 patients waiting to be seen. Patients scheduled to see a specialist may be pushed back due to a more urgent referral. This combination of triage and limited resources can render a waiting list long and increase patient dissatisfaction with the healthcare system. It also impedes timely care of patients who are suffering. Some patients wait for over a year to get to see their specialist.

Consider the second waiting list. This is divided into two parts: those patients who are placed on "the board" and those who are on an elective waiting list. The "board" is for emergency surgeries that are constrained by limited resources. When the day's scheduled surgeries are completed,

Table 2.

Countries	#CT Scanners Per 1000 Pop.	#MRI Scanners Per 1000 Pop.	Health Expenditure % GDP	Practicing Physicians Per 1000 Pop.	Male Life Expectancy at Birth	%Public Asking for Complete Rebuild of System
Canada	12	6.2	9.8	2.1	78	12
United States	33.9	26.5	15.2	3.7	75.2	34
United Kingdom	7.8	5.6	8	2.9	77.1	15

the patients on the board get their turns. Due to limited resources again, only one or in rare cases two operating rooms are allowed to run to clear the board. Board surgeries can fall under three categories: E1, E2 and E3. An E3 surgery has to be called within 24 hours. An E2 surgery has to be called within 8 hours of booking and an E1 has to be called within 1 hour of booking. In practice though an E3 can have patients waiting several days for their surgeries and, in some instances, patients have walked out of the hospital in frustration against medical advice. In addition, an E3 surgery cannot be started after midnight. An E2 surgery can only be started after the day's cases are done and an E1 case can "bump" a scheduled elective surgery usually from the same surgical specialty. A patient may join the board as an emergency arrival at the Emergency Room. That patient may be a new patient, a patient not on the scheduled waiting list or one who is already on the scheduled waiting list and his condition has deteriorated.

The second part of the second waiting list is the patients who are placed on a scheduled waiting list for elective surgery. This list is generated by the degree of urgency of the patient's ailment requiring surgery. Patients on this waiting list are called on a specific date to come for surgery. However, there is a chance that on the day of their scheduled surgery, they may be refused surgery because of limited resources on that day. They would they go back on the scheduled waiting list and once again, wait their turn. It is easy to see that the system has been patched up with disjoint solutions that disregard patient suffering while waiting and inappropriate use of limited resources.

The keys to the inefficiency in the system are the limitation of resources that is blind to demand and the sharing of these limited resources by all the surgical specialists. A surgeon may be given, for instance, 3 or 4 operating days per month. Thus, if he has 70 patients waiting for surgery, some of the patients would have to wait for 6-8 months provided none of the scheduled patients

is "bumped" by non-availability of resources on the day of surgery or none is "bumped" by a more emergent patient who entered the system through the emergency room.

CONCLUSIONS

The analysis above suggests that surgical waiting times are generated from a lack of addressing the mechanisms underlying the generation of waiting lists. Statistical studies done in each of the three countries in this chapter appear to show different independent factors affecting waiting times. Specifically, in Canada, limited number of hospital beds, limited number of specialists, limited operating times, limited medical technologies and a system operates under economic externalities can all contribute to long waiting lists and increased patient suffering. In comparing the three countries and their healthcare systems, the issues are not the relative superiority of one system versus the others. It is the degree to which each country lacks the proper incentives to achieve efficiency within its system. The issue therefore is the inadequacy of ad hoc incentives in a system without a formal modeling-based understanding of the healthcare delivery. One cannot blame a given system for the inefficiencies generated by inappropriate or inadequate contracts and incentives.

REFERENCES

Chaoulli v. Quebec (Attorney General) (2005). 2005 SCC 35. 1 S.C.R. 791, Para 123, Docket 29272, Supreme Court of Canada.

Conner-Spady, B. L., & Sanmugasunderam, S. (2005). Patient and physician perspectives of maximum acceptable waiting times for cataract surgery. *Canadian Journal of Ophthalmology*, *40*, 439–447.

DeNavas-Walt, C.B.P., & Smith, J. (2007, August). *Income, poverty, and health insurance coverage in the United States: 2006.* U.S. Census Bureau.

DeNavas-Walt, C.B.P., & Smith, J. (2008, August). *Income, poverty, and health insurance coverage in the United States: 2007.* U.S. Census Bureau.

Esmail, N., Hazel, M., & Walker, M. A. (2008). *Waiting your turn: Hospital waiting lists in Canada* (18th ed.). Fraser Institute.

Fuchs, B.C., & Sokolovsky, J. (1990, February). *The Canadian health care system, CRS Report for Congress.* Congressional Research Service: Library of Congress.

Health Data, O. E. C. D. (2001). *A comparative analysis of 30 countries CD-ROM.* Paris: OECD and CREDES.

Hurst, J., & Siciliani, L. (2003). *Tackling Excessive Waiting Times for Elective Surgery: A Comparison of Policies in Twelve OECD Countries.*

Laing, W., & Buisson, C. (2001). *Private Medical Insurance: UK market sector report 2001.* London: Laing & Buisson.

Lewis, S., & Donaldson, C. (2001). The future of healthcare in Canada. *BMJ (Clinical Research Ed.)*, *323*, 926–929. doi:10.1136/bmj.323.7318.926

Martin, R., Sterne, J. A. C., & Gunnel, D. (2003, January). NHS waiting lists and evidence of national or local failure: analysis of health service data. *BMJ (Clinical Research Ed.)*, *326*, 188. doi:10.1136/bmj.326.7382.188

Martin, R. M., & Sterne, J. A. C. (2003). NHS waiting lists and evidence of national or local failure: analysis of health service data. *BMJ (Clinical Research Ed.)*, *326*, 188–192. doi:10.1136/bmj.326.7382.188

Milgrom, P., & Roberts, J. (1992). *Economics, Organization and Management.* Englewood Cliffs, NJ: Prentice Hall.

Mohan, R., Mirmirani, S. (2007, December). *An assessment of OECD health care system using panel data analysis.*

Province of Alberta. (1994). *Regional health authorities act.* Edmonton: Queen's Printer for Alberta.

Siciliani, L., & Hurst, J. (2003). *Explaining waiting times variations for elective surgery across OECD countries.*

Statistics Canada, Estimates of Population, Canada, the Provinces and Territories (Persons), CANSIM Table No. 051-0001, Ottawa.

Chapter 2
Economic Efficiency and the Canadian Healthcare System

Asha B. Sadanand
University of Guelph, Canada

ABSTRACT

In this chapter the authors examine the compatibility of the objectives of universality and public funding which are two important pillars of the Canadian healthcare system, with the objectives of cost effectiveness and more generally economic efficiency. The authors note that under some very innocuous conditions, markets and other economic based mechanisms such as second price auctions are characterized by economic efficiency and cost effectiveness. For the particular case of healthcare, some additional features that must be considered in the design of the mechanism are that healthcare services and products are valuable if, when taken together they constitute the components of a needed procedure, and otherwise they are worthless to the individual; and timely completion of procedures is what is valued, delays and waiting not only prolong suffering but may eventually prove to be more costly to the system if the condition worsens. They recommend a market-based mechanism, encompassing these features, that utilizes mobile agents representing patients and their medical needs. In order to incorporate the basic goals of universality and public funding, the agents will participate in virtual auctions using a needs based ranking as the currency for making bids.

INTRODUCTION

A universal, publicly funded healthcare system, such as the one in Canada, has many attractive features that have general appeal. The belief that healthcare is a basic necessity, which must be provided by the state for all the citizens, is the underlying principle for universality. Public funding ensures that all people, no matter how wealthy or poor, can rely on the government for their healthcare needs.

The system has been a source of great pride for Canadians, and a reason for envy by other nations. For decades, it has served the Canadian people well in taking care of their health needs in a timely fashion

DOI: 10.4018/978-1-60566-772-0.ch002

and without a large financial burden. However, recent times have witnessed some dissatisfaction as the Canadian population is beginning to age and health costs have burgeoned. The costs, that have throughout been creeping upward, have now threatened to overtake the budget and the system has responded by lengthening waiting lists. In the case of some procedures the waiting lists have reached such proportions that patients are needlessly suffering by prolonged waiting, during the course of which, their conditions have often worsened, at times to the point where they must be treated on an emergency basis. Indeed, many patients have contracted further complications in addition to their original illness, and in rare cases died from the complications. Allowing the patient to worsen generally has irreversible implications on treatment, and ultimately on outcomes; quite perversely, it can also increase the total cost of treatment for the patient, further aggravating the budget problem of healthcare provision. This escalation of both cost and suffering for the patient could have been prevented had the patient been treated in a timely fashion.

In effect, the much touted public healthcare system is now forcing Canadians to accept a compromised level of service by requiring protracted waiting followed by late treatment, and possibly at higher cost. This is certainly not fitting of a world class standard of care, and it is certainly not what was envisioned by the founders that first drafted this policy.

In trying to find solutions, three main strategies arise, and ideally, all three strategies should be used in forming and maintaining the best healthcare programs. The first and most obvious is to increase the budget. This has proven to be quite difficult when taxpayers are already burdened with fairly high taxes. Nevertheless, a somewhat higher budget does seem inevitable in the present situation. Indeed, it should be expected that supplying healthcare for an aging population, should cost more. However, in the future, such demographics should be anticipated. A scheme should be insti-

tuted whereby rather than burdening the current work force of younger individuals with the large healthcare costs of the top heavy aging cohort, the healthcare system avoids periods of crisis and recovery as the population demographics swing from aging to youthful populations. To achieve this steady cost for healthcare, a fund must be developed which would accumulate a total for each person summing to the average expected lifetime healthcare costs. An important part of developing such a system would be to have access to accurate data on average lifetime health costs, and to be able to make accurate predictions of future average lifetime health costs.

Another direction is to reduce the demand for healthcare by urging the public to adopt healthier lifestyles. There are certainly many initiatives being taken in this direction by both private individuals and organizations, as well as through Canadian public policy. There is currently greater awareness in the general public about maintaining a healthy active lifestyle than ever before. The government has also been promoting healthy living through massive advertising campaigns and economic incentives, such as preferential tax treatment or deductions for the cost of children's fitness participation. However, these are long horizon initiatives, and the benefits of these efforts in terms of improved health and lower medical costs will only be realized much farther in the future.

Finally, there is the strategy of ensuring that, given the limited budget that does exist for healthcare, it is allocated in a manner that achieves the maximum benefit at the lowest possible cost. In this chapter we will focus on this last strategy. This is not to say that the other two directions are not worthwhile, but rather that we do not expect to see much immediate relief by utilizing them, although they definitely have a necessary role in the proper long term functioning of a carefully crafted healthcare program.

The concept of a universal publicly funded healthcare system is very idealistic, and as such there are some inherent difficulties that must be overcome in order that the scheme works smoothly. The first and foremost issue has to do with the limited budget. The reality, of a budget that is limited, is that we are immediately confronted with the difficult questions of choices: Which treatments are to have a priority, which procedures are covered and which ones are not; among all the different needy patients, which shall we treat first and which patients will be treated later, all become very relevant questions.

These difficult questions that must be answered, are not exclusively encountered in the healthcare sector, but are issues that arise for most goods and services. We are accustomed to resolving these questions (in the other contexts) by allowing markets to determine the allocation of who gets how much of each good. Individuals decide whether to buy a certain good based on the price and whether, given the price, it is worthwhile to buy the good as compared to the next best alternative purchase. Suppliers are willing to provide quantities of the goods at different prices based on their costs; generally prices cover cost and more because suppliers who may be providing specialized goods or services often have incurred some set-up costs that must be covered in the long run. It is competition that keeps in check the suppliers' motivation to obtain prices that exceed their costs. The price for a good adjusts depending on demand until the amount demanded is exactly equal to the amount that can be supplied at that price. At that point the market is said to be in equilibrium. Once the market is in equilibrium, the people that end up buying are those that value the good more than the price, and those who do not buy, value the good less. Thus, the market achieves an allocation where the people are neatly divided into two groups; the high valuation people who consume the good, and the low valuation people who do not; and we notice that this maximizes the sum over all people, of the value of having this good. Further, if we extend the market to all goods, then the overall value to all people for all goods is maximized.

We are interested in knowing whether the market allocation is a good allocation: that is, whether the right people end up with the right amounts of goods or whether one could redistribute to achieve a better allocation. Economists have explored this issue and come up with the notion of economic efficiency.[1] The idea here is that an allocation is good (efficient) if it is impossible to alter the allocation and find that all people are at least as happy with their situation as before, and some strictly happier. This is called allocative efficiency. Starting with an arbitrary allocation, if we had to go from person to person, asking about alternative allocations, to verify allocative efficiency of the initial allocation, it would be an almost impossible undertaking, particularly if the number of people were large: the sheer volume of people that must be consulted and the number of questions that must be asked about all the possible alternative allocations will be endless.

Happily there is another way to verify efficiency. Economic theory shows that given certain conditions[2] market equilibrium is always efficient.[3] To see this intuitively, suppose that initially the market determined the allocation of all goods. Now suppose one attempted to reallocate by taking a unit of a good away from a person and returning the price to them, and at the same time allowing another person who did not initially buy, to buy the one unit of the good at the market price. The first person would be able to spend the money on something else if they liked. But since they did not originally buy any alternative good, it must have been that their value for the alternative good was not as high as that for the good they actually bought, leaving them worse off as compared to how they were before the reallocation. Similarly, the new person to whom the good is being reassigned would not find it worthwhile to pay the price for the good, since, if instead they had found it worthwhile they would have bought it in the first place. We can see how the second person is also worse off from our reallocation. Any other attempt to reallocate will suffer the same fate. It can then be concluded that markets must achieve allocative efficiency.

In addition to allocative efficiency, one might be interested in productive efficiency: whether, for a given cost of production, the maximum amount of goods has been produced. Here, again, economic theory indicates that markets result in productive efficiency,[4] since producers wish to make the highest possible profit. If production were not efficient, producers could simply modify their choices of inputs, produce more, earn more revenue, while throughout, keeping their cost the same.

Finally, even if all existing products are allocated efficiently, and all production of these products is efficient, there can still be room for improvement. If our economy was producing the wrong sorts of goods that people didn't particularly want, for example, this would be an area for improvement. In very simplistic terms, if a list of goods was being produced, but the consumers would be willing to pay more if only there was a different mix of goods available, it will improve things to change to the different output mix. Now, in a market economy where firms are motivated to earn profit, if there could be more profit made by modifying the line up of products offered, then naturally firms would change their product lines to avail themselves of the higher profit.

Thus, we see that under certain required conditions[5] the market (price system) does result in allocations that satisfy all the different aspects of efficiency. And this maximization of efficiency as it turns out, is equivalent to the notion that markets maximize the sum of the value to all individuals of all the goods in the market.

Why can we not apply this approach to healthcare? The greatest stumbling block in utilizing the efficiency properties of the market for healthcare is that we would lose the claim to universality. Some people would not be receiving even basic healthcare because they cannot afford it. While we can enjoy the benefits of the market system, namely the efficiency, we see that simultaneously we must accept the vagaries of the market.

However, as it happens, the market system outcome leads us to only one of many possible economically efficient outcomes. To see what extreme situations are admitted as efficient, consider a situation where we allocate all the goods and services available in an economy to a single individual. This one individual has everything and all the others have nothing. We notice that this satisfies the definition of economic efficiency and indeed would be economically efficient, because there would be no possible reallocation that would improve or leave *everyone* as well off, since if we change anything, the one person that had everything will become worse off. Once we see that this is efficient, we can also see that all the other allocations where we give everything to another of the people and nothing for the rest would also all be efficient. And then we can imagine that there will be all the possibilities in between that gradually distribute more among all people in the economy, but at the same time maintain economic efficiency. How can we choose between all these different efficient allocations?

We know that the market system chooses one particular allocation from all of these possible efficient outcomes, and that allocation depends on the wealth distribution of the people. The drawback of such an allocation is that, although it would be efficient, the wealthy can afford much healthcare, and the poor, very little. Universal healthcare instead requires that all people have equal access to healthcare, whenever the need arises.

The main question that this chapter addresses is whether the efficiency qualities of the market can be harnessed while at the same time preserving the universality of healthcare. This will be a measure of how well we are able to achieve the maximum benefit for the greatest number of people, with a fixed healthcare budget.

A number of schemes have been proposed to utilize the market system in the context of healthcare. One such plan gives each person an equal sum of healthcare dollars annually that can be saved to form a fund, from which they can draw as a health need arises. Being market based it does have potential for being efficient. However, the argument against such a plan is that it *equalizes spending* rather than equalizing access to treatment. In particular then, if an individual was very unlucky in their health problems, through no fault of their own, they may risk running out of funds; while another person who is relatively healthy may have a surplus in their account. Therefore, this plan in biased in favor of individuals with a good genetic endowment in health factors and as well as individuals that have been lucky in their health outcomes. Another similar possible approach is to allow individuals to save tax-free in order build a fund to be used for health needs, much like an RRSP. Individuals who know that they are predisposed to certain conditions would have the ability to prepare for such a contingency and would benefit form the tax-free treatment of these funds. However, like the open market, this has the problem that wealthier individuals will be able to save more, and afford more healthcare than the less wealthy. Moreover, in our current fluctuating financial climate, bad luck or unwise investment decisions may render an entire lifetime of saving earmarked for healthcare completely worthless. Thus, in addition to the inherent uncertainty about health outcomes, we may end up imposing even more uncertainty on individuals with this scheme.

In addition, both of these policies have the problem that if individuals are not farsighted enough they may have long spent their budgets on negligible health issues, and underestimate their future healthcare needs. There are a few other variations on these basic themes, but the general conclusion about the market based policies that have been proposed is that they have some important drawbacks with regard to universality as well as farsightedness, but in their favour, they do have the efficiency properties gained by utilizing the market system.

In this chapter we propose an entirely new market based mechanism. The plan proposed here uses the efficiency of the market system and simultaneously allows the system to be needs based. In order to have a market based system, we need to have a virtual market working in the background that signals the cost and the value of each procedure. At the same time if we want the system to be needs based, we need to establish a priority of medical procedures, and also have a needs based sense of which patients should be treated first, and the order in which the rest would receive treatment.

For the system to be truly needs based, patients must be ranked according to which ones have the more serious need. In the Canadian system there is some rudimentary ranking of the patients belonging to a single specialist, and this is the waiting list. Patients are mostly ordered according to their arrival into the system. The specialist has some discretion in modifying rankings based on his/her own reassessment of the changing of urgency of the patients. However, there is no sense in how one physician's patients compare with another physician's patients. For a market type system to work, there must be something akin to a "master" waiting list that ranks patients nationwide (or at least within a region that is served by a geographic cluster of medical care facilities) for urgency and priority of treatment. Compiling such a list itself is a major undertaking, and approaches to how this can be effectively achieved will be discussed further and in greater detail in a later section.

Once the ranking has been established, it will influence how patients will propagate through the system. The actual scheduling will be done with mobile agents, each representing a patient in the system. The agents will participate in a mechanism that is similar to a market, which will allow the system to realize the efficiency properties of markets. Moreover, because need alone govern the capability of the agents to secure treatment in the schedule, there is no connection between the timing, or quality of treatment, and the patient's wealth. The allocation is not based on ability to pay, but rather on need, thus satisfying the goal of universality.

THE MECHANISM

The mechanism for scheduling elective procedures that we propose here will be achieved by representing each patient by a mobile agent. The agent will have assigned to it the detailed description of the patient's malady, and will be updated as there are changes in the patient's information. Based on the description of the patient's case, physicians will have some input in arriving at a ranking between 1 and 100, indicating the urgency for treatment of this patient. The mobile agent will be given this ranking and it will also be given information about the treatment the patient needs, including all the hospital and medical equipment and types of personnel necessary for the treatment. With the treatment information and the rankings the computer agent will search and obtain treatment for the patient as early as possible. The agent will essentially participate in a mechanism that is very similar to a market or auction. We will discuss in depth both the ranking process and the auction.

The system will have information about the availability of all the hospital facilities and staff at each point in time. These are the items that are being auctioned in our fabricated market. Each agent will have a list of items that are needed to complete their procedure. For example the procedure may be a hip replacement. In that case the agent needs to secure adequate surgery time in an operating room, find an orthopedic surgeon that is available at that time, enough nurses to assist, an anesthetist and any specialized equipment and medical supplies that will be needed. The ranking, which reflects the urgency of its case, will be the amount that the agent has to spend to secure all the items on its list. How this ranking, or budget, is determined will be discussed in a later section; for the present we will simply assume that the budget gives a true representation of the urgency of the case.

The agent will bid on each needed item in virtual auctions that will be conducted on an ongoing basis, competing with other agents representing other patients who may seek different procedures and place bids for a somewhat different list of needs. The actual method for determining which agents will obtain the items is quite involved. The agents participating in our large-scale auction will together form an economic game. In designing the game, the objective will be for the equilibrium to be characterized by all items going to the agents that have the highest willingness to pay. A simplified version of the mechanism to be used is the second price or English auction[6]. In this setting, for any particular item, the agent with the highest bid will receive the item, and pay the second highest bid price. Since each agent's valuation for the items on his list depends on the urgency of his own situation, this is called a private values auction.[7]

There is a large literature on second price private values auctions. Essentially it is an economic game; a situation where a number of people are all taking actions and everyone's action affects each person's outcome. Here, the agents are acting in the place of people. The outcome is generally thought to be a Nash equilibrium for the game: a stable set of choices where, if we fix what everyone else is choosing, each agent will not want to change their choice. Another way to state the Nash conditions is that no agent will unilaterally want to change its choice, given the choices of all the other agents.

To understand the Nash equilibrium for second price private values auctions, we initially simplify by supposing that all bidders know each others' valuations. In such a situation, economists have established that although there can be many equilibria, the most compelling one[8] is where the each agent bids his true value. The agent with the highest valuation wins and pays the second highest valuation. In the case of private information, that is, a situation where the agents do not know each others' valuations, the case for truthful bidding by each bidder is even stronger. With unknown valuations, agents will not want to bid a lower price than their own valuation, for fear that there might be another agent with a valuation that is between the amount bid and the agent's valuation, that could outbid it. The agent will not want to bid any higher than what it is worth because of the negative payoff earned it the agent wins the auction. Thus, in the private or unknown values situation, each agent will bid his true value and the highest valuation agent will win.[9]

In the auctions, agents are trying to buy all the components needed for the treatment, and they try to schedule the treatment for the earliest date possible. Consequently, the same procedure at an early date will have a higher price than for a later date. Since all agents are searching at once, only the most urgent cases—where the representing agent can bid higher than anyone else—will succeed in obtaining all the necessary items at an early date.

Just as we have found with markets, it has been shown that private values second price auctions are also always economically efficient. Economic efficiency requires that the object should go to the bidder with the highest valuation. Since in the most compelling Nash equilibrium all agents will bid truthfully, we find that the agents representing the patients with the highest needs (as determined by physicians) are served first, which is the efficient outcome.

Economic literature has established the basic result of the efficiency of private values second price auctions in allocating a single item that is being auctioned by a seller. Things become a little more complicated when there are several items, and multiple units. Further, the literature distinguishes between situations where buyers are interested in purchasing only a single item and where each buyer buys a set of items. Situations where each buyer eventually buys something, are referred to as the assignment problem. A distinction is also made for situations when the value of acquiring one item maybe affected by the entire set of items acquired. This is clearly the case in our setting, since the items are only valuable to the patient if all the necessary ingredients for the

required procedure are obtained. Distilling all this literature[10], it seems that an efficiency preserving mechanism that generalizes the second price auction in all these various dimensions can be created. Such a mechanism would constitute our virtual market where the mobile agents would interact, and economic efficiency would be attained.

Ranking by Colleagues

Finding the best way to rank patients is quite a major undertaking. In the Canadian system, a physician maintains his own waiting list by using his/her assessment of his/her patients. Occasionally physicians working in a group may request their colleagues to accommodate early treatment for a particularly serious patient if they will not fit in their own schedules. However, for the most part the waiting lists are not integrated across physicians.

As a result there is no proper ranking across lists to determine the absolute urgency for a patient. This integrated waiting list is a very important aspect of our mechanism. One way to achieve integration is to have a system of multiple ranking. Each physician will periodically be given anonymous information about a list of patients and be asked to rank them impartially. The lists will include not only some of the physician's own patients, but also some patients belonging to other physicians that are also in the system. The list of patients to be ranked by a particular physician will be randomly generated by the computer with the specification that a fraction, such as say at least a three quarters, will be another physicians' patients, and we can also require that every patient is ranked by at least by a certain number of physicians, say a minimum of four.[11] The actual ranking that each patient is assigned will be an average of all the various physicians' rankings, and this will serve as the currency, utilized by the agents representing the patients, in obtaining from the virtual market the various scarce resources required for the needed procedure.

One sentiment raised by the medical profession in our current world of very scarce resources, is that patients also have a role in affecting their health outcomes. In keeping with this line of thinking, patients that have been following prescribed lifestyles and taken all the preventative measures but have nevertheless contracted some illness that needs medical attention should be more deserving of higher rankings[12] than others who may not have been as conscientious. If there was a strong consensus that these factors were to be taken into consideration, such information could also be contained in the anonymous patient profiles.

To the extent that some resources will be common across many procedures, patients from each of these areas would all need to be in a common auction. This will mean that each physician will be ranking patients not only from his own speciality, but also some from other specialities. There may be some apprehension among doctors about having to rank cases outside their respective areas, but if we consider the alternatives, there is no one better qualified to rank than impartial (and unbiased by speciality) physicians themselves; without such a fully universal ranking, we cannot guarantee efficient use of resources that are common to several specialities.

Clearly, the universal ranking that will be produced using this method may initially be somewhat contentious, and perhaps there can be a built in adjustment procedure to allow for over riding corrections of any result that is too anomalous. However, in time we expect that this procedure will provide generally acceptable results. Perhaps over time there will be some adjustment of approaches to ranking as the doctors see how their own choices are connected to the final ranking. If there is a worry that doctors may recognize their own patients from the anonymous profiles that they are asked to rank, and may inadvertently be motivated to rank their own patient higher, the ranking protocol can be adjusted to accommodate such issues by having a lower fraction of the profiles to be ranked be the doctor's own patients,

diluting the impact of the own patient ranking. In the end, if this continues to be a serious problem, we can even have that no patients to be ranked will be the doctor's own patients.

Economists have studied incentives in making choices. It is known that there are many incentive compatible mechanisms and they mostly rely on achieving truth telling by not allowing an individual's choices to affect matters that are important to the individual. Thus, a situation where the ranking involves only the patients belonging to other doctors, the outcome will not be biased by any incentive to alter the rankings.

THE DYNAMICS AND PRACTICAL ISSUES OF SCHEDULING

What we have described so far will work for allocating resources at a single moment in time. However, we know that healthcare allocation is an ongoing process. Therefore we need to discuss how the auctions will be held in a dynamic time setting.

It is quite reasonable to think that schedules will be fixed a certain amount of time in advance of the actual date of the procedure; this will be for the convenience of all involved. Such a lead-time may be a couple of weeks or perhaps a month, or it could also be dependent on the specific procedure. All bidding would be finished in advance of this time, and the participants (both patients and medical practitioners) would be informed of the schedule; all people will stick to the schedule unless something completely unexpected happens that forces them to cancel.

If, after the schedule is fixed, an even more urgent patient arrives, they would have to be dealt with as either on an emergency basis or may be able to be accommodated in the regular schedule, if someone has cancelled at the last minute. Until the point at which the schedules are fixed, new agents could be joining the auction. Agents, who could not afford to purchase their treatment requirements at a particular point in time, will automatically start making bids on components for procedures scheduled for a later time. In the meantime, having waited the extra time, their ranking will be higher, and so, all other things being equal, they will have a greater chance of securing the requirements for their procedure. Instead of having to re-rank a continuing patient, perhaps (if the medical profession endorses it) there can be an automatic inflation factor in the ranking of patients that do not secure treatment in a week and must be carried over to another week. The automatic ranking adjustment can be overridden if there is some important change in the patient's health status that requires physicians to revisit the needs ranking of the patient.

The agents can also be given extra information of a non-medical nature such as the patient's scheduling preferences (availability of dates and times, possibility of travelling to nearby locations, and any other relevant aspects for scheduling). An issue that we find in the current system, which can be easily addressed, is that of surgeons and other specialists working and or being on call continuously for extended periods of time, that may be deemed as excessively long. With the agent system, we can easily include system checks that record the duration of work for the various specialists, and we can easily institute regulations such as mandatory breaks after a certain duration of work. This might ensure that specialists performing critical procedures are well rested, and best able to exercise the care and precision needed for good results.

Shadow Prices and Other Incidental Benefits

Besides giving us economically efficient outcomes, there are further advantages associated with our mechanism. The mechanism and the prices therein provide us with some much needed, valuable information.

The prices, at which all the various medical

facilities trade, are very significant. They represent the current relative value to the system of each medical component. In situations where there is an opportunity to expand the available facilities these shadow prices will specify which facilities are most in need, as indicated by the highest auction price. Specifically, if more money becomes available and there is a plan to expand the healthcare facilities in the locality, the most efficient use of the funds at the margin is to invest in the particular items that have the highest difference between relative prices and relative real dollar cost. For example if a new hospital bed costs $100 per night and new MRI equipment costs $400 per use[13], say, we compare that to the shadow prices for the same amount of use for each equipment coming from our auction. Suppose the auction prices were 12 and 20, respectively, say, then it would be better to spend on more beds, since the cost ratio of beds to MRI is ¼, but the ratio of valuations of hospital beds to MRI equipment is 3/5. The beds are valued relatively higher in the auction than their relative dollar cost. Of course, this type of analysis is valid only at the margin. If there is a large infusion of funds, the relative shadow prices will no longer be accurate.

In addition, the whole aspect of being able to computerize all use of the medical system in a constellation of hospitals and medical facilities allows the generation of valuable data about many issues. Of primary importance to the whole business of healthcare provision is that the data from this mechanism will allow us to estimate the lifetime real medical costs of an individual, controlling for any number of characteristics that could be relevant. This would allow for precise and sophisticated forecasting of future healthcare costs for the system as whole, allowing for demographic trends and any other trends that could be relevant.

There will be a huge wealth of other data (of course respecting the understood rules of patient anonymity[14]) that could be useful for medical research; such as in the success rate of various procedures in the treatment of different conditions, the incidence of certain conditions in different populations, better documentation of past treatments of a given patient (instead of relying on the patient's memory) that might be significant for their current ailment. This could lead to a better level of service for the patient, as well as a better understanding of the success of treatments and thus greater progress in development of appropriate treatments.

CONCLUSION

Economists have been pivotal in devising many currently adopted mechanisms for allocation, where the goal is to find the best match, or in other words maximize the economic efficiency of the allocation. An example of such a mechanism is the matching system for medical residents to hospitals.[15] Markets and also auctions are known to maintain economic efficiency, but have the problem that the efficient outcomes are tied to individual wealth, and do not result in an equitable allocation. We have devised a mechanism here to overcome his drawback, by allowing representative agents to be traders in markets for healthcare products and services utilizing a fictitious currency that is equitably distributed according to the medical need of the patient, as determined by physicians. The mechanism further has the potential to provide valuable information about many aspects of healthcare provision, such as trends, estimation of costs, utilization rates of various equipment, and these data can be employed to give precise projections of the future based on demographics, and other relevant information about the population. Also of importance is the feature that the shadow prices arising form the mechanism will point to the areas that have the most benefit from investment and expansion of facilities. Thus, we have the means to develop a mechanism that maintains all the principles underlying a universal publicly funded healthcare system.

REFERENCES

Amoros, P., Corchon, L., & Moreno, B. (2002). The Scholarship Assignment Problem. *Games and Economic Behavior*, *38*, 1–18. doi:10.1006/game.2001.0852

Anderson, M., & Sandholm, T. (1999). Leveled Commitment Contracting among Myopic Individually Rational Agents. [Special Issue on Agent-Based Computational Economics.]. *Journal of Economic Dynamics & Control*, *25*, 615–640. doi:10.1016/S0165-1889(00)00039-7

Bansal, V., & Garg, R. (2001). Efficiency and Price Discovery in Multi-item Auctions. *ACM SIGecom Exchanges*, *2*(1), 26–32. doi:10.1145/844309.844314

Bikhchandani, S., & Haile, P. (2002). Symmetric Separating Equilibria in English Auctions. *Games and Economic Behavior*, *38*, 19–27. doi:10.1006/game.2001.0879

Bikhchandani, S., & Ostroy, J. (2002). The Package Assignment Model. *Journal of Economic Theory*, *107*, 377–406. doi:10.1006/jeth.2001.2957

Clarke, E. H. (1971). Multipart Pricing of Public Goods. *Public Choice*, *11*, 17–33. doi:10.1007/BF01726210

Demange, G., Gale, D., & Sotomayor, M. (1984). Multi-Item Auctions. *The Journal of Political Economy*, *94*(4), 863–872. doi:10.1086/261411

Gilpin, A., & Sandholm, T. (2007). Information-theoretic Approaches to Branching in Search. *Proceedings of the International Joint Conference on Artificial Intelligence (IJCAI)*.

Groves, T. (1973). Incentives in Teams. *Econometrica*, *41*, 617–631. doi:10.2307/1914085

Groves, T., & Ledyard, J. (1977). Optimal Allocation of Public Goods: A Solution to the 'Free Rider' Problem. *Econometrica*, *45*, 783–809. doi:10.2307/1912672

Leonard, M. (1983). Elicitation of Honest Preferences for the Assignment of Individuals to Positions. *The Journal of Political Economy, 91*(3), 461–479. doi:10.1086/261158

Milgrom, P. (1985). The Economics of Competitive Bidding: a Selective Survey. In L. Hurwicz, D. Schmeidler, & H. Sonnenschein (Eds.), *Social Goals and Social Organization: Essays in Memory of Elisha Panzer*.

Roth, A. (2003). The Origins, History and Design of the Resident Match. *Journal of the American Medical Association, 289*(7), 909–912. doi:10.1001/jama.289.7.909

Sandholm, T. (1996). Limitations of the Vickrey Auction in Computational MultiagenSystems. *Proceedings of the International Joint Conference on Artificial Intelligence (IJCAI)*.

Sandholm, T., & Lesser, V. (1997). Coalitions among Computationally Bounded Agents. [Special issue on Economic Principles of Multiagent Systems.]. *Artificial Intelligence, 94*(1), 99–137. doi:10.1016/S0004-3702(97)00030-1

ENDNOTES

[1]   This idea of efficiency was first introduced by Pareto, and it is called Pareto efficiency. It includes many components of efficiency, such as allocative efficiency, production efficiency and efficiency of product mix, which are discussed later.

[2]   There are several conditions necessary to guarantee efficiency of markets. First all participants must be competitive, and this is typically assured if there are large enough numbers so that the choices of any one agent alone do not affect prices. Next all participants must have full information about the available choices. Now in this auction all that they really need to know is which components they need. Lastly, there are no externalities, which means that one agent's benefit from obtaining a particular item is unaffected by what items other agents have obtained.

[3]   This idea was first developed by Adam Smith in 1776 in his famous book, *The Wealth of Nations*.

[4]   Markets result in productive efficiency under the same conditions as required for allocative efficiency.

[5]   See footnote 2.

[6]   The English auction is the one with which we are the most familiar. Bidding begins at a starting or reserve level, set by the seller. Buyers will sequentially offer higher and higher bids until finally no one bids any higher. The winner is the highest bidder, and he pays his winning bid price. As it turns out this formulation can be shown to be identical (in terms of the underlying game and its Nash equilibrium) to the second price (or Vickrey) auction where players simultaneously submit sealed bids; the agent with the highest wins and pays the next highest bid price.

[7]   Private values refer to a situation where each agent can have a different valuation for the item being auctioned. This is in contrast to the alternative scenario, termed common values, where all participants have the same value for the item being auctioned. The latter best describes auctions where an asset is being auctioned, all participants value it the same, since their main purpose in buying it, is for investment; the critical issue in such auctions is whether all participants are fully informed about the what the common value is. In our setting the agents are buying the item for the patient's personal use, and so it is very plausible that different agents have different valuations.

[8]   The dominant strategy, as it is called, is to always bid truthfully when playing this game. This is because for each possible choices

that the other people make, agent will be no worse off by being truthful, as compared to any other action.

[9] The reader, who may not be familiar with the economics literature, may wonder why we use second price instead of first price auctions. We note that the actual price paid is not important since no real currency is spent; of greater importance is who wins the auction, and whether the allocation was efficient. Since the highest valuation agent wins the second price auction, efficiency is achieved. It turns out that the first price auction can also be efficient, but the argument is more involved.

To provide just a rough idea of the argument, in a Nash equilibrium of the first price auction, there must be an agent that bids just below the winning bid, to prevent the agent with the winning bid to shade his bid lower. Thus, the highest valuation agent can bid anywhere between his own valuation and the next highest valuation and win. In particular, then, he could bid just above the second highest valuation, giving a result which is not too different from the second price auction. Indeed there is a technical result known as the revenue equivalence theorem, which states that the expected social surplus from first and second price auctions is the same.

[10] The early economics literature is on the Clarke-Groves mechanism, where is purpose is to elicit truthful information about individuals' valuation. See Clarke (1971), Groves (1973), Groves and Ledyard (1975), and Leonard (1983). This is not a main concern in this application, since the valuations are known as the rankings are actually assigned by groups of physicians. Instead our focus is on whether the assignment can be implemented by a decentralized process where participants (the agents representing the patients) can arrive at the scene whenever their condition presents itself, and expect to join a process that has already begun with earlier participants. Examples of the literature examining various decentralized mechanisms begin with the simple auctions and branch out to multi item auctions, assignment problems, and package assignment problems. See Milgrom (1985), Demange, Gale and Sotomayor (1986), Bansal and Garg (2001), Amoros, Corcheon and Moreno (2002), Bikhchandani and Ostroy (2002),. Some of the literature is due to computer scientists and is particularly focused on automatic bidding, or agents bidding. See Sandholm (1996) and Sandholm and Lessor (1997), Anderson and Sandholm (1999), and Sandholm and Gilpin (2007). One important idea discussed in some of the recent literature, is the notion that agents may want to renege their contracts with a penalty (cost) if they are not able to obtain all the remaining items needed to complete their list.

[11] The precise values to be used here are not known at this stage. Fine-tuning of the system will be necessary and possible as more experience is gained.

[12] The question of whether a patient's illness is due their own neglect of health or whether it arises through no fault of their own is a very slippery surface. Recently some medical practitioners have advocated that a healthy lifestyle naturally resulting in healthy outcomes should be rewarded, while illness arising from unhealthy lifestyles should not be as readily treated, particularly for repeat offenders. Of course the worry is that in many instances there cannot be definitive proof that a particular lifestyle choice lead to a particular illness. We suppose that the medical profession is best informed in these matters, and if such consideration is included in rankings all necessary precautions to avoid unfair rankings would be taken.

13 These numbers are completely hypothetical and do not in any way represent the real costs of any of the medical equipment discussed. Similarly the auction prices are purely fictional and in particular have not been produced from any simulation of the mechanism.

14 Computer systems are generally very good for maintaining anonymity of data, as it can simply be programmed into the system that all names and other identifying references be dropped when information is being used for purposes other than the patient's own treatment.

15 The combined work of many economists such as Starr, Ludmerer, Gale and Sahpley, and Roth and Sotomayer has shaped the current system of resident matching programs. See Roth (2003) for a survey of this topic.

Chapter 3

A Review of Recent Contribution in Agent Based Healthcare Modeling

Simerjit Gill
University of Regina, Canada & TRLabs Regina, Canada

Raman Paranjape
University of Regina, Canada & TRLabs Regina, Canada

ABSTRACT

This chapter reviews and summarizes eight selected paper in the area of agent-based healthcare systems. The objective of the summaries is to provide an overview of recent research work in the area and to examine the characteristics of agent-based healthcare applications. The chapter also briefly discusses reasons for adopting agent-based simulation and modeling over traditional modeling techniques.

INTRODUCTION

Agent-based modeling and simulation is a modern approach to model complex systems. Agent-based simulation systems are comprised of autonomous agents that interact with each other to create a working dynamic model of a real world system. Today, applications of this new paradigm of modeling and simulation can be found in variety of domains ranging from modeling the stock market and supply chains behaviours to modeling the complexities of the human immune system and predicting the spread of epidemics (Macal & North, 2006). Traditional modeling techniques are no longer sufficient in dealing with the complexities of real world systems as they are becoming increasingly more sophisticated. Software agents can break a large problem or task to smaller tasks and distributes the work over number of agents to provide an optimal solution. The operation of healthcare is complex as it involves large numbers of staff and other resources that work together to deliver healthcare services to patients. The agent-based modeling and simulation approach is increasingly attracting researchers who exploit the capability of agent system in order to explain the complex behaviour of healthcare systems.

DOI: 10.4018/978-1-60566-772-0.ch003

Software agents can be defined in numerous ways. Each definition varies depending on the context and the application. However the main attributes are common to all the definitions. The common attributes of software agents are: autonomy, pro-activity/re-activity, communicativity, collaborative problem solving and mobility. The mobility attribute refers to the ability of an agent to travel across different platforms to achieve its goal. Autonomy pertains to the ability of an agent to act autonomously with limited or no user interaction and to completely represent an object or entity. Pro-activity/re-activity implies the ability to react to the environment and adapt its behaviour accordingly. Communicativity refers to the capability of agents to exchange messages between each other and with the external users and systems. The collaborative problem solving attribute pertains to the ability of agent to collaborate and work together to accomplish a common goal which no single agent is able to attain on its own.

Software agents should only be used to develop applications for systems which require some or all of the above attributes of agents. Most of these attributes are required in order to create effective and accurate simulations and models of healthcare systems. In this chapter, we review and summarize eight recent papers to provide an overview of the state of research in agent-based healthcare modeling system. Agent-based modeling and simulation is a relatively new approach in healthcare modeling. We observe three common themes in the work presented in this chapter - these are: (i) support for patients and medical professionals; (ii) effective and efficient communication between health professionals; and (iii) optimization of healthcare delivery services.

We provide a brief introduction on each selected paper to give a high level picture of the content of the summaries before proceeding to the actual summaries.

A Multi-Agent Approach to the Design of an E-Medicine System

This paper proposes a multi-agent based framework for the development of an e-medicine system. E-medicine integrates information communication technology with medical technology to deliver healthcare to geographically distributed areas. The paper presents a case study on telemedicine for diabetes to illustrate the development of an e-medicine system.

Building Agent Based Corporate Information Systems: An Application to Medicine

In this paper, author proposes an agent-based framework for supporting collaborative work among human and software agents. The proposed framework is applied in the field of telemedicine to build complex and cooperative decision support systems (DSS) within the context.

A Framework for Building Cooperative Software Agents in Medical Applications

This paper focuses on improving the cooperation and interoperability among different health care professionals engaged in the process of delivering health care services with the aid of software agent technology. This paper experiments the management of patients affected by acute myeloid leukemia (AML) with the help of developed prototype.

HealthSim: An Agent-Based Model for Simulating Health Care Delivery

This paper introduces an agent-based simulation model, called HealthSim, which facilitates users understand various health care delivery issues in a hospital environment through simulations. The system is primarily designed for managers and planners of hospitals who want to identify the effectiveness and efficiency of health care services that are being provided to patients. HealthSim has a potential to address several aspects of health care operations that deals with procurement, distribution, maintenance, and replacement of medical equipment and personnel. It also helps in the management of the details of medical operation.

Mobile Software Agents for the Support of Chronic Illness: A Case Study in Diabetes Management for Rural Areas

This paper presents a framework for managing diabetes particularly in rural areas using mobile agents. This paper presents a framework which has a potential to manage and control diabetes in remote areas that lacks diabetic specialists.

Nature-Inspired Planner Agent for Health Care

This paper presents an agent-based human thinking reasoning model based on past experience. The main purpose of the development of this model is to facilitate elderly people with disabilities, in particular with Alzheimer.

Mobile Agent-Based Framework for Healthcare Knowledge Management System

This paper presents a framework for effective management of information and knowledge in healthcare sector using mobile agents. Authors sense the necessity of transposing stored healthcare data and information into knowledge so that it can serve as a facilitator for making critical decisions during healthcare operations. This paper presents various components that can work together to create an effective knowledge management system (KMS).

A Multi-Agent Security Framework for e-Health Services

This paper presents a multi-agent security framework for e-health services. It describes and categorizes various type of communication into different levels that takes place among health care professionals. Subsequently, the paper identifies security requirements associated to each level of communication and introduces a multi-agent based security approach for e-health services.

REVIEW

Title: A Multi-agent Approach to the Design of an E-medicine System
Authors: Jiang Tian, Huaglory Tianfield
Source: Multiagent system technologies. German conference, Erfurt, ALLEMAGNE (22/09/2003) 2003, vol. 2831, pp. 85-94
Publisher: Springer-Verlag Berlin Heidelberg

This paper proposes a multi-agent based framework for the development of an e-medicine system. E-medicine integrates information communication technology with medical technology to deliver healthcare to geographically distributed areas. The paper first explores the functional and non-functional requirements of e-medicine system and then presents a structural design of agent-based e-medicine system. In the end, the paper presents a case study on telemedicine for diabetes to illustrate the development of e-medicine system.

The four basic functions of medicine presented in the paper are disease prevention, disease diagnosis, disease treatment, and health consultation. According to these functions, authors have divided requirements of an e-medicine system into functional and non-functional requirements. Distant medical services such as telemedicine, e-healthcare, teleconsultation; distant clinical practices such as telesurgery, telementoring, and training patient; establishing medical databases and exchanging medical information are included in the functional requirements of e-medicine systems. On the other hand, security and privacy, efficiency, convenience and reusability are considered as non-functional requirements.

This paper adopts a multi-agent approach to align the complex requirements with the design of an e-medicine system. Design itself is broken into two parts: design of agents and design of multi-agent society. Designing an agent includes the proper identification of roles and responsibilities of each agent in e-medicine systems. And, design of multi-agent society focuses on the architectural design of multi-agent system and interactions between the agents. Authors believe that the general set of requirements provided in the paper can serve as a reference guide to build any kind of e-medicine system.

The proposed framework of an e-medicine system involves a large number of agents. Each agent carries out specific task and may interact with other agents to complete the assigned task. Agents in the e-medicine systems are categorized into three groups: the Control group, the Implementation group, and the Interface group. The interface group consists of agents responsible for providing the user with graphical user interface, initiating a search, or showing the results of a query to the user. The interface group may contain interface agent, search agent, or any other agent responsible for keeping the link between patient and other e-medicine systems. The second group, which is the control group, contains the controller agent, administration agent and department agent. The controller agent controls the whole e-medicine system and resolves the conflict among agents. The administration agent assigns tasks and helps cooperate between departments and agents. The department agent has knowledge of certain medical department and manages the internal department affairs. The third group is the implementation group. The implementation group implements the monitoring, diagnosis, therapy, consultation, and archival function to achieve the goals. The implementation group contains most

number of agents namely the monitoring agent, data processing agent, diagnosis agent, therapy agent, archival agent, education agent, decision support agent, training agent, consultation agent, surgery agent, and database wrapper agent.

The interaction in e-medicine systems is divided into the internal model and external model. The internal model is responsible for internal communication while external for external communication. Control group, implementation group, and interface group carry out internal communication. External communication takes place when agents belonging to the implementation group and interface group interact with an external environment.

To illustrate the framework proposed for e-medicine systems, the paper present a case study of telemedicine for diabetes. The Telemedicine system provides diabetic patients with real-time health monitoring and can also provide immediate therapy. After a complete requirement analysis of telemedicine for diabetes, the paper listed down several services that a telemedicine system must provide on a daily basis. These services are visiting the patient and providing individual therapy, monitoring the patients in real time and processing the monitored data immediately, diagnosing the patients in term of monitored data and making a proper therapy for the diabetic patients, training the diabetic patients to monitor themselves and educating the physicians to update their skills, maintaining patients record/database, providing consultations to patients and the system must have a functionality to interact with other systems in e-medicine systems.

The diabetic telemedicine system makes use of several agents in order to fulfill the identified requirements. Agents in the implementation group are monitoring agent, data processing agent, diagnosis agent, therapy agent, consultation agent, decision support agent, training agent, archival agent, department agent, and interface agent. Each of them is responsible for certain task and interacts with other agents. The monitoring agent is responsible for real time monitoring of diabetic patient and transmits the data to the data Processing agent. The data processing agent integrate the data and process it for diagnosis agent. The diagnosis agent plays an important role in implementation group as diagnosis is a complex process. It examines the situation and makes and accurate judgement for the patient. The diagnosis agent not only interacts with other agents in implementation group but also communicate with decision support agent, clinic agent, education agent, and consultation agent. Depending on the decision made by the diagnosis agent, the therapy agent determines a proper therapy method for the diabetic patient. The consultation agent provides consultation to the enquiry of patients. The decision support agent, as name implies, provide decision support. Both consultation agent and decision support agent interacts with diagnosis agent. The Training agent trains patient by giving instructions on the proper intake of medicine and self care. The Archival agent maintains the patient record and used therapy methods. It encrypts the information and links it to the medical database. Control group and Interface group, contains department agent and interface agent respectively. Department agent is responsible for the control of the telemedicine system while interface agent provides the interface with search services and information services.

This paper presents a multi-agent approach to the design of an e-medicine system. The paper examines various functional and non-functional requirements that must be considered in e-medicine system. Based on that, it presents a general structural design of an e-medicine system composed of many software agents. To illustrate the application of the system in the real world scenario, the paper adapts a general design of an e-medicine system to a more specific diabetic telemedicine system.

Title: Building Agent Based Corporate Information Systems: An Application to Medicine
Author: Tung Bui

Source: European Journal of Operational Research 122 (2000) 243-257
Publisher: Elsevier

In this paper, author proposes an agent-based framework for supporting collaborative work among human and software agents. Bui's (2000) framework enables geographically dispersed organizations to distribute the task across the internet and work collaboratively. The system is embedded with the intelligent software agents that are capable of making decisions facilitating the implementation of complex and distributed decision making process. The proposed framework is applied in the field of telemedicine to build complex and cooperative decision support systems (DSS) within the context. Telemedicine is an application of clinical medicine where medical information is transferred via telephone, the internet or other networks for the purpose of consulting, and sometimes remote medical procedures or examinations (AbsoluteAstronomy, 2009).

The paper presented taxonomy of an agent characteristics and the proposed taxonomy can facilitate in identifying different types of agents to support different type of decision tasks. Furthermore, this paper proposed a development lifecycle for building agent-based systems. Author sensed the need of adopting a new approach for the development of an agent-based system. The new methodology supports a two-tier approach to design a given system. The first tier functions as an assignment model which is primarily responsible for searching, identifying and selecting the agent(s) that are believed to be most appropriate to perform required tasks. It covers the first three phases of the lifecycle. The second tier manages a coordination and collaboration strategy for all the participating agents to work together and makes the last two phases of the lifecycle.

The first phase of a software-agent development lifecycle begins with analyzing the problem task. It consists of all the elements necessary for examining the problem task such as decision support requirements and detailed breakdown of all decision processes. The decision processes are collections of partially ordered steps that are required to reach a particular goal. The next phase involves searching of eligible agents in an iterative manner or creation of new agents that meets the requirements determined in the preceding phase. Agents are selected on the basis of their competence, reliability, and cost to perform the given task. The third phase specifies agent's behaviour. Instructions are pre-set for showing identifications, following protocols and utilizing web-resources in a cost effective fashion. The last phase involves assigning appropriate tasks to selected agents. The execution plan to solve the entire problem is sketched in this phase.

The proposed framework is adopted to build a web-enabled telemedicine. Referring to the first phase of software-agent development life cycle where the problem task is analyzed, problem solving associated to the healthcare is categorized into four processes. The processes are (i) medical examination, (ii) diagonosis, (iii) treatment recommendation (Dx), and (iv) treatment plan/prognosis (Tx). In the real world scenario, people involved in the telemedicine are patients, advice nurse, doctors on duty, and other specialists. And in the proposed agent-based web-enabled telemedicine, duties of above people are supported by software agents named as (i) the Exam Manager, (ii) Dx/ Tx Manager, (iii) Session Manager, (iv) Speciality Problem Solver, and (v) Negotiation Manager.

In this experimental set up, the Exam Manager gathers the subjective data such as patient's description of symptoms, feelings and other biographical data through web form via internet at the patient site. The data may also be collected through sensors/health monitoring equipments as well. The data is then passed down to the Dx/ Tx Manager. The Dx/Tx Manager examines the received patient data and decides which Speciality Problem Solver should take part in generating treatment recommendations. Once all Speciality Problem Solvers are identified and selected, the Session Manager initiates the communication and

administers it throughout the session. Problem can be executed, independently or interactively with a human specialist, by the Speciality Problem Solvers to come up with recommendations. Recommendations made by various Solvers are then received by the Negotiation Manager and the Negotiation Manager facilitates in reaching a single consensual solution. Subsequently, the solution is transmitted back to the Dx/Tx Manager and then presented to the field provider through a human interface.

The next phase of the software agent development lifecycle decides whether or not a software agent should be developed to implement that process and if so then selects which would be the most appropriate profile of that agent. The selection of agents is based on the cost-benefit analyzes. Profile of each agent is created through examining each of the agents attributes and gives the most suitable value for it. Intelligence, Mobility, Lifetime, Interaction, Task-specificity, and Initiative are the attributes of agents. Once agent profile is determined, agents are ready to be embedded into workflow.

According to Bui (2000), there are lot of benefits of the proposed system. The biggest benefit is that the data can be collected seamlessly and cost effectively with relatively low investment of the internet infrastructure. Internet provides adequate communication support to carry out the task of medical information system connectivity. Other benefits include that the system has a potential to provide anytime anywhere healthcare as the patient is always in touch with his/her primary care provider no matter where in the world he/ she is.

Title: A Framework for Building Cooperative Software Agents in medical applications
Authors: Lanzola G.; Gatti L.; Falasconi S.; Stefanelli M.
Source: Artificial Intelligence in Medicine, Vol. 16, Number 3, July 1999, pp. 223-249(27)
Publisher: Elsevier

This paper focuses on improving the cooperation and interoperability among different health care professionals engaged in the process of delivering health care services with the aid of software agent technology. It is evident that during the course of medical process, a variety of information and knowledge traverses among number of health care staff. This information may range from a simple biographical data of a patient to sensitive contagious disease information. Although there might be different communication channels available to heath care workers, the primary medium of conveying information is typically through phone calls or face-to-face talks. Frequent interruption is very common in this sort of interactions. The interruption may occur in any form such as if a doctor is attending a patient and nurse calls him and asks him to urgently attend another patient which is in a serious condition, the doctor may pass the health related information of the current patient to a nurse and advices her to take necessary steps for the betterment of the patient. Since, it is an emergency situation, a nurse may not be able to comprehend all the information bombarded by the doctor at her and there is a very good chance that a nurse may make wrong assumptions. Authors believe that this may cause serious consequences if some sensitive information is lost or misinterpreted. Such situations arises primarily because of the intrinsic nature of hospitals which are highly event driven environments where professionals are required to regularly move across several departments and sometimes even off campus.

As described in the paper, the process of delivering health care services involves large number of people like clinicians, nurses, laboratorists, etc. and features a high distribution of expertise, knowledge and physical resources. Thus the effectiveness and proficiency strictly depend both on the skills of the professionals involved as well as on the level of cooperation and coordination reached by them within the clinical context. As such authors insist that there is a need of improvement in the clinical communication infrastructure. A careful deployment of the information technol-

ogy will have a great impact on improving the interoperability among people working together in the health care settings and minimizes the problems associated to it. In this paper, an information technology tool called Software Agent has been proposed to achieve effective and efficient flow of information among health care professionals.

Software Agents have the tendency to act on behalf of some entities and make intelligent decisions based on the working environment. They may also interact with each other to achieve their goal. This paper tends to simulate the real world interaction of different health care professionals through Cooperative Software Agents. These Agents are equipped with the Task Specific Knowledge and Cooperation Knowledge. The Task Specific Knowledge handles information required to achieve a certain task. For instance, if it is an optometrist agent then it is responsible for providing instructions pertaining to eye related illness. The Cooperation Knowledge, on the other hand, tells an agent how to cooperate with other agents to perform a specific task. It also constitutes Agent Communication Language module which implements communication protocol and administers agent-interaction over the network. Each Agent is linked to the Knowledge-Based System. The Knowledge-Based System is an information repository which has a reference to a database of knowledge of any particular subject. Thus, in the given computational model one section is concerned with the interconnection among Software Agents and enabling of the exchange of information and knowledge among them through a suitable Agent Communication Language (ACL), while other one addresses the problem of effectively modelling and representing cooperation knowledge within each Agent. Authors have followed KQML specifications to develop a tool that has a tendency to achieve a high-level communication between Software Agents. KQML is declarative, syntactically simple, extensible and easily readable by humans. This framework facilitates in developing a generic communication model which could be coupled with pre-existing legacy systems or other available applications, thereby helping them converting into Software Agents while preserving much of their internal coding and functionality.

The paper also states that even though ACL is powerful tool that has a capacity to provide a solid foundation for exchanging information and knowledge among agents, the ability to interoperate with other agents and to exploit some kind of social behaviour demonstrated by each agent in the environment cannot be accomplished by the language alone. Authors sensed the need of enhancing task specific knowledge already available within agents with a set of suitable primitives that should be able to contour their behaviour to be adopted while interoperating with others.

This paper experiments the management of patients affected by acute myeloid leukemia (AML) with the help of developed prototype. Several Software Agents were implemented tailoring the specific need of a particular health care professional and enforcing his/her cooperation with others involved in the treatment of a patient suffering from AML. Participating agents in this experimental set up are the General Practioner, Hospital Administration, Hematologist, Nurse, Donor Bank, BMT Unit, and Oncologist. These agents interact with each other and may get multiple task requests from different agents at a given point of time. Agent allocates resources to different task on the basis of its importance and priority. The information collected by these agents in the course of this process is stored in the database and can be fetched for a later use.

This paper provides a framework that has a potential to achieve an effective and efficient communication among agents. Old legacy systems and other standard applications utilized by Hospitals may be converted to agents following the given framework. Moreover, it also opens the door for many other researchers to exercise the idea and develop agent based information system for hospitals for their specific needs.

Title: HealthSim: An Agent-Based Model for Simulating Health Care Delivery
Authors: John H. Christiansen and A. Peter Campbell
Source: Argonne National Laboratory, Chicago, Illinois

This paper introduces an agent-based simulation model, called HealthSim, which facilitates users understand various health care delivery issues in a hospital environment through simulations. The system is primarily designed for managers and planners of hospitals who want to identify the effectiveness and efficiency of health care services that are being provided to patients. HealthSim is flexible enough to be deployed in a small to large scaled organizations. It can be used in a small department in a hospital, for a single-practioner surgery, or in a major medical centre with hundreds of thousands of patient each year.

HealthSim has a potential to address several aspects of health care operations that deals with procurement, distribution, maintenance, and replacement of medical equipment and personnel. It also helps in the management of the details of medical operation.

HealthSim runs various models with thousands of agents in a single simulation to understand the relation of different dynamic behaviours associated to health care. These behaviours may include human physiological processes such as beginning and progression of disease, development of signs and symptoms, and effects of interventions; human cognitive behaviour such as response to symptoms and making and keeping appointments; clinical/logistical processes such as clinical practice guidelines, office procedures and personnel policies; and medical monitoring equipment response.

The system has a potential to address various health care management issues depending on type of simulation performed. For instance, the response to various perturbations in health care delivery service can be investigated by simulating the inpatient and outpatient loads for a hospital unit within a health care system. Inpatient is a patient who is admitted to the hospital and stays overnight in hospital for quite some time depending on the illness. Outpatient on the other hand is not hospitalized overnight but regularly visits a doctor for diagnosis or treatment. In this simulation, the main inputs are service provider's schedules, outpatient visit rates for each type of visit, inpatient visit rates for each diagnostic related group (DRG), and call center operator schedules. The main outputs are appointment wait times, average phone waits, costs, revenues and many more. These outputs help the management in making critical decisions. The system can also be used to examine the effects of new technology or equipment, efficiency of new treatment paths, cost effectiveness of new drugs, and consequences of changes to management procedures or policies.

HealthSim accepts number of adjustable inputs from the user to perform the simulation providing a great deal of flexibility. The input and output items of the system can be easily replaced, added or deleted with no or minimal effect on the overall simulation structure. The paper has listed down several results that can be obtained from the simulation. Few of them are average appointment length (in minutes) by department, average appointment wait (in days) by department, admittance trends report, average length of stay by DRG, average phone waits (in seconds), inpatient bed-days per month by DRG, hospital financial report by month and year, daily number of beds occupied, and number of appointment by department.

HealthSim is an agent-based framework that is based on the Dynamic Information Architecture System (DIAS) and the Framework for Addressing Cooperative Extended Transactions (FACET). Both DIAS and FACET are developed at Argonne National Laboratory (ANL). HealthSim is largely implemented in SmallTalk with some of key functionalities coded in C++. The system runs on Unix or Windows platform and may be configured to run in a distributed environment.

DIAS executes time-ordered event simulations where event objects and associated data structures are distributed to the appropriate objects. All event posting are managed by the DIAS global even manager. Each object response to the even posted by itself or by another object. DIAS object class definition supports abstraction where abstraction description of object behaviour is given with no implementation details. As it is indicated in the paper, DIAS is a general framework for building simulation systems which consists of many models. In DIAS, objects are interlinked to other objects appropriately in the system during their activation depending on the state of the simulation. These factors make DIAS ideal for simulating the complex operations involved in health care delivery.

In HealthSim, models of social behaviour patterns are constructed with the aid of FACET. It is composed of several software objects that can be used to build and run complicated and cooperative behaviour models of agents. In FACET, complex operations are broken into several courses of actions (COA's), and these courses of actions are further sub-divided into COA steps. Each step of COA represents an action or series of actions which are tied to some constraints and negotiate with participating entities for their cooperation. In case the condition does not meet, COA step is broken down further until all the conditions are met.

Both DIAS and FACET are incorporated into HealthSim. There are various Objects and Processes that are modeled in HealthSim. The general classes of the objects include Persons such as patients, doctors, nurses, administrators etc; Organizations such as different medical departments, Infrastructure such as rooms, utilities etc; any equipments either medical, safety or administrative; medicines and supplies; and financial and usage records. The classes of the processes that are modelled in the system are normal physiological processes in each patient, disease processes in each patient, diagnostic equipment response and behaviour pattern models for patients, staff, and organizations. Models of normal physiological processes and pathophysiology behaviour are embedded in Person objects. Pathophysiology is the study of the disturbance of normal mechanical, physical, and biochemical functions normally caused by a disease (NationMaster, 2009). Sofware Agents in HealthSim represent patients, healthcare workers of all type, administrative/management personnel and hospital departments. Each patient agent has a detailed physiological model and a set of disease model. Disease model is heavily based on the differential-equation-solver model that simulates the beginning and progression of the disease, development of signs and symptoms of the disease, and physiological response to interventions. Furthermore, the progression of any existing disease will alter the physiological state for other disease as the disease models are linked through common risk factors.

HealthSim is a flexible event simulation tool which contains numerous models and agents to represent different entities involved in the health care delivery mechanism. Authors believes that the system can be used for various kinds of applications ranging from small work flow involved in a single surgery to the management of complex operations in large hospitals. The tool can be very useful to executives and administrator of medical centres in various decision-making processes.

Title: Mobile Software Agents for the Support of Chronic Illness: A Case Study in Diabetes Management for Rural Areas

Authors: Tarapornsin, V.; Ray, P.; Chowdhury, A.

Source: e-Health Networking, Applications and Services, 2006. HEALTHCOM 2006. 8th International Conference on Volume, Issue, 17-19 Aug. 2006 Page(s): 72 – 77

This paper presents a framework for managing diabetes particularly in rural areas using mobile agents. As stated in the paper, diabetes is one of the serious and most widely spread diseases. Approximately 150 million people are affected with this chronic illness and their numbers are growing rapidly. Diabetes can result in a variety of complications if it is not properly managed or left untreated. These complications include heart disease, kidney disease, eye disease, impotence and nerve damage. Diabetes can be managed by doing exercise, eating healthy food, measuring blood glucose levels on a regular basis, and having a regular consultation with the doctor. According to authors, most patients in rural areas do not have the advantage of having their blood test regularly due to lack of facilities and diabetic specialists. This factor lowers the treatment of diabetes in rural areas. This paper explores the possibility of mobile agents to address this problem assuming the availability of internet in rural side.

The paper points out several efforts in the past to control diabetes by designing tools and models for monitoring and managing diabetic patients. Among them are "Fit for Life" programme by Ministry of Health in Singapore, "Check Your Health" programme of Alexandra Hospital, An Ontology-driven Multi-agent approach for Diabetes Management (Ganendran G. et al, 2002), A multi-agent Healthcare System- An Example for Diabetes Management (Vivian, A., Venky, S., & Y.Y.Zhu., 2001), and 3G Network Oriented Mobile Agents for Intelligent Diabetes Management: A conceptual Model (Li, M., & Istepanian, R.S.H., 2003). This research focuses on the improvement of diabetes in rural areas where most of the diabetic care is provided by generalists. The paper addresses the challenge of creating a system where a patient, generalist and a diabetic specialist coordinate and work together to improve the care of diabetic condition. The authors implements mobile agents to improve the quality of diabetic care in rural areas. They also affirm that with the aid of mobile agents, patients can receive better consultation on time no matter where a diabetic specialist is physically located.

The paper deploys the mobile agent system to address this problem as the mobile agent technology has a capacity to travel across network which may help health care professionals such as diabetic specialists, general practitioner, clinicians, and patients locate one another and transact diagnose electronically. Furthermore, authors have specified that the implementation of mobile agents in health care to control diabetes will allow the interconnection and interoperation of multiple existing systems such as legacy patient health information, patients decision support systems, or other e-health systems; improve scalability of the system as agents have the capability to deal with dynamic environments; and provide solutions withdrawn from distributed information sources.

According to the architecture presented in the paper, each village (node) is connected to a city hospital (speciality hub) with adequate number of diabetic specialist. Village generalist registers the patient details to the diabetic support system by entering the medical data and history such as blood glucose measurements and other symptoms of his/her patient in it. The data is carried to the speciality hub, which in this case is a city hospital, where diabetic specialists can access the medical data. In this way, diabetic specialists may view medical record of all the patients suffering from diabetes from various villages on a single site and coordinate the intervention of all available diabetic specialists to response to symptoms of rural patients throughout the year. To make the system more effective, villages located within the region are connected to their Regional Hub. There can be number of regional hubs such as northern hub, southern hub etc. Each Regional Hub is further connected to various diabetic specialists through several Central Agencies. Each central agency contains adequate number of diabetic specialist agents. Each central agency containing diabetic specialist agents are linked to the database wrapper which first retrieves internal medical information from the diabetic departmental database and then stores in its database. Central Agencies are also connected to each other to provide coordination. Village patient and central agencies connects to the Regional Hub, which serves as a centralized information repository, at each state to provide and

receive medical treatments and follow -ups.

Mobile agents involved in the system are the Village Agent and Diabetic Specialist Agent. When a patient is registered in the system by a local generalist, the Village Agent is created which hold medical information of the patient. Patient's medical information contains the name of the patient, patient identification number, address, date of birth, allergies, medical history which contains information about medical examination, date of visit, problem description, medical centre ID, generalist ID, and Specialist ID. Specialist ID is not available until the completion of the first cycle of the diabetic support system. Once the village agent is created and loaded with the required information, it travels across the network from a village health care centre to the regional hub and wait for the central agency to provide list of available diabetic specialists. The regional hub holds general information of each central agency such as list of diabetic specialists in each centre in the area. It also checks the availability of each diabetic specialist in that area and directs the village agent to available specialist in a timely fashion. The diabetic specialist agent is responsible for maintaining the schedule of the specialist and holding his appointment times. Once the diabetic specialist is chosen, the regional hub directs the village agent to meet the diabetic specialist agent at the central agency. After the completion of interaction between the village agent and diabetic specialist agent, the village agent goes back to the village health centre and provides the obtained recommendations and consultations to the village generalist.

According to authors, the idea of keeping a centralized database in each region brings numerous advantages such as huge amount of data of patients can be compacted for easy storage, data processing becomes faster, easier maintenance of patient data, and better availability of information. This paper presents a framework which has a potential to manage and control diabetes in remote areas that lacks diabetic specialists.

Title: Nature-Inspired Planner Agent for Health Care

Authors: Javier Bajo, Dante I. Tapia[2], Sara Rodríguez, Ana de Luis and Juan M. Corchado

Source: Computational and Ambient Intelligence, 2007, Volume 4507, pages: 1090-1097

Publisher: Springer Berlin / Heidelberg

This paper presents an agent-based human thinking reasoning model based on past experience. The main purpose of the development of this model is to facilitate elderly people with disabilities, in particular with Alzheimer. Alzheimer is a progressive and fatal brain disease in the form of dementia (loss of memory and other intellectual abilities serious enough to interfere with daily life) with no current cure (Alzheimer's Association, 2009). The paper presents an autonomous deliberative Case-based Planner agent named AGALZ or Autonomous Agent for Monitoring Alzheimer Patients. AGALZ integrates with an environment aware multi-agent system called ALZ-MAS to improve health care of aged people. ALZ-MAS exploit RFID technology which is mounted on bracelets worn on the patient's wrist or ankle to learn about the environment. The RFID technology uses radio waves to automatically identify people or objects (Webopedia, 2009).

Authors incorporates the Case-Based Planning (CBP) mechanism (a derivative of Case-Based Reasoning architecture) together with the BDI (Believe, Desire, Intention) architecture to develop nature inspired deliberative agents, AGALZ, which have a capability to respond to events, take the initiative according to their goals, communicate with other agents, interact with users, and make use of past experience to identify best plans to achieve goals. The CBP helps AGALZ generate plans using past experiences and planning strategies. CBP cycles through four stages. The function of each stage is as follows: the retrieve stage to recover the most similar past experience to the current one; the reuse stage to combine the retrieved solutions in order to obtain a new optimal solution; the revise stage to evaluate the

obtained solution; and the retain stage to learn from the new experience. Each cycle of CBP is implemented through goals and plans. AGALZ implements multi-agent system to work co-ordinately with other agents to solve problems in a distributed fashion.

AGALZ formulate plans in such a way that each plan is composed of a sequence of tasks. These tasks have to be carried out by a nurse to execute a plan. A task creates a problem description for a nurse to carry out, resources available, and times assigned for their shift. Similar problem descriptions with an original problem are recovered during the retrieve stage of AGALZ. To achieve this, AGALZ applies various similarity algorithms and upon the selection of most similar problem description, it recovers the solutions associated to these problems. A solution contains all the plans and these plans are combined later in the reuse stage to determine available resources that are needed to fulfill the global plan. The resources that are required to complete some of tasks can be food, equipments, rooms and some other. Availability of time of nurse can be a problem restriction.

In this paper, the model is tested in the Alzheimer Santisima Trinidad (ST) Residence of Salamanca to improve the current services being offered to its patients. This residence is build for elderly people, specifically over 65 years old. The residence offers variety of services and facilities such as TV, room, geriatric bathroom, hairdressing, salon, medical service, religious attention, occupational therapy, technical assistance, terrace, garden, laundry service, clothes adjustment, infirmary, reading room, living room, visitors' room, cafeteria, social worker, chapel, elevator, customized diet, and multipurpose room. Authors selected 30 patients from the residence to test the system. They also installed 42 ID door readers, one on each door and elevator, 4 controllers, one at each exit, and 36 bracelets mounted with RFID one for each patient and nurses. The ID door readers get the ID number from the bracelets and send the data to the controllers which send a notification to the Manager Agent. Manager agent is located in a central computer. For the purpose of testing, authors instantiated 30 Patient agents, 10 AGALZ agents, 2 Doctor agents, and 1 Manager agent. Together these agents make a framework called ALZ-MAS Each one of these agents is explained below.

The Patient Agent runs on a central computer and manages the personal data of patient and its behaviour such as monitoring location, daily tasks, and anomalies. According to authors every hour a patient agent validates the patient location, monitors the patient state and sends a copy of its memory base, which is patient state, goals and plans, to the manager agent for the backup purposes. At the time of execution, the patient state is created as a set of beliefs. These beliefs are controlled through goals that must be achieved or maintained. These beliefs define the general state of the patient at residence. The beliefs are in the form of weight, temperature, blood pressure, feeding (diet characteristics and next time to eat), oral medication, parenteral medication, posture change, toileting, personal hygiene, and exercise. The paper also states that the beliefs and goals set for every patient depend on the treatment plan or plans that the doctors prescribe. The state of the patient is known by the patient agent by means of accomplished or failed goals. To track whether the goal has been accomplished or has failed, the patient agent maintains continuous communication with the rest of the ALZ-MAS agents especially with AGALZ. AGALZ can send the result of nurse agent's assigned tasks to the patient agent. Authors also state that the communication between the patient agent and the nurse agent must take place at least once per day depending on the corresponding treatment.

The second agent involved in ALZ-MAS framework is the Manager Agent. It also runs on a central computer. The paper lists down two roles of the Manager Agent: the security role and the manager role. In security role, the manager agent controls the patients' location and manages locks

and alarms and during the manager role, it manages the medical record database and the doctor-patient and nurse-patient assignment.

The Doctor agent is the third agent of ALZ-MAS. In simple words, Doctor agent treats patients. The doctor agent interacts with all the agents of ALZ-MAS. It sends treatment to the patient agent and receives periodic reports. It communicates with the manager agent to consult medical records and assigned patients and it transact with AGALZ agent to determine patients' evolution.

The fourth and the last agent of the proposed framework is the AGALZ. As it is discussed above the main responsibilities of the AGALZ include scheduling the working day of nurse, managing nurse's profile, tasks, available time and resources. The AGALZ agent runs on a mobile device so that each nurse can see her plans task by task. System has placed a limit of 8 hour working time for any nurse.

Upon the implementation of the system, authors have derived some useful results. According to authors, the workers have reduced the time spent on routine tasks. Activities of the patient and staff are also monitored and the monitored data can be used for the purpose of analysis to further improve the quality of health care to patients. Authors further affirms that the system also improves the security of the residence as it monitors the location of the patients which guarantees that there are in the right place and secondly, only authorised personnel can gain access to the residence protected areas.

Title: Mobile Agent-Based Framework for Healthcare Knowledge Management System
Authors: LEE Sang-Young, LEE Yun-Hyeon
Source: Mobile ad-hoc and sensor networks, International conference, Wuhan, China, December 13-15, 2005, vol. 3794, pp. 1103-1109
Publisher: Springer Berlin / Heidelberg

This paper presents a framework for effective management of information and knowledge in healthcare sector using mobile agents. Authors sense the necessity of transposing stored healthcare data and information into knowledge so that it can serve as a facilitator for making critical decisions during healthcare operations. The architecture has a number of components which are further divided into sub-components. Each component is responsible for carrying out specific task. The Knowledge Identification Agent and the Knowledge Interchange Agent are the two main agents that are implemented in the proposed healthcare knowledge management system. The system is further supported by the knowledge organization agent, knowledge reusability agent, knowledge query agent, knowledge visualize agent, new knowledge discovery agent and mobile dynamic planning agent.

Proposed healthcare knowledge management framework is primarily divided into two areas: the application area and the service area. The application area is responsible for tasks such as acquisition, identification, organization and reusability of knowledge. It consists of the knowledge acquisition tool which facilitates healthcare experts to insert basic information into the system. It is also equipped with the identification and interchange tool which is useful in sharing knowledge, provided by healthcare professional, with others or for personal use with the aid of mobile agents. Another tool that is a part of application area of the system is the organization and reusability tool. This tool provides systematization and reformatting of information for special purposes.

The second area of the proposed healthcare knowledge management system is the service area. This area is in charge of making strategic plan and assessment, and consists of three tools. The first tool is the dynamic healthcare knowledge visualize tool. As the name implies, the main functionality of this component is to visualize healthcare knowledge acquired from repository for better understanding. The second tool is the dynamic healthcare planning tool with customization feature which is intended for personal use. The third and the last tool which is a part of service area is the healthcare coalition information tool.

This tool exercises plans, schedules, and resources to formulate the optimal team to execute work in healthcare administration.

The application area of the framework is based on mobile agents and, as discussed above, is composed of three tools: the knowledge acquisition tool, the identification and interchange tool and the organization and reusability tool. Basic functionalities of these tools are summarized above however the paper further breaks down each of these tools into its sub-components.

The first tool which is the knowledge acquisition tool is composed of three components: the mail server, the application server, and the mail repository. The mail server is responsible for handling email transactions, email forwarding and formulation of an auditor group (specialized for health issues) controlled by intellectual email administrator, and the re-formatting of emails before they are stored into the database or forwarded to a receiver. The application server component is in control of receiving services required by users and evaluation of emails in the form of usage, accuracy and pertinence. The last component of knowledge acquisition tool is the mail repository which is the main mechanism for saving mails into database.

The knowledge management framework of mobile agent base, the knowledge identification agent and the knowledge interchange agent are part of the knowledge identification and interchange tool. The knowledge management framework of mobile agent base provides basic and general architecture to mobile agent sub-components. The knowledge identification agent implements a search protocol which facilitates the non-professional healthcare people to perform their queries effectively and fetches the most proximate healthcare related results. The Multi-query acquisition, query optimization, knowledge delivery and knowledge matching are the sub-components of the knowledge identification agent. These components are linked together to provide the most efficient results to the user. The last element of the knowledge identification and interchange tool is the knowledge interchange agent. This agent is equipped with three components: the interchange knowledge detection, knowledge formatting, and knowledge interchange delivery component. The knowledge interchange agent carries out various tasks such as detecting knowledge through searching documents and emails, providing formatting, and sharing knowledge by transmitting it to other platforms.

The third tool is the knowledge organization and reusability tool. It consists of two agents: the knowledge organization agent and the knowledge reusability agent. The knowledge organization agent organizes the stored knowledge autonomously and keeps the database up-to date and removes unnecessary data from the repository. The second agent is the knowledge reusability agent and it is responsible for the effective re-use of healthcare knowledge. It has an ability to apply the existing healthcare knowledge for solving new problem. It also personalizes the solutions based on the user of the system.

The service area of the proposed healthcare knowledge management framework is in charge of providing tools for knowledge visualization, healthcare planning, and healthcare coalition. The knowledge visualization tool includes knowledge discovery engine, knowledge query agent, knowledge structure engine, knowledge structure DB, graphic rendering engine, knowledge visualize agent, knowledge delete engine and new knowledge discovery agent. All of these components work together to provide efficient knowledge visualization services.

Another tool in the service area of the proposed system is dynamic healthcare planning tool which provides support for healthcare planning. The subcomponents of this tool are: the general planning repository, resource and schedule repository and mobile dynamic planning agent which are responsible for healthcare plan storage, individual health condition and information resource storage, and dynamic planning with the help cooperation with

other two components respectively.

This paper presents various components that can work together to create an effective knowledge management system (KMS). Authors believe that this framework has a potential to address issues with regards to the management of knowledge in healthcare.

Title: A Multi-Agent Security Framework for e-Health Services
Authors: Sulaiman R., Sharma D., Ma W., Tran D.
Source: A Multi-Agent Security Framework for e-Health Services. Knowledge-Based Intelligent Information and Engineering Systems and the XVII Italian Workshop on Neural Networks on Proceedings of the 11th International Conference, Vol. 4693, (pp 547 – 554).
Publisher: Berlin / Heidelberg: Springer

This paper presents a multi-agent security framework for e-health services. It describes and categorizes various type of communication into different levels that takes place among health care professionals. Subsequently, the paper identifies security requirements associated to each level of communication and introduces a multi-agent based security approach for e-health services.

The paper begins with the thought that the internet is not a secure place to communicate and share sensitive information. Computer systems are often compromised for illegitimate purposes and organizations that transact business through internet must make sure that their systems are secured. For example, e-health exercises information technology to deliver its services to people. During this process, sensitive information is communicated among users in e-health either through wired or wireless media. Thus, it is necessary to safeguard the communication mediums between medical professionals and patients to ensure the confidentiality and integrity of the transmitted information. To address this, the paper presents a security framework for e-health services based on the multi-agent system.

Communication occurs among various actors

or users over network in e-health settings. To demonstrate this, authors present a scenario in e-health where a doctor in a hospital communicates with another doctor from another hospital through internet and a paramedic at an accident spot communicate with a system coordinator at the hospital to update current status of a patient using his personal data assistance (PDA). Authors identify seven actors which may participate in the given scenario. These are the Doctor, Patient, Nurse, Social Worker, Paramedic, System Coordinator, and System Administrator. In addition to that the type of communication among these actors are identified as (1) Doctor <=> Doctor, (2) Doctor <=> Patient, (3) Doctor <=> Nurse, (4) Nurse <=> Patient, (5) Paramedic <=> Social Worker, (6) Social Worker <=> Doctor, (7) System Administrator <=> (Doctor, Nurse, Patient, Social Worker, System Coordinator, and Paramedic).

Each of the above communication paths requires different level of protection depending on the sensitivity of information involved in the communication process. For instance Doctor <=> Doctor and Doctor <=> Patient communication exchange more sensitive information compared to Doctor <=> Social Worker interaction since social worker does not have to know all the details of the patient illness. Taking this into account, the paper categorises these communications into five levels on the basis of the sensitivity of information transmitted. Level 1 is classified as Extremely Sensitive Communication and requires highest protection which includes Doctor <=> Doctor, Doctor <=> Patient, Doctor <=> Nurse, Nurse <=> Patient communications. Level 2 is classified as Highly Sensitive Communication that involves System Coordinator <=> paramedic communication as information on patient's current condition is exchanged which is considered highly sensitive as well. Level 3 being a Medium Sensitive Communication only involves general information which does not require a great deal of protection but a medium security protection would suffice. Social Worker <=> Doctor can be considered a

level 3 communication. Then comes the level 4, also referred as Low Sensitive Communication, which engages low sensitive information but high in confidentiality such as communication regarding user accounts or passwords. Interaction between the System Administrator and all other users falls under level 4 communication. The last type of communication is Level 5, named Public, and is open for public. Broadcasted announcements and seminars is an example of level 5 communication.

From this point, the paper identifies distinct security requirements associated to each communication level in order to design a secure system environment. Authentication to enter the system, confidentiality to prevent disclosure of sensitive information, and anonymity are the general requirements listed in the paper for a system used in health care. It further states that, these requirements can be met by securing the communication processes among users, analyzing and monitoring the network to protect against security breaches, and organization security policies. These policies include but are not limited to access control policy, site policy, hardened host policy, incident and disaster response, and auditing policy. Furthermore, authors concerns about the client and server communication and urge that the messages must be encrypted or digitally signed before transmission. Web servers can be compromised easily if they are physically accessible therefore all authorized users must follow the access control policy to access data and all the actions of users must be logged for auditing purposes. Authors also recommend that the email client must support digital certificate technology and signs and encrypts the message before sending it. With that, all activities from the firewall, intrusion detection system, and software patches and updates should be logged in to analyze any irregularity in the system. At last but not the least, authors insist that all the security policies of organization must be enforced for suitable results.

Taking all the security requirements into account, the paper presents a multi-agent based security framework for e-health. The framework is structured into three main components which are the Organizational Policies, Communication Manager Agent (CMA), and Network Analysis and Monitoring Agent (NAMA). The framework also has an Interface Agent and Authentication Agent. The Interface Agent gets information from the user such as ID and password and passes down to the Authentication Agent which is responsible for authentication process. The Communication Manager Agent manages other agents such as Multi-level communications agent, Message Encryption/Detection Agent, and Email Agent based on services needed. Multi-level communication agent determines the level of communication for a user based on the user's role such as doctor, nurse, patient, etc. The Communication Manager Agent makes sure that all the types of communications adhere to the standard security processes as encryption algorithm required in level 1 is stronger than level 3. The Email Agent also plays an important role in the proposed framework as it assures that there is certificate installed at the user's machine to encrypt the message before sending it out to the network. The Network Analysis and Monitoring Agent monitors and track agents such as Intrusion Detection System Agent, Firewall Agent, Patch Server updates Agent, and Anti-virus Agent. These Agents communicates with Network Analysis and Monitoring Agent to provide on-going state of the system to analyze the network traffic for any malicious activity.

This paper presents a multi-agent based security framework for e-health at a superficial level. It introduces a multi-level communication approach to provide more effective and efficient security to the network. Authors believes that this framework will be implemented in future to study the capability of agents to coordinate and cooperate together to improve the performance of the security processes.

REFERENCES

AbsoluteAstronomy. (2009). Retrieved February 25, 2009, from http://www.absoluteastronomy.com/topics/Telemedicine

Alzheimer's Association. (2009). Retrieved February 7, 2009, from http://www.alz.org/alzheimers_disease_what_is_alzheimers.asp

Bajo, J., Tapia, D., Rodríguez, S., Luis, A., & Corchado, J. (2007). Nature-Inspired Planner Agent for Health Care. *Computational and Ambient Intelligence, 4507*, 1090-1097. Berlin/Heidelberg: Springer

Bui, T. (2000). Agent Based Corporate Information Systems: An Application to Medicine. [Elsevier.]. *European Journal of Operational Research, 122*, 243–257. doi:10.1016/S0377-2217(99)00231-3

Christiansen, J., & Campbell, P. (2003). *Health-Sim: An Agent-Based Model for Simulating Health Care Delivery*. Chicago, Illinois: Argonne National Laboratory.

Ganendran, G., Tran, Q., Ganguly, P., Ray, P., & Low, G. (2002). An Ontology-driven Multi-agent approach for Healthcare. *Proceedings of the Health Informatics Conference (HIC2002)*, Melbourne.

Lanzola, G., Gatti, L., Falasconi, S., & Stefanelli, M. (1999). A Framework for Building Cooperative Software Agents in medical applications. [Elsevier]. *Artificial Intelligence in Medicine, 16*(3), 223–249. doi:10.1016/S0933-3657(99)00008-1

Li, M., & Istepanian, R. S. H. (2003). 3G Network Oriented Mobile Agents for Intelligent Diabetes Management: A conceptual Model. *Information Technology Applications in Biomedicine* (pp. 31-34).

NationMaster. (2009). Retrieved March 2, 2009, from http://www.nationmaster.com/encyclopedia/Pathophysiology

Sulaiman, R., Sharma, D., Ma, W., & Tran, D. (2007). A Multi-Agent Security Framework for e-Health Services. *Knowledge-Based Intelligent Information and Engineering Systems and the XVII Italian Workshop on Neural Networks on Proceedings of the 11th International Conference, 4693*, 547-554. Berlin/Heidelberg: Springer.

Tarapornsin, V., Ray, P., & Chowdhury, A. (2006). Mobile Software Agents for the Support of Chronic Illness: A Case Study in Diabetes Management for Rural Areas. e-*Health Networking, Applications and Services; 2006 HealthCom 2008. 10th International Conference* (17-19, 72-77)

Tian, J., & Tianfield, H. (2003). A Multi-agent Approach to the Design of an E-medicine System, *Multiagent system technologies, 2831*, 85-94. Berlin/Heidelberg: Springer.

Vivian, A., Venky, S., & Zhu, Y. Y. (2001). A Multi-agent Healthcare System-An Example for Diabetes Management. [Aquila, Italy.]. *Proceedings of IEEE Healthcom, 2001*, L.

Webopedia (2009). Retrieved February 10, 2009, from http://www.webopedia.com/DidYouKnow/ Computer_Science/2005/rfid.asp

Section 2
Healthcare Modeling Systems

Chapter 4
Agency in Health Care System Modeling and Analysis

Raman Paranjape
TRLabs Regina, Canada & University of Regina, Canada

Simerjit Gill
TRLabs Regina, Canada & University of Regina, Canada

ABSTRACT

This chapter examines the paradigm that a health care system's behavior may be examined using an agent simulation in order to illuminate its macroscopic characteristics and the effects of policy on its over all operation. Further, if the individual components are well articulated, the component behavior may be also studied. Health care systems in North America are generally regulated by various processes and mechanisms in order to provide orderly access to, and control of, the health care system. While all processes are designed to be fair and equitable, in many ways the system can not be examined or optimized because the risk, that making changes to the system might result in degraded services, is too great to permit making even simple changes. In this context we propose the development of a health care system model in which agents mimic the behavior of the key components of the system. These components interact and engage each other in a manor analogous to the operation of the health care system. The formulation of such a system is, by its very nature, an extremely complex process, and necessitates development in components or units. In this chapter we present the first components of such a system. Each component has unique and complex behaviors. These components will, with additional development, form the basic structure of a health care system model. Specifically we present results from the development of a diabetic patient agent model, the development of an agent-based neurosurgery ward bed allocation system, and the development of an agent-based scheduling system that may be used to allocate resources within the health care system.

DOI: 10.4018/978-1-60566-772-0.ch004

INTRODUCTION

The modeling of health care actors, components and systems in order to develop a complete understanding of component interactions and system reaction is one of the more challenging simulation and modeling problems for software agent systems (Moreno, Isern & Sanchez, 2001). There are many benefits to this approach, which may be summarized by simply stating that through development of a good understanding of the mechanics of the system, optimal, or more realistically closer to optimal, operation of the system may be possible, with reduced cost, greater efficiency, reduced pain and suffering, and a healthier population. For example, better allocation of resources in health care management may be possible by modeling each component in the system with the goal to clarify inefficiencies in the system. By testing and evaluating the various scheduling techniques and policies used, enhancing patient outcomes are possible. A second example may be the modeling of disease in the human population. If the evolution of disease can be modeled, the expected impacts on the health care system over time and as population's move, age, etc. may be come more predictable, allowing for better planning.

We propose to build a working model of the healthcare system, which will accurately depict its current operation and function, and in addition will enable physicians, hospital administrators, and government officials to test various new policies to characterize how effectively they deploy the available resources or to see if the implementation of these policies will result in better patient outcomes. The goal being to move the health care system closer to an optimal operation so that, the use of hospital resources will be efficient, there will be a decrease in waiting periods for patients for services, there will be a reduction in the cost of delivering health care services, and to use existing systems will be at maximal efficiencies.

This type of work attempts to answer a number of important questions regarding the use of health care resources: First, can we construct a faithful macro-model of healthcare system behavior? Second, can we implement this model using distributed software and agent systems? Third, can this model be used to evaluate the present operation of the healthcare system particularly with respect to resources allocation? Fourth, can these models be used to propose new and improved ways to allocate scarce resources in order to improve efficiency, reduce costs, and most significantly reduce human suffering?

An agent model of the health care system requires the formulation of agents that will be programmed to mimic the behaviors of key components of the health care system. The process of applying health care policy to these agent components, which form the system model, is manifested in the behavior and function of the agents, and in the interactions between agents. Mechanisms to monitor and observe the behavior of the system will then allow us to examine the performance of the system.

In this work we propose the use of a uniquely symmetric modeling structure in which we identify four foci around which the model may be centric. These four foci are: (1) the patient, (2) the physician, (3) the nurse, and (4) the hospital infrastructure. Our structure embeds a high degree of connectivity between each of these foci, and in fact allows the model to be seen as centered about any one of these foci depending on which focus is specifically being tracked or analyzed. The foci themselves are typically more than a single agent and may represent be a set of agents with similar goals, objectives or expectation of the operation of the health care system,

Software agents have specific and unique characteristics, and if these can be harnessed in addressing this modeling and simulation problem, it is expected that significant benefit may be obtained (Wooldridge & Jennings, 1995). These unique characteristics of agents include: autonomy, social ability, pro/re-activity and mobility (in the case of mobile agents). These unique characteristics map naturally into the attributed of human systems, organizations, and even societies. Thus software agents based modeling can be highly effective in representing actual component behavior which is typically autonomous, and socially proactive and reactive. These components can then be further evolved and modified with time to create components with dynamic and time varying characteristics. Software agents can make certain choices or decisions based on a given set of rules for decision-making. The agents can interact with other agents that are linked by a network, they can negotiate and exchange information with these agents based on the criteria that have been programmed into them. Thus we see that basic agent characteristics map accurately into real world processes, systems, components, and even individuals.

In modeling individual components of the health care system we base our development on the key characteristic of agent autonomy. For example, in the case of modeling a patient within the health care system, we consider the agent as fully representing all the characteristics of the patient. The patient agent is a model of an archetype human patient who has specific needs for nutrition and activity etc.; it has specific outputs (as relevant to the health care system) such as heart rate, blood pressure, etc., and has specific attributes such as age, gender, ethnicity, etc. The time evolution of the patient agent can then be expressed as dynamic output variables, with the potential within the system model to select an arbitrary time rate and period (next 24 hr or next 5-10 years).

As another example, we model hospital services by studying the process of bed allocation in a small urban hospital ward. In this example we have used actual health record data (with names and other identifications removed) to track hospital bed allocation and usage. Using the actual bed usage information we examine the flow of patients through the hospital ward from the perspective of the hospital service. If we further provide a mechanism through which to alter

patient in-flows to the ward and out-flows from the ward we begin to create a simulation environment that might be relevant to the demographical chance of an ageing population, for example, or other system wide change such as the increased in obesity or diabetes. This component is seen as hospital service centric and allows the behavior of the hospital service to be examined in various hypothetical conditions.

An important aspect of the health care system is the efficient allocation of resources in a constrained environment. For example, the allocation of operating room time for elective surgeries is a case in point. Funding constraints, in countries with socialized medicine, have resulted in long elective surgical waiting lists, some as long as one year. During this time, many patients with chronic illnesses slowly deteriorate and bear the burden of worsening pain and physical discomfort. Some eventually make it to the operating room on an emergency basis. Some develop other illnesses while waiting and may even die from them. It may be short sighted to blame the funding and resource framework for the waiting lists without questioning the mechanisms in place for resource allocation.

Ineffective scheduling may be seen as part of the problem in the current design of the health care system. The scheduling within the health care system model can be developed as a Constraint Satisfaction Problem (CSP) (Yang, Paranjape & Benedicenti, 2005; Paranjape, 2006; Yang, Paranjape & Benedicenti, 2006) The constraint satisfaction problem is considered to be NP complete and therefore it is not feasible to solve this type problem analytically. Patients, and medical and clinical staff and even equipment are difficult to schedule because of their complex, varied, and time changing (evolving) characteristics. These complex characteristics are overlaid upon health care queuing and scheduling problems. Beyond this, health care processes often involve multitasking and non-interchangeable skill and capabilities in the real and agent populations. Queuing theory

(Tse & Paranjape, 2005) also has other important features such as the rate of reneging (withdrawing from the queue). Finally, as queue sizes increase, the reneging rate increases and people (agents) on the list leave for service elsewhere, become more seriously ill (and join other lists) or even die waiting (withdraw completely from the system).

The goal of hospital scheduling is to efficiently utilize limited resources such as physician and surgeon staff time and specialized equipment, within a framework of patients who are enduring pain and suffering while carrying their ailments. This schedule must be found while simultaneously satisfying other constraints such as avoiding idle, resources, convenience to staff, etc. We have applied agent technology (Benedicenti, Paranjape & Yang, 2004; Benedicenti, Paranjape & Yang, 2006) to solve specific scheduling problems previously and feel that although health care scheduling is much more intricate than simple logistical scheduling there is significant potential to dynamically address scheduling problems in the health care field.

METHODS

Agent Execution Environment

In this work, the agent technology is based on TEEMA platform. TEEMA stands for TRLabs Execution Environment for Mobile Agents (Gibbs, 2000; Liu, 2002). It has been developed jointly by TRLabs Regina and the University of Regina, and it is a relatively standard Agent Execution Environment (AEE) or agent platform. TEEMA provides addressing and naming, messaging, mobility, security, logging, and a procedure for the addition of services like many AEE. TEEMA and all the agents on this work are programmed with Java. While TEEMA is used in this work because of its familiarity to the authors, no unique or special features are required of the AEE, and any other AEE with these same basic functions could be used in this work.

The Model Structure

The high-level architecture of the system is described in Figure 1 below. The four key foci for this Health Care system model are: (1) the patients, (2) the physicians, (3) the nurses, and (4) the hospital infrastructure. This model maps directly into the physical or real world, and each focus of the model can developed in order to create a microscopic internal view of the component, or a macroscopic view of the interactions between the foci.

Each focus defines a type of entity in the system and may be implemented using an agent model, a compound agent model, or can be most effectively implemented as a number of interacting or independent agents. For example, the Patient focus may be a single agent representing a single human patient with needs, expectations, heath conditions, treatment plans, etc. Equivalently, the Patient focus may include a collection of agents representing the individual human patients as well as the other forces directly and emotionally involved in the patient such as his family, or other interested parties (for example- recipient of an organ donation). The Patient focus can, at certain resolutions, even include a set of patients with similar expectations of the health care system (for example – all patients waiting for access to a specialized piece of equipment such as an MRI machine, or all the patient with a specific type of illness).

The Physician focus, similarly, may represent a single physician with his or her own unique skill set and methods of operation, etc. It might equally be a type of specialized physician such as all neurosurgeons with equivalent expertise at some resolution. It might be all physician involved in treating a specific patient represented as a set of agents, or even multi-agents functioning a certain resolution of the system with similar expectations of the health care system function. Thus the Physician focus may be manifested in the model as a single agent, a compound agent,

Figure 1. General architecture of Health Care Component Model with four foci. Each focus of the model is a software agent or set of agents. The model is symmetric and can be centered on any focus.

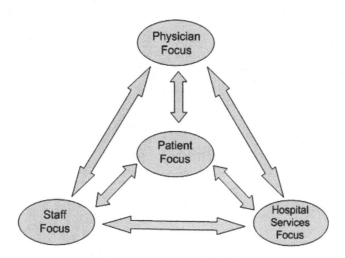

or a set of agents. Similar to the Physician focus, the Staff focus identifies a class of agents, which work to supply the patient with critical but support-oriented services. Typically, nursing staff is the primary mechanism of interaction with the patient in terms of meeting he/her basic needs. This includes providing the patient with the basic needs of sustenance, bedding etc., as well as the primary levels of the patient health care support such as monitoring, testing and interaction. The Staff focus is also in principle striated into various levels of service and care such as critical care, emergency care, and on-going care. The Staff focus may be implemented in the system as a single or a set of agents depending for example on what focus the model is centered upon.

The Hospital Services focus is diverse grouping of agents and is typically not created using a single agent. There can be similarities between Hospital Staff and Hospital Services foci however, the Hospital Services focus is oriented more around equipment and specialized settings rather than human action based services although there will necessarily be the need for staff to maintain or support the Hospital Services also. For ex-

ample, a specialized type of equipment such as a MRI unit, a type of operating theater and all of the equipment with in, or even a critical care or neurosurgery ward it might be best identified as a Hospital Service.

A key observation about this model is that it is a tetrahedron. This means the base is an equilateral triangle and each of its sides is identical to the base. The model has six edges and four sides that are all the same shape. This symmetry allows the model to be equally centered or directed on any of the components of the model with equal levels of resolutions.

A complete delineation of the health care system model with the typical variation within each of these foci is an immense task. Although we have been developing components of this model structure for some years, we are still a long way from finishing the complete system. In this chapter, we examine only a subset of the components of this model. While all foci of this model are extremely important to the faithful creation of the health care system model, we demonstrate a limited number of foci of the model. Our goal is to show both microscopic level and macroscopic

Figure 2. Generalized diagram of attributes, inputs and output for the archetypical patient agent.

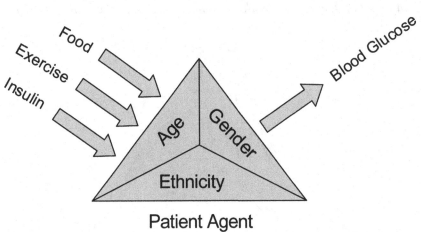

DIABETIC PATIENT MODELING

level interactions. Specifically we present microscopic views of the patient focus and macroscopic views of various hospital services.

DIABETIC PATIENT MODELING

An example, which illustrates the patient focus, is work we have done on the development of a Diabetic Patient Agent (Ghoreishi-Nejad, Martens & Paranjape, 2008). The basic idea is to create a representation of a set of archetypical diabetic patients using agent models. The patient agents then interact with other components and actors of the health care model in order to examine the system behavior. Some determinable fraction of the population of cases dealt with by a local health system is, for example, healthy middle-aged men with type II diabetes. The patient agent is the actor, which mimics the characteristics of one of the individuals in that faction of the population. In order for the patient agent to represents an arbitrary class of individuals, characteristics of this group of patients must be known and well understood. A single agent represents the human patient, and this single agent captures all the attributes and expectations of that patient.

Agent Design

The basic architecture of the patient agent is presented in Figure 2. We present typical inputs and outputs as arrows entering and leaving the body of the agent. Figure 2 also shows examples of the patient agent's fixed attributes such as age, gender and ethnicity, however, other variable attributes such as general health, condition or progression of the disease, and lifestyle are also important attributes, which must be considered. The diabetic patient agent essentially converts inputs such as food, exercise and medication into outputs such as heart rate, blood pressure and blood sugar. Figure 2 is specific for the diabetic patient agent; however, other patient agents will have a different formulation in terms of the exact type of inputs, output and key parameters that affect their function.

A simple example of the use of the Diabetic Patient Agent is to examine the effect of changes in the inputs on the observed outputs; such as modifying the amount of patient's food intake and observing the effects on his/her blood glucose level; or including/ excluding an exercise program in his/her lifestyle and observing the effects.

For a typical diabetic patient, there can be two types of factors to consider. The first type is described as parameters and are considered as risk factors for diabetes such as age, ethnicity, and gender. Depending on their value, the patient is more or less likely to be influenced by diabetes (Canadian Diabetes Association, 2006). People in different age groups have different risks of developing diabetes. For example, people aged 40 or over are more prone to be diabetic. In addition, diabetes is more common in some ethnic groups, such as Aboriginals, or African-Americans. In addition, typically more men are affected by diabetes than women (CDC, 2006).

The other type of factor is considered a variable and will directly have an impact on the medical test results -- immediately and over the short term. Examples of this type of variable are food (particularly carbohydrates), medications (insulin intakes), and exercise.

A number of models exist for diabetes (Boutayeb and Chetouani, 2006; Kuang, Li, and, Makroglou 2005) and in order to transform the input parameters and variables into output signals, using agent simulation, the following equation has been applied (Wu, 2005)

$$x(t) = \frac{F}{\omega} e^{\frac{-\beta t}{2}} \sin \omega t$$

In this equation, the output variable, x(t), represents the blood glucose level, F is a measure of the food intake, β shows the effects of exercise and medications, ω is the frequency of the system, and *t* is time (Wu, 2005). In order to have a measure of the food intake, its Glycemic Index is calculated. Glycemic Index is a numerical index that classifies carbohydrates depending on their rate of glycemic response, or their conversion to glucose within the human body (NutritionData, 2006). The model variables have been shown to be independent of each other (Wu, 2005). However, parameters that affect the human response to diabetes, affect all of these variables. In other words F is not simply Glycemic Load but is instead some combination

of GL together with functional relationships to ω and β and parameters of the individual such are state of general health, level of fitness, progression of disease, life style, level of stress, etc. While we have not calibrated this equation, we propose that the relationship between output and these input variables may be derived from future comparisons of the model output to existing physiological data for each archetypical patient category. A moderate daily exercise program is included in our Patient Agent model as modifying the value of β.

Single Agent Behavior

Figure 3(a, b) shows the Blood Glucose over a 24 hr period for an archetypal "normal" and "middle age type 2 diabetic" patient. The curves have three major peaks, which represent meals or carbohydrate intake. Over night the Blood Glucose reaches a low level before it again moves up because of the morning meal. In Figure 3(b), we see that the three peaks representing three daily meals are of greater height and width than the peaks of Figure 3(a). The position, height and width of the peaks changes depending of the condition and behavior of the patient and create the possibility of the effects of one meal overlapping with the effects of the next meal and ultimately influencing the amplitude of the patient's system response. While this "Diabetic" Patient Agent output still represents a patient with "good" control of this Blood Glucose, many actual human patients do not demonstrate the necessary discipline and the values of Blood sugar can be as high as 30 mmol/L which results in significant potential for vascular damage.

Multi-Agent Interactive Outputs

A key agent-modeling strength in simulation comes from the agent's ability to incorporate dynamic system component behavior, where each component represents a complete physical unit in the physical system. We can thus examine not only individual actor behavior, but also interaction

Figure 3. (a) Blood Glucose level of Normal Patient Agent over a 24-hr period. (b) Blood Glucose level of Diabetic Patient Agent over a 24-hr period.

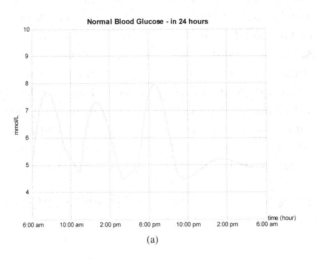

(a)

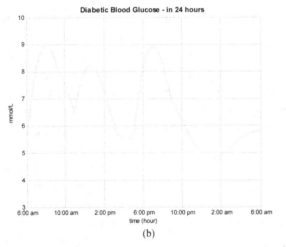

(b)

based on system and other actor interactions.

The function of the diabetic patient agent can change based on user input and/or interaction with a Physician Agent actor. For example, the Physician Agent can simply require the Patient Agent to change its behavior in some way, which ultimately impacts the output variable, the Blood Glucose. These types of effects are observed in specific scenarios in which the diabetic patient is first monitored for 60 days after which the physician agent requires a change in the patient agent's behavior. The first 60 days are represented using a complex of curves showing Blood Glucose levels

as seen in Figure 4. This complex of curves is generated using the short-term formulation of the diabetic patient agent for a middle-aged male with type 2 diabetes. These curves are analogous to the single curve presented in Figure 3(a). Figure 4, however, presents 60 curves that represent 60 days of monitoring in a 3-dimensional presentation. The patient consumes three meals each day. The meals are distributed in time as a random distribution around fixed points – 6:00am breakfast, 11:30am -1:30pm for lunch, and 5:00pm – 7:30pm for dinner. The patient's level of exercise activity is also distributed randomly but in a binary formulation

Figure 4. Typical daily curves of Diabetic Patient Agent Blood Glucose over a 60-day trial. The vertical axis shows the Blood Glucose in mm/L while the horizontal axis shows the time of day, and the axis into the page show the date of the experiment for day 1 to day 60.

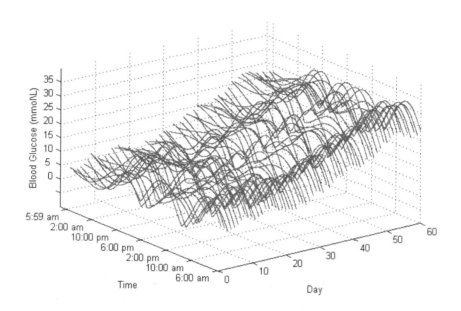

of either doing exercise or not. The patient has a fixed need for medication that he takes on a regular basis and is represented in our formulation, in terms of β.

The data in Figure 4 is shown in a compressed format in Figure 5. In this figure, the range of the Blood Glucose is shown as a vertical line for each day of the simulation. This vertical line representation allows easier comprehension of the range of the data and trends in the data over the days of the trial. For example, it may be observed from Figure 5 that the range of values of Blood Glucose begin with a range of 0-14 mmol/L on the first day of the trial and finish on the last day of the trial (60th day) with a range of 17-32 mmol/L. There is clearly a trend in the data of the Blood Glucose range climbing higher over the run. One may conclude from observing these figures that the Patient Agent's lifestyle and behaviors are not leading to good control of his/her Blood Glucose levels.

The Patient Agent's overall output Blood Glu-

cose can be described in a summary formulation as a table. The table format is most effective in examining the effect of interactions between the Physician Agent and the Diabetic Patient Agent. The Physician Agent prescribes particular behavioral modifications after 60 days of monitoring the Diabetic Patient Agent. Each row of Table 1 shows the distribution of Blood Glucose of the Patient as a daily average, before and after each meal, and then the number of times the Blood Glucose hits particular thresholds of 30, 20 and 15 mmol/L. The first row of Table 1 shows typical values for the Diabetic Patient Agent for the first 60 days. An examination of the first row of Table 1 shows that the Diabetic Patient Agent clearly does not have good control over his/her Blood Glucose. There are instances of Blood Glucose levels that are both too low and too high. Ideally, the Patient's Blood Glucose should remain between 5 and 8 mmol/L at all times.

The subsequent rows of Table 1 show the change in these values for specific physician agent

Figure 5. This curve shows the range of values of Blood Glucose on each day of the 60-day trial. The vertical axis shows Blood Sugar while the horizontal axis shows day of the trial from 1-60 days. Points when the Blood Glucose is too low or too high are marked with red.

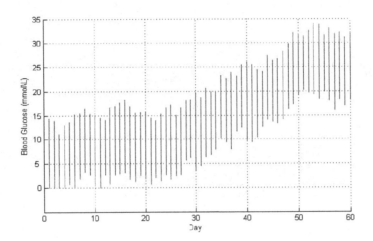

instructions. The physician instructions can be to control: (1) time of exercise, (2) amount of food intake (30% less food at specified meal), and/or (3) reduction in time variation for food intake. Each of these factors has a significant impact on the Blood Glucose. Each of the methods to control Blood Glucose recommended by the Physician Agent has a positive effect on the Diabetic Patient Agent but does not ultimately provide sufficient regulation of the Blood Glucose individual. The last row of Table 1 displays results for the compound instruction of limiting food intake at all three meals and also the results of controlling the time variation for these meals. Interestingly, with these multiple restrictions on amount of food at each meal and a restriction in the variation in the time of the lunch and dinner meals, the Diabetic Patient Agent has a 60 day period with all Blood Glucose levels between 5 and 8 mmol/L.

An Assessment of the Diabetic Patient Agent

As the results over the 24-hr trial and the 120-day trial demonstrate, there is a substantial potential in the Diabetic Patient Agent to express the functional behavior of the human diabetic patient's Blood Glucose activity. Even more interesting is that the Diabetic Patient Agent has the capability to demonstrate the dynamic effects of behavioral activity, physical activity, and medication change in the patient's function and how this is manifested in Blood Glucose level. The Blood Glucose levels may be further stratified to count the number of excursions over fixed thresholds in order to quantitatively assess the degree of compliance of the patient to expected norms for Blood Glucose.

Ultimately, however, in these results the focus is not on the registration of the Diabetic Patient Agent to the particular type or category of human patient, but rather to show the potential of this simulation and modeling system to represent the human patient and to then examine the effects of hypothetical modifications in the behavior of the Patient Agent dictated by a Physician Agent. The level of detail captured by the Diabetic Patient Agent transformation of input variables and parameters is currently very limited, however, it is interesting to see how this limited representation nevertheless has dynamic and appropriate changes

Table 1. Summary of Blood Glucose levels in Diabetic Patient Agent with behavioural modifications.

Condition	Average daily Blood Glucose (mmol/L)	Breakfast Pre/ Postprandial (mmol/L)	Lunch Pre/ postprandial (mmol/L)	Dinner Pre/ Postprandial (mmol/L)	# of time over 30 mmol/L	# of time over 20 mmol/L	# of time over 15 mmol/L
Diabetic Patient Agent-Baseline	15.1452	13.171/ 21.59	9.3247/ 17.414	10.909/ 18.204	12	27	51
w/ morning exercise	5.3194	3.4188/ 11.485	0.8301/ 8.3481	0.34818/ 8.1558	0	0	10
w/ afternoon exercise	9.8173	7.8461/ 16.113	3.536/ 12.551	5.9952/ 12.209	0	2	46
w/ evening exercise	7.0271	5.0443/ 13.521	1.1507/ 9.1821	3.28/ 9.6993	0	0	16
w/ controlled morning diet	4.3012	2.6736/ 7.0909	0.68933/ 9.7442	0.6893/ 7.5898	0	0	15
w/ controlled afternoon diet	10.5042	8.5511/ 16.866	4.6476/ 13.055	6.3411/ 13.24	0	1	53
w/ controlled evening diet	8.5457	6.6407/ 14.87	2.9216/ 11.208	4.4365/ 10.594	0	0	21
w/ controlled afternoon eating time	5.5185	3.5898/ 11.819	0.4204/ 7.8589	0.82139/ 8.3776	0	0	4
w/ controlled evening eating time	8.0062	6.096/ 14.534	2.2768/ 10.434	2.9942/ 11.19	0	1	26
w/ controlled eating time and diet (breakfast, lunch, dinner)	5.8143	5.6718/ 6.8386	4.5661/ 7.7263	3.3797/ 7.7323	0	0	0

*Note: The first row of the table provides baseline data for the Diabetic Patient Agent for the first 60 days. In the subsequent rows — the Physician Agent instructs the Diabetic Patient Agent to follow a specific regime for food intake and/or exercise. The summary information shows how the Blood Glucose level is controlled by the specific instruction. We see that the last row of the table in which the instructions are to control food intake at each meal and limit the variability of the time for food intake has the greatest effect in terms of limiting Blood Glucose variations and forcing these levels closest to a 'normal' range.

in the output variable.

The configuration of the Diabetic Patient to fit into various archetypical patient categories is specified by the system designer and may be tailored to the population and local demographics. The characteristics of the patient behavior in terms of variability in food intake for timing and volume carbohydrates consumed are also within the control of the system designer. The output curves, on the other hand, are generated by a functional relationship between the input variables, parameters and the output variable and are based on empirical formulation.

In order to transform this simple modeling system into a useful tool, for prediction and system testing, much work will be needed to calibrate and register the attributes of the Diabetic Patient Agent with those of the Human Diabetic Patient. However, for the simulation results as presented, it is clear that a complex system like the human response to lifestyle factors, can to some extent be captured by the patient agent.

The Diabetic Patient Agent presents a novel and dynamic model of illness using software agents. Thus we begin to confirm that indeed it is possible to generate dynamic active components of the health care system using software agents.

In this model, we specifically concentrated on Diabetes Mellitus. The continuous output signals generated in this model can predict outcomes for patients with diabetes, based on their behavior and lifestyle. Thus model can be useful in a larger model of the health care system and as an effective educational tool on its own. The model can help patients explore their prognosis if they are not meticulous in controlling their blood sugar and insulin levels. Diabetes is an interesting disease in that its manifestations on Blood Glucose can be relatively easily impacted by the human patient's behavior and actions. Regular exercise, smaller meals spaced more uniformly throughout the day and appropriate administration of medication can very dramatically alter the level of Glucose in the patients system. Thus this Patient Agent model can be used as part of an education and teaching protocol, which allows Patients to graphically and visually see the impacts of relatively simple decisions about their life style.

The Patient Agent Model has to be further developed in order to more fully connect the model variables to the input variables. Specifically, model variables are dependant on each other therefore relationships between input variables and model variables need to be explored and clarified.

The patient agent model can also be used as a component in a complex model of a complete health care system. The system model would be populated with a statistically distribution of patient agents with similar but not identical curves. The distributions of the patient agent population would be taken for the actual population of patients visiting the health care system. By sampling various inputs and outputs, Patient Agents can simulate different illnesses. Then dependent on the behaviors of these patient agents, a certain fraction may enter the health care system and demand access to specific resources such as physicians, hospital beds, hospital services such as operating rooms, and hospital services. The specific manner in which they interact will characterize a particular

scheduling system. These components interact with each other and engage in a manor analogous the operation of the health care system.

HOSPITAL SERVICES MODELING

The proper and well-organized administration and deployment of health care services is an important issue in health care management and organization. We attempt to model the operation of a neurosurgery ward with the goal of attempting to describe and define the current function of the ward and then extrapolate from the current operation to the future to predict new demands and expectations of the ward as operational and demographic changes are simulated (Paranjape, Ogrady, & Ghoreshi-Nejad, 2008).

Proper provisioning of medical care requires effective decision-making (Harper, 2002). Nicholls and Young (Nicholls & Young, 2007) have observed that an essential part of successful and ethical health care management involves managing the existing hospital beds effectively and ensuring their occupancy levels to be high but also in control. The assignment of empty beds to incoming patients is a daily challenge for hospital staff. Management inefficiencies continually result in practical and financial frustration for hospital staff as well as patients. Hospital managers need to be able to forecast future activity on the wards, such as the number and length of time for which beds are needed, the type of beds and the various related staffing levels required (Marshall, Vasilakis & El-Darzi, 2005). However, hospital managers are constrained by economic and financial issues when making such predictions (Marshall, Vasilakis & El-Darzi, 2005). Beyond daily utilization, they have to consider fluctuations in demand because of population growth or decline, demographic changes, improvements such as changes in health care practice, and changes in hospital policy (Marshall, Vasilakis & El-Darzi, 2005).

Data Analysis, Clean-Up and Re-Code

In order to connect closely to the current operation of the neurosurgery ward, actual usage data from the Regina General Hospital was collected. The data records from the neurosurgery ward included information on 1029 admitted and discharged patients, for the period from March 01, 2005 until March 29, 2006. There were three physicians attending the patients in the ward known as Physician B, Physician C and Physician D. Physician B attended 241 patients, Physician C attended 383 patients and Physician D attended 405. If the population of patients entering the ward was assumed to be in a Normal distribution, the mean value for the rate of entry into the ward was 3.13 and the Standard Deviation 1.78. Patients were diagnosed by the physicians with 241 different diagnoses and subsequently they underwent 162 different treatment procedures depending on their specific diagnoses.

After analyzing this original data, it was concluded that the original data had too much variability in order to be seen as a consistent population and some form or re-coding was required in order to reduce variability. The diagnoses were therefore re-coded into 40 groups and the procedures were re-coded into 29 using contextual information to identify similar diagnosis and treatments. Patient categories could then be recognized with a triplet of information; Diagnosis, Procedure and Physician (Diagnosis-Procedure-Physician). Within the category, each patient's information included a Length of Stay (LOS) record. Patients with the same triplet of Diagnosis-Procedure-Physician could have a different LOS. The total number of patients having the same triplet (and thus in the same category) was also noted and used to capture the probability of each sequence within a population of 1029 patients. LOS was included for each triplet, as a separate record and the file included as many records as were available. The mean exit rate was 3.09 and with a Standard Deviation

of 1.85. It is observed that the entry rate and exit rate are sufficiently close. It should be noted that there maybe more patients in the ward at the end of the simulation than at the beginning and that the assumption of normal population entry and exit from the ward is only approximate.

Agent System Implementation Model

Figure 6 presents the framework of the implementation model used to simulate the flow of patients within the neurosurgery ward. An empty shell of a patient agent is created based on the user input that defines the rate at which patients enter the system. The patient attributes are obtained from the re-coded database and loaded into the patient agent. The patient agent then enters the neurosurgery ward and obtains a bed if it is available. It may go through the regular neurosurgery ward or to the overflow if there are not sufficient beds in the regular ward. However, if the overflow is also full the system simply notes the unavailability of space and removes the agent from the system and the simulation. More typically, the agent stays within the neurosurgery ward or overflow for the number of days that it is assigned as it entered the system. When the number of days has passed the patient agent signals that it has completed the required duration of time in the ward and exists the system.

Three different software agents are specified in the implementation model: Administrator Agent, Patient Agent, and Observer Agent.

The Administrator Agent performs the majority of the functions of the model. These tasks include: (1) generates Patient Agents at the user specified rate, (2) assigns each Patient Agent a triplet of Diagnosis-Procedure-Physician and selects a LOS from the category, and (3) assigns a bed to the Patient Agent in the neurosurgery ward or the overflow. If there are insufficient beds in the hospital system (actual ward beds and overflow beds) the Patient Agent is required to leave the system and is removed from the simulations as

Figure 6. Implementation flow diagram for the movement of agents through the neurosurgery ward.

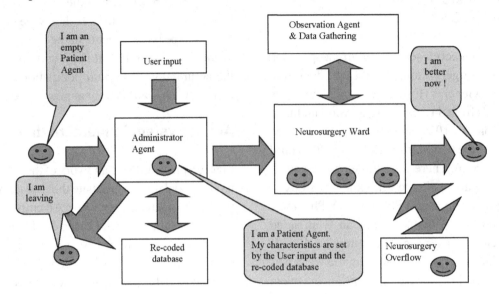

it is assumed that the Patient is moved to another hospital. This event is defined as a Critical Over Flow (COF).

The system runs on a 24 hour cycle with each second is considered equivalent to one hour. At the beginning of each cycle, a random number is generated from a Normal population with a specific Mean and Standard Deviation. For example, if the generated random number is 4, the Agent Administrator generates a Patient Agent every 6 seconds; after 24 seconds (the next day)

another random value is generated to specify the number of Patient Agents to enter the system on the following day. Administrator Agent defines each Patient Agent with a Diagnosis-Procedure-Physician triplet and then from this category, a LOS is selected.

Patient Agent is actually a shell or stub only in the Hospital Service centric focus as a detailed implementation of the patient characteristics is not necessary. The Patient Agent maintains its existence within the modeling system for the

Figure 7. Daily Bed Usage over 1ˢᵗ month of baseline year

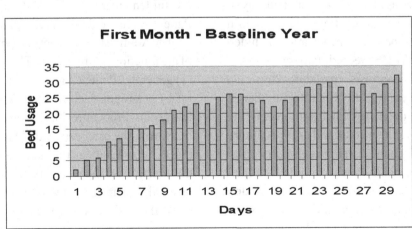

Figure 8. Daily Bed Usage over 2ⁿᵈ month of baseline year

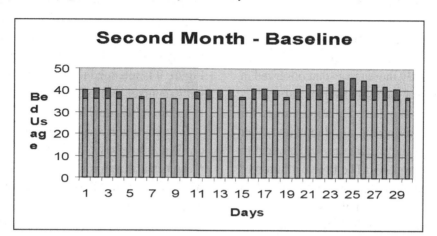

period of its particular assigned Length of Stay (LOS). After the LOS is completed, the patient agent informs the Observer Agent and exists the simulation.

The Observer agent is responsible for keeping track of Patient Agents who entered and exited the system, and publish a summary of the bed utilization.

Results and Discussion

Graphical and tabular representations of the hospital bed usage illustrate the behavior of the simulation. Bed usage numbers are presented for both daily and weekly usage over the year. In order to observe the system under various hypothetical conditions, the baseline behavior of the system is first defined.

Figure 9. Weekly bed utilization in the baseline experimental year

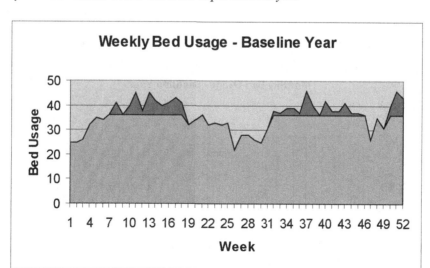

Baseline System Behavior

The system baseline is defined as the behavior of the simulation when the generated patient agent rate is exactly the same as that observed in the actual hospital data set. System parameters of the mean and standard deviation values for the population entering the simulation and other characteristics of the system are set identical to the physical data records. The time evolution of bed utilization in the neurosurgery ward is then simulated for an experimental baseline year.

Figures 7 and 8 show the first and second month of daily bed utilization in the neurosurgery ward for the experimental baseline year. The first month shows a ramping up of bed utilization because of system start-up. The system appears to reach a steady-state by the second month. The second month also shows a small oscillation about a mean value of approximately 40 beds being used on average. An arbitrary level of 36 beds is assumed in the ward and an overflow capacity of 10 beds or 27% is identified in grey in the graph.

Figure 9 shows the variations of bed usage on a weekly bases. It is interesting to note that the resolution with which the utilization data is observed can have a profound impact on the observed number of overflows and that summary information for the full year may not show the complete level of variation. For example, Figure 9 only shows the number of beds in use on the last day of the week and any overflows which occur on a daily or hourly bases are not observable. Thus Figure 9 is intended to show the bed utilizations with a courser level of granularity than that shown in the monthly graphs.

Figure 10 presents the average bed utilization on a monthly basis. We see an apparent lower mean bed utilization value in the first month after which the mean utilization stabilizes at a somewhat higher level. This baseline data can be used to compare and contrast system behavior under various operating conditions.

Manipulating the Rate of Patient Daily Arrivals

The hypothetical condition of increasing the average number of patient daily arrivals to the ward can be now considered. This situation may arise naturally, if for example, the population of the city goes up (but otherwise remains the same in terms of demographics), and thus the rate of patients entering the system also goes up by a similar rate. One can then examine the behavior of the system in the number of overflow events, number of critical overflow events and patient transfers. In this example we assume the ward

Figure 10. Monthly Mean and Standard Deviation for Bed Usage in Baseline Year

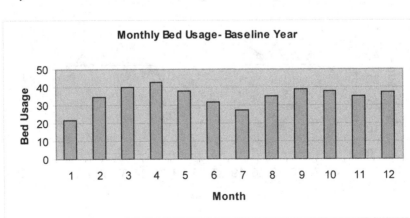

Figure 11. Time evolution of Neurosurgery Ward Bed Utilization with markers for possible Full Ward, In-hospital Overflow and Critical Overflow for the year (note actual thresholds are set arbitrarily). The number of Critical Overflows is nine in this year.

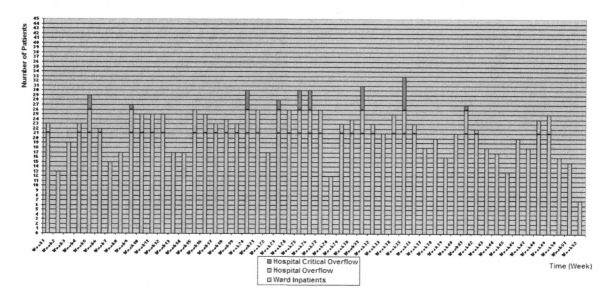

size to be 21 beds and the overflow size to be 5 beds and an overflow capacity of 24%. In this example, unlike the baseline example we allow the system to have critical overflows with patients required to leave the simulation. In this situation, for the initial year there are 9 weeks in which the ward and the overflow are not able to hold all the patients needing services. A graphical representation of the weekly bed usage for the full year with ward beds, overflow beds and critical overflows are shown in Figure 11. Interestingly, when the rate of patients entering the system is increased by only 12%, the number of times critical overflow events occur increases dramatically to 36 weeks. This is an increase by a factor 3 of the number of overflow events from the previous year, but is generated by a very modest (12%) increase in the rate of patients arriving at the ward. Figure 12 shows a graph of the bed usage for the increase arrival rate year. The figure shows the increase ward overflow events, and the number of times the health care model hit a critical overflow condition and patients are required to exits the health care system. Thus we see that through

this type of simulation, hospital administrators and planner can more clearly understand if their facility is operation close to a threshold and the consequences of simple changes in the operation of the health care system.

Manipulating the Physician's Behavior

The hypothetical condition of a modification of the amount of time a physician keeps his patients in the ward was also examined. This is a simulation of the evolution of treatment practice and an attempt to examine the effect that this type of evolution might have on the operation of the ward. It was assumed Physician D (who typically attends the largest number of patients) decided first to extend patients' Length of Stay (LOS) 50% more than before, then by 100% and finally all physicians in the model increase LOS by 50%. Table 2 shows the effects of these changes in the behavior of the physicians on bed utilization.

In these results we see that the effect of physician behavior has a very significant impact on the bed utilization. The progression in the mean value

Figure 12. Simulation generated with a hypothetical 12% scale up of the population entering Neurosurgery Ward. It is interesting to note that the number of time Critical Overflows is 36 in the scale up year.

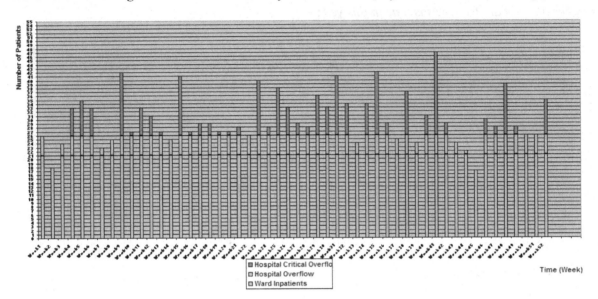

Table 2. Mean and Standard Deviation Values for LOS Extension Hypothetical Conditions on an annual basis.

Condition	Mean	Standard Deviation
Baseline	37.4	6.5
Physician D-50% LOS Increase	43.02	5.76
Physician D-100% LOS Increase	46.19	8.49
All Physicians -50% LOS Increase	51.65	7.68

of bed utilization is as expected with the Physician D-50% LOS Increase having higher mean values of bed utilization than the Baseline. This is followed by Physician D-100% LOS Increase and then All Physicians-50% Increase, which has the highest level of bed utilization. We also see that there is a general increase in the standard deviation however, this is less consistent than that for the mean.

An Assessment of the Hospital Service Focus Simulation

In this section we have presented initial results from the development of a bed allocation model for a neurosurgery ward. The model is based on software agents. The agents are used to create software patients, which exist with in the model claiming use of beds for specified duration. The model allows evaluation of the dynamics of the hospital ward under various conditions, such as increase in patient population which may be the result of a general increase in the local population of the city, and changes in physician protocol such as increased duration of stay for particular procedures, etc. The model could allow hospital administrators to identify the limitations of the system, the number of overflow beds, which should be available, etc.

This system is developed using the concepts

of software agents. The fundamental attribute of Agent autonomy is used in the representation of the patient agent, which is an autonomous entity. It should be noted however, that the true benefit of the agent paradigm in this system will only be achieved when the model is made even richer with more complex behavior in the patient agents and the ability of the patient agents to interact with hospital staff agents etc. Thus the future work in this area will be to develop a more complex and rich environment in which the patient agents can exist.

SCHEDULING OF HOSPITAL RESOURCES

We have developed a comprehensive room scheduling system using agent technology (Paranjape, 2006; Tse & Paranjape, 2007; Tse, Paranjape & Joseph, 2008; Yang, Paranjape & Benedicenti, 2005; Yang, Paranjape & Benedicenti, 2006; Yang, Paranjape, Benedicenti & Reed, 2005; Yang, Paranjape, Benedicenti & Reed, 2006). The focus of this room scheduling system is to provide a mechanism where by resources within the health care system can be allocated efficiently and effectively. This scheduling system provides a framework primarily around the hospital services focus but as it also schedules patients and physicians, and as such it connects to all of the foci of the health care system model. The system essentially schedules events using an agent to represent each event. The event could for example be a specific surgery for a specific patient. Each event is unique and has a set of non-exchangeable participants which include for example the patient, the physician/surgeon, the anesthetist, etc., and a certain number of important but non-specific or exchangeable actors or components such as surgical nurses, equipment, surgical theaters, etc.

Agent System Design

The basic approach is to give each resource (can be a service, equipment, agent actor, etc.) in the system its own timetable. The event then contacts each resource and checks its timetable for free slots into which the event can be scheduled. There are various rules put into place to ensure that race conditions and system blocks such as competing events reserving the last element of a set of resources so that neither can complete the reservation, does not occur. These mechanisms include limiting the number of times an event can request the same resource and in the eventuality of unavailability release of all associated resources. The system is essentially a constructive timetable building process which builds most of the schedule (without conflict) and then a local search with events requesting resources in fixed intervals with limited cycles and time out conditions.

The system is very general and can be used for multiple kinds of events, from booking operating theaters to booking examinations in diagnostic facilities such as MRI or CT scans. The system essentially identifies resources, which are needed in order to schedule an event, and then allows the event to reserve in the resource's timetables until the event is scheduled.

Using this approach means that resources uninvolved with an event are not affected by the event and other events can run simultaneously in effect breaking the scheduling problem up into a set of smaller parallel sub-problem that can be solved simultaneously.

The actors and components needed in scheduling an event (such as an operating theater) are shown in Figure 13. The figure shows an event being scheduled by the event agent contacting various required resources to request empty time slots in the timetable and negotiating with other event agents that may be requesting the same resource. Another strength of this type of approach is that it is highly suited to dynamic scheduling where queues and events are continuously changing and

Figure 13. Schematic showing the scheduling process for events within the Health Care System Model. Events are autonomous agents that interact with various exchangeable resources and non-exchangeable resources to schedule themselves into the timetables of each resource [R(n)]. Event agents will negotiate with other event agent to cooperate and share resources effectively.

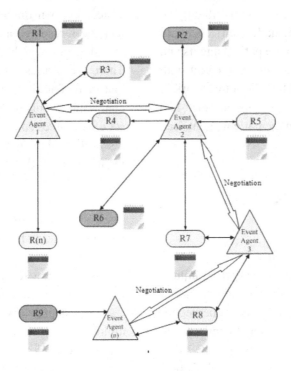

it is necessary to adjust and evolve the final time table almost continuously.

Assessment of Scheduling System

The scheduling system presented here is a significant departure from the current practices in most health care systems. Typically in most health care systems, scheduling is done manually by informed parties though a system of queues and priorities. This system is typically highly consultative and attempts to be fair and equitable on the broadest level. Unfortunately, this also means that it is typically inflexible and can not rapidly adjust to a fluid and continuously changing environment. Schedules are formed with the best available information at the time of formation, but once defined, serious and well established changes must occur before schedules can be re-adjusted.

In the approach presented in this section, we do not attempt to model the current scheduling system. We do not attempt this because the current system is derived primarily from the expertise of the individuals doing the scheduling and their process is likely to be ad hoc and experience-based rather then algorithmic or rule based.

While we plan to create a representation of the existing real-world system, it is our belief that resource allocation is one of the major limiting factors in the efficient use of resources in health care.

DISCUSSION

As seen in the preceding sections, we have generated a number of realistic and reasonable actors and components of the health care system in a simulation model. Each of the components developed, is independently useful but can also be use as a part of a large health care system simulation model. The Diabetic patient agent for example can be used as a teaching tool to allow human diabetic patients to examine their outcomes on a short term based on food/carbohydrate intake. Within the health care system simulation, the diabetic patient is one of an ensemble of patient actors in the system. They move through the system interacting with other components in an asynchronous and spontaneous fashion. Doctor/physician agents read the patient agent's vital statistics and make decisions for the patient including the need for hospital services including surgeries, etc.

The hospital bed allocation system also demonstrates a very great potential to be used independently of a larger health care simulation model. As indicated in the results section, the bed allocation system can be used for planning and policy testing. By using an up-to-date data sets for the system, a very accurate modeling and simulation facility is produced. The capability to then extrapolate to changes in physician practice, population demographic and numerical change, etc. can be accurately and carefully examined. On the other hand, within the health care system simulation model, the bed allocation system represents the orderly flow of patients through the relevant part of the model. As patients comes into the system and need to be processed by the system, physicians and nurses need to do various tests, read various typed of data, requisition various types of procedures and allow the patient agents to either recover and leave the simulation healthy and cured or in other, less desirable states.

The scheduling system we have developed has applications well beyond the health care simulation model also. The system develops a constructive scheduling paradigm which builds the schedule one event at a time and can continuously re-schedule as higher priority events enter the system. By developing this dynamic model it is expected that various inefficiencies in the system

will be identified and scheduling system itself may show mechanisms to alter the work flow in the operation of various health care services.

Returning now to some of the general questions posed in the introduction of this work, we see that clearly agent and agent systems can play an important role in modeling the health care system. We have demonstrated actors and components that we have constructed using agent technology show great promise in modeling different aspects of the system. The second question, that of demonstrating an improvement is efficiency, is reserved for the future. It can only be addressed once a complete model containing all the focus components of the health care system has been constructed. However, based on initial results, we do not anticipate any difficulty in assembling the model; the efficiency of alternative management strategies can then be easily assessed, based on the various objectives of the hospital management, the government, or even the general public.

We believe that the strength of this approach to system modeling in that if each component can be faithfully represented then the complete system behavior will naturally evolve as an extension of the collective behavior. This agent based approach is more appropriate for modeling the health care system than a deterministic and interrelated model which may be developed without using the agent methodology. Thus, by mapping agent autonomy into the autonomous representation of components, we ensure independence of the final system behavior from any preconceived notions of health care system interaction which are not specifically prescribed for individuals in the system.

While the actual complete physical system is incredibly complex to develop and still some years away from completion, we believe we have demonstrated that it is possible to model components of the system. Moreover, each component is itself quite important and has potential for many useful applications beyond the larger health care system model. We believe that by developing each component individually the actual factors that purely affect the component can be identified. The system, without external factors, must be well understood in order to optimize its behavior by adjusting component behavior and interaction. If there is going to be any ability to maximize effectiveness of the health care investment and to minimize patient suffering and distress, agent based systems, such as the one proposed here, will have to be developed.

CONCLUSION

We have proposed a comprehensive, broad-spectrum, health-care-system modeling, paradigm using agent technology. We have presented a general framework for the health care system model. We have examined three aspects of the system; the patient focus, the hospital services focus, and a scheduling system, which helps connects these focuses. We believe that this type of agent model can identify weaknesses, bottlenecks and inefficiencies in the health care system which will allow optimization of health care investment. We have shown that effective agent models for a diabetic patient (as an example of the patient component), for hospital services, and for hospital scheduling can be developed. We believe that such modeling can have a profound impact on predicting outcomes for individuals and for the system, based on their behavior and operational patterns.

ACKNOWLEDGMENT

This work is financially supported by grants from TRLabs and NSERC. Access to patient data provided by the Regina Qu'Appelle Health Region.

REFERENCES

Ackerman, E., Rosevear, J., & McGuckin, W. (1964). A Mathematical Model of the Glucose-tolerance test. *Physics in Medicine and Biology*, *9*, 203–213. doi:10.1088/0031-9155/9/2/307

American Diabetes Association. (2006). Retrieved December 12, 2006 from http://www.diabetes.org

Boutayeb, A., & Chetouani, A. (2006). *A Critical Review of Mathematical Models and Data used in Diabetology*. Retrieved December 6, 2006 from http://www.biomedical-engineering-online.com/

Canadian Diabetes Association. (2006). Retrieved December 12, 2006 from http://www.diabetes.ca/

CCHBPC. (2006). *Canadian Coalition for High Blood Pressure Prevention and Control*. Retrieved December 12, 2006 from http://hypertension.ca/bpc/

CDC. Centers for Disease Control and Prevention (2006). Retrieved December 11, 2006 from http://www.cdc.gov/diabetes/statistics/prev/national

Chun, A., Wai, H., & Wong, R. (2003). Optimizing agent-based meeting scheduling through preference estimation. *Engineering Applications of Artificial Intelligence*, *16*, 727–743. doi:10.1016/j.engappai.2003.09.009

Gérard, P., Massin, M. M., Maeyns, K., Withofs, N., & Ravet, F. (2000). Circadian Rhythm of Heart Rate and Heart Rate Variability. *Archives of Disease in Childhood*, *83*, 179–182. doi:10.1136/adc.83.2.179

Ghoreishi-Nejad, S., Martens, R., & Paranjape, R. (2008). An Agent-Based Diabetic Patient Simulation, KES-AMSTA. In N.T. Nguyen (Ed.), *Lecture Notes in Artificial Intelligence, 4953*, 832–841.

Gibbs, C. (2000). *TEEMA Reference Guide, Version 1.0.* Saskatchewan: TRLabs Regina.

Harper, P. R. (2002). A Framework for Operational Modelling of Hospital Resources. [Kluwer Academic Publishers.]. *Health Care Management Science, 5*, 165–173. doi:10.1023/A:1019767900627

Health Canada. (2002). *Diabetes in Canada* (2nd ed.). Center for Chronic Disease Prevention and Control, Population and Public Health Branch, Health Canada

Hertz, A., & Robert, V. (1998). Constructing a course schedule by solving a series of assignment type problems. *European Journal of Operational Research, 108*, 585–603. doi:10.1016/S0377-2217(97)00097-0

Kuo, P. C., Schroeder, R. A., Mahaffey, S., & Bollinger, R. R. (2003, December). Optimization of operating room allocation using linear programming techniques. *Journal of the American College of Surgeons, 197*(6), 889–895. doi:10.1016/j.jamcollsurg.2003.07.006

Liu, Q. (2002). *Master Degree Thesis: A Mobile Agent System for Distributed Mammography Image Retrieval.* Regina, Saskatchewan, Canada: University of Regina.

Makroglou, A., Li, J., & Kuang, Y. (2005). Mathematical Models and Software Tools for the Glucose-Insulin Regulatory System and Diabetes: An Overview. [Elsevier.]. *Applied Numerical Mathematics, 56*, 559–573. doi:10.1016/j.apnum.2005.04.023

Marshall, A., Vasilakis, C., & El-Darzi, E. (2005). Length of Stay-Based Patient Flow Models: Recent Developments and Future Directions. [Springer Science + Business Media, Inc.]. *Health Care Management Science, 8*, 213–220. doi:10.1007/s10729-005-2012-z

Moreno, A., Isern, D., & Sanchez, D. (2001). Provision of Agent-Based Healthcare Services. *Proc. of AIME 2001.*

Nicholls, A. G., & Young, F. R. (2007). Innovative Hospital Bed Management Using Spatial Technology. *Spatial Science Queensland* (pp. 26-30)

Nutrition Data. (2006). *Glycemic Index.* Retrieved December 12, 2006 from http://www.nutritiondata.com/glycemic¬index.html

Paranjape, R. (2006, May 9-12). Macroscopic Modeling of Information Flow in an Agent-Based Electronic Health Record System. *Fifth International Workshop on Agents and Peer-to-Peer Computing (AP2PC 2006) Fifth International Joint Conference on Autonomous Agents and Multi Agent Systems (AAMAS06)*, Hakodate, Japan.

Paranjape, R., Ogrady, M., & Ghoreshi-Nejad, S. (2008, August 18–20). A neuro-surgery ward bed-allocation modeling system using software agents. *Internet and Multimedia Systems and Applications*, Kailu-Kona, Hawaii, USA.

Saenchai, K., Benedicenti, L., & Paranjape, R. (2004, May). The design of an architecture for software agents on mobile platforms. *Canadian Conference on Electrical and Computer Engineering* (CCECE04), *3*, 1389-92. Niagara Falls, Canada.

Saenchai, K., Benedicenti, L., & Paranjape, R. (2005, May 1-4). A Dynamic Extension of the Asynchronous Weak-Commitment Search Algorithm. *Canadian Conference on Electrical and Computer Engineering* (CCECE05), Saskatoon, Canada (pp. 1112-1115).

Saenchai, K., Benedicenti, L., & Paranjape, R. (2006). Solving Dynamic Distributed Constraint Satisfaction Problems with a Modified Weak-Commitment Search Algorithm. *Lecture Notes in Computer Science, 3910*, 130–137. doi:10.1007/11734697_10

Schaerf, A. (1999). A Survey of Automated Timetabling. *Artificial Intelligence Review*, 87–127. doi:10.1023/A:1006576209967

Tse, B., & Paranjape, R. (2005, May 1-4). Mathematical Analysis of Agent Swarm Behavior in an Agent-Based Electronic Health Record System. *Canadian Conference on Electrical and Computer Engineering*, Saskatoon, (CCECE05) (pp. 996–1001), Saskatoon, Canada.

Tse, B., & Paranjape, R. (2007). Macroscopic Modeling of Information Flow in an Agent-Based Electronic Health Record System. In H. Lin (Ed), *Architectural Design of Multi-Agent Systems: Technologies and Techniques* (pp. 305-334). Information Science Reference.

Tse, B., Paranjape, R., & Joseph, S. (2008). Information Flow Analysis in Autonomous Agent and Peer-to-Peer Systems for Self-Organizing Electronic Health Records. In J.S.R.H., Despotovic, G. Moro, & S. Bergamaschi (Eds.), *Agents and Peer to Peer Computing, Lecture Notes in Artificial Intelligence, 4461*, 1-20.

University of Virginia Health System. (2006). *Diabetes and High Blood Pressure*. Retrieved December 12, 2006 from http://www.healthsystem.virginia.edu/uvahealth/adult_diabetes/hbp.cfm

Web, M. D. (2006). *Heart Disease Health Center*. Retrieved December 12, 2006 from http://www.webmd.com/hw/heart_disease/hw233473.asp

Wooldridge, M., & Jennings, N. (1995). Intelligent agents: theory and practice. *The Knowledge Engineering Review, 10*(2), 115–152. doi:10.1017/S0269888900008122

Wu, Hsin-I. (2005). *A Case Study of Type 2 Diabetes Self-Management*. Retrieved January 22, 2005 from http://www.biomedical-engineering-online.com/

Yang, Y. **P**aranjape, R., & Benedicenti, L. (2004). An Examination of Mobile Agents System Evolution in the Course-Scheduling Problem. *Proceedings of the 2004 IEEE Canadian Conference on Electrical and Computer Engineering* (pp 5782-5785)

Yang, Y., Paranjape, R., & Benedicenti, L. (2006). A Hierarchical Multi Agent Architecture For The University Course Timetabling Problem. *Autonomous Agents and Multi-Agent Systems (AAMAS05)*, Hokodate, Japan.

Yang, Y., Paranjape, R., Benedicenti, L., & Reed, N. (2005, December). A Mobile Agent System for University Course Timetabling. *Proceedings of the Second Indian International Conference on Artificial Intelligence* (IICAI 2005) (pp. 2926-2937), Pune, India.

Yang, Y., Paranjape, R., Benedicenti, L., & Reed, N. (2006). A System Model for University Course Scheduling using Mobile Agents. *Multiagent and Grid Systems - . International Journal (Toronto, Ont.), 2*(3), 267–275.

Chapter 5
Operating Room Simulation and Agent–Based Optimization

Q. Peng
University of Manitoba, Canada

Q. Niu
University of Manitoba, Canada

Y. Xie
University of Manitoba, Canada

T. ElMekkawy
University of Manitoba, Canada

ABSTRACT

Healthcare systems are characterized by uncertainty, variability, complexity, and human roles. Simulation can test scenarios of changes in processes, resources, and schedules without major physical investment or risk. Agent-based technology can model systems with autonomous and interacting activities. This chapter introduces the method of using simulation and agent-based technologies to enable a better understanding of the patient flow to improve the process performance in healthcare. The proposed method is used to identify the existing problem and to evaluate proposed solutions for the problem of the operating room (OR) at Winnipeg Health Sciences Centre. Issues are identified including patient flows, operation schedules, demand and capacity of the system and the configuration of resources required. An optimum scheduling is proposed for the OR operation to shorten the patient waiting time.

INTRODUCTION

Healthcare systems provide health-related services by the medical, nursing, and allied health professions. Healthcare is an enormous part of the economy

DOI: 10.4018/978-1-60566-772-0.ch005

as it consumes average 6.7 percent of GDP in the high-income countries (WHO, 2008). Healthcare in Canada is funded and delivered through a publicly funded healthcare system. Canada spent an estimated $142 billion on healthcare in 2005, or $4,411 per person. It was projected to reach $160 billion, or 10.6% of GDP, in 2007 (CBC, 2006).

A common problem of Canadian healthcare systems is a long waiting list of patients, which may result from the inefficient utilization of human resources and facilities, or the failure to eliminate non-value added activities. It is critical to improve the performance and productivity of the national healthcare system.

Winnipeg Health Sciences Centre (WHSC) is a healthcare centre serving residents of Manitoba, Northwestern Ontario and Nunavut. The operating room (OR) department is one of the most demanding departments in WHSC based on the statistical data. The problems of the OR are the long waiting list of patients and the inefficient utilization of resources.

This chapter introduces the use of computer simulation and agent-based methods to analyze and improve performance of the OR department in WHSC. Computer simulation is an efficient way to imitate real-world problems over time for analyzing and describing the behaviour of the real-system (Mahapatra, 2003). One of the main capabilities using simulation is to analyze what-if scenarios, which allows a significant exploration of multiple options, without spending enormous amounts of expense on staff, training, and equipment (Barnes, 1997). The term *agent* has been used for an entity in a system with key properties autonomy, social ability, reactivity and pro-activeness. A multi-agent system is a group of agents that interact with each other to solve complex problems (Mes, 2007). Multi-agent technology offers a convenient platform to represent real units for optimization and visualization of flows of material, work, and information. It has features of scalability, modularity, flexibility, and online reconfigurability (Garcia, 2008). Therefore, the computer simulation and agent-based optimization are used in this research for the performance improvement of healthcare systems. The simulation model is used to identify existing problems and to evaluate proposed solutions. The agent-based optimization is applied to model the system and find solutions of the problems.

Following parts of this chapter will first describe the research background of healthcare system simulation and agent-based optimization. Details of the simulation modeling for the OR department at WHSC will then be discussed. Different healthcare variables and constraints are considered in the system modeling. The agent-based method is introduced based on the analysis of the simulation solution. The conclusion and further work will also be discussed.

BACKGROUND

Simulation in Healthcare

Great efforts have been made for performance improvement of healthcare systems in the worldwide area. Computer simulation has been an effective tool for operational analysis of the stochastic processes of healthcare delivery (Lowery, 1994). Computer modeling and simulation enable users to better understand the patient experience, process performances and staffing inter-relationships. An open and proactive communication is always the best way to ensure the success of any project. Computer simulation models and analyzes real-world problems that cannot be successfully approached by other types of analytical techniques. In the last two decades, the use of computer simulation as a planning and decision making tool has been spreading rapidly in the healthcare arena. Simulation in healthcare has been applied with success. Specialized applications targeting emergency rooms and other operation issues at large institutions are well documented (Centeno, 2003). Testing scenarios of changes in process methods, equipment locations, resources, and schedules without major physical investment and risk is a key objective in the application of healthcare simulation (Morrison, 2003). There are many successful simulation applications in healthcare. For example, a simulation model was built for the emergency department in a general hospital to examine patient flows and the patient waiting time (Takakuwa, 2004); the simulation was used to estimate the maximum level of demand in an emergency room and the configuration of resources required (Baesler, 2003); a discrete event simulation model analyzed the renal transplant waiting list and reduced the size of the waiting list (Abellán, 2004); a patient scheduling simulation model was built to capture four components of outpatient clinic scheduling systems including external demand for appointments, supply of provider timeslots, the patient flow logic and the scheduling algorithm (Guo, 2004); and a computer simulation model of the hospital layout was used for the efficient use of resources (Osidach, 2003).

Simulation is more effective than analytical solutions for complex models, where the state of the system changes over time (Miller, 2004). Healthcare systems are characterized by uncertainty, variability, complex, and human role (Brailsford, 2007). It must be noted that the simulation only allows potential solutions to be relationally quantified. Without the involvement of healthcare professionals, and experienced personal in the operation and management, a meaningful and successful simulation would not be possible (Lowery, 1994). Since human in healthcare systems are not machines, human factors are necessary to account for unanticipated ergonomic problems (Osidach, 2003). Other important problems in simulation modeling include: the scope of the simulation model is easily lost in the decision-making process of a system, which can create a complex and sophisticated model which adds little or no value to the output of the simulation (Ferrin, 2004); the model in a high abstraction level may not match the need of the real-world, and developing simulation models becomes a complex, tedious and time-consuming task (Sinreich, 2004). Agent-based technology is an option for the solution of these problems.

Agent-Based Technology

Much research has been done in the development of agent-based systems. Agent-based systems have been applied in different areas for the solution of problems that may not be solved by conventional computing methods. Manufacturing is one of these areas. For example, a multi-agent based tool, called flexible and adaptive scheduling tool, was developed for a flexible, fault tolerant, and scalable manufacturing scheduling system (Garcia, 2008); An agent-based architecture with a three-layered structure was developed based on the intelligent agent technology to support resource integration and scheduling (Wang, 2007); An agent interface was used to encapsulate distributed manufacturing functional entities as resource agents and to connect them with the agent community. Mok et al modeled humans and machines as agents for workflow problems that do not have existing computer-based solutions (Mok, 2006). A multi-agent approach was proposed by Zhang (2007) to dynamically integrate production planning and control decisions with systems reconfiguration and restructure. The approach promises hierarchical structure modeling of complex systems and avoids centralized control in classical hierarchical frameworks. The system structure and configurations also be evaluated through a discrete event simulation.

The agent-based system provides a variety of strategies for decision-making and operation control. A multi-agent approach can be integrated with a filtered beam-search-based heuristic algorithm for the dynamic scheduling problem in a FMS shop floor with multiple manufacturing cells (Wang, 2008). A scalable agent-based approach can meet scheduling problems with the distributed and dynamic needs (Hassine, 2007). A collaborative agent-based intelligence system can control and resolve dynamic scheduling problem of distributed projects (Chen, 2007). An agent-based dynamic scheduling can meet the need of various products, processes, and disturbances in manufacturing systems (Xiang, 2008). Ant colony intelligence can be combined with a local agent to make autonomous agents adaptive to changing circumstances for the efficient global performance. The multi-agent workload control methodology can work for the due date setting, job release and scheduling in manufacturing (Weng, 2008). The agent-based technology is also a useful tool for the support of collaborative process planning. A proper agent-based computer-aided process planning (CAPP) system has become a vital task to improve the performance of modern manufacturing systems (Zhang, 2007).

The agent-based approach was also used for intelligent vehicle route scheduling (Mes, 2007) and for patient-centered healthcare management (Rodríguez, 2005). The vehicle agents interact with job agents for minimum transportation costs and easy schedule adjustments in reaction to information updates. An ambient intelligence system uses autonomous agents to provide capabilities of intelligence in healthcare environments furnished with ubiquitous computing and medical devices.

A multi-agent system uses independent intelligent control units linked to physical or functional entities for a flexible, stable and robust planning system. It is a promising solution for controlling complex systems to provide flexibility, reliability, adaptability and reconfigurability. Agents act autonomously by pursuing their own interests to interact with each other, such as the use of information exchange and negotiation mechanisms.

In the healthcare system, each operation and resource can have its own goal-directed agent. For example, a doctor agent may focus on on-time operation against the lowest possible time delay, and a bed agent may strive for utilization. The key issue is to configure agents for their self-interested behavior to yield an optimal solution for the whole system. The objectives of our research are to reduce the length of patients stay and to improve the utilization of resources in the OR department of WHSC. The bottlenecks will be identified. The suggestions for the improvement will be provided.

A visualized environment is used as the simulation interface in this research, which provides an efficient interaction between users and systems. Using visualized simulation and agent-based technology, human behaviours and model levels of details can be integrated to accommodate modeling of healthcare systems. Rather than to view recommendations as "black-box" answers to complex problems which use the notion of the mystery of statistics, the integration of the simulation with agent-based optimization will provide an effective tool to manipulate different scenarios in the healthcare delivery. A full understanding of the complex patient flow would be achieved. Based on such understanding, a detailed guide on the improvement of the healthcare system can be generated.

SIMULATION MODELING AND SYSTEM EVALUATION

The simulation modeling is based on data collected from WHSC. The system evaluation is based on the model built for the OR department. The purpose of the simulation is the improvement of the OR operation through the test of different scenarios. Options to test the performance improvement are supported by patient scheduling, resource scheduling, physical resource requirements, and operating procedures. The simulation modeling and system evaluation include following major phases of work:

- Data collection of the OR department at WHSC.
- Simulation modeling.
- Verification and validation of the simulation model.
- Experiment with scenarios.
- Analysis of the simulation result.

Table 1. Resources in the OR department

No.	Resource items	Quantity
1	Operating Rooms/beds	13
2	Front desk	1
3	Holding Area (Music room)	6 chairs
4	PACU (Post anaesthesia care unit)	12 beds
5	Operating Room Nurses	36
6	Perioperative Aides (Pas)	3
7	Transport Personnel	2
8	Anaesthetists	12
9	IHA (Backup Anaesthetist)	1

It is important to have correct and enough data for the system modeling as solutions resulting from the simulation model are dependent upon the data very much, As shown in Figure 1, the patient flow related to the OR department starts from the registration. Patients can be either day patient, same day admission patient or inpatient. The patient is picked by Pre-operative Unit and is sent to Inpatient Ward or other units after the surgery. The unit may be Post Anaesthesia Care Unit (PACU) or Surgical Intensive Care Unit (SICU). Only elective patients are considered in the modeling. The elective patients' types include Same Day Patients (SD), Same Day Admission Patients (SDA) and Inpatients (INP). The elective hours are 07:30 to 15:30, Mondays to Fridays, with 10-12 staffed operating rooms.

Most patients are tested in Pre-operative units, such as X-ray and blood test units. The patient is also interviewed by an OR nurse, and is assessed by the anesthetist in the hold area, or called music room, before the surgery. After the operating room is ready, the patient is moved in the operating room. The OR nurse and anesthetists place the patient in the position for sleep. The patient is taken to the PACU or SICU to recovery after the surgery. The OR has the link with many other departments, such as Pre-operative units and Inpatient departments. There are many factors influencing patients' surgery. If, for example, there are not enough beds in MS3, a pre-operative unit in the hospital, the patient will not be arranged for the surgery.

The OR resources included in the modeling are operating rooms, beds, front desk, holding area and others as listed in Table 1. Table 2 lists resources related to the OR in WHSC. There are 13 rooms or beds in the OR department that are located in one floor as the layout shown in Figure 2.

The simulation model is built based on the layout and collected data in the OR department of WHSC. The details data related to the OR operations are as follows:

Data related to patients:

• Type of patients;
• Stay time of different types of patients in the hospital;
• Number of patients per day;
• Percentage of each type of patients;
• Arrival time of each patient;
• Leaving time of each patient.

Table 2. Resources related to the OR

No.	OR resources	Quantity
1	Admitting	1
2	MS3	6 Beds
3	B3	4 Beds
4	Inpatient ward	164 Beds

Figure 1. The patient flow

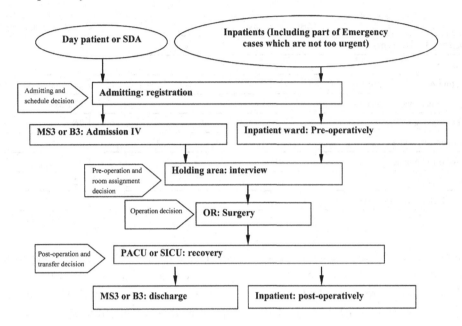

Data related to staff:

- Types of staff, such as doctors, nurses, and technicians;

- Number of each type of staff in different departments;
- Total number of each type of staff;
- Shifts of staff in different departments;

Figure 2. Layout of the OR department at WHSC

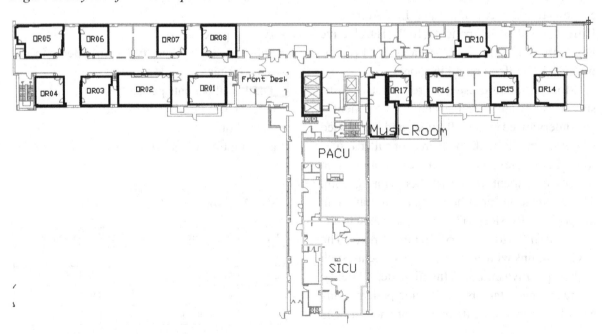

• Coffee break time.

Data related to other resources:

• Number of OR rooms;
• Number of beds;
• Number of vehicles;
• Number of receptions;
• Number of holding areas, such as: music area;
• Other places in the area;
• Rules of the bed use.

Data related to work in processing:

• Processing time of operations;
• Processing time of tests;
• Processing time of moving patients from one place to another place;
• Processing time of admission, assessment, discharge, and cleaning;
• Working flow between different departments;
• Types of tests;
• Test required for the patient;
• Priority of the operations.

A database is built with five weeks data collected from elective patients. The data listed in Table 3 are used for simulation modeling based on the data available, operations and problems to be modeled. Figure 3 shows the data tables used in the database. The system variables used in simulation modeling are shown in Table 4, which are used for the system performance analysis.

Figure 4 is a histogram that shows the distribution of the surgery processing time based on the collected data of five weeks from the OR including 740 patients. Figure 5 shows the length of stay of same day patients. Distribution functions are used to generate the processing time based on the analysis of the collected data and the statistical test. The distributions used in the modeling are listed in Tables 5 and 6.

There is a variety of simulation modeling systems available such as Witness (Lanner, 2006), Flexsim (Flexsim, 2008) and Delmia Quest (DS Group, 2008). They are commonly used in the simulation of manufacturing and logistics systems. Our simulation model was initially modeled using Witness simulation system. Witness provides the basic functions required for the proposed research. Flexsim is used later for the model extension to the 3D visualization and for the need of agent-based optimization.

The patient models are built with different types. Attributes are utilized in collecting and

Table 3. The data used for the simulation modeling

No.	Items
1	The admitting time
2	The arrival time to pre-op units which are MS3, B3, Inpatient ward
3	The leave time from pre-op units
4	The arrival time to OR
5	The leave time from OR
6	The arrival time to post-op units
7	The discharge time
8	The start time of OR setup
9	The end time of OR setup
10	The start time of OR cleaning
11	The end time of OR cleaning

Figure 3. Tables in the database to record the collected data

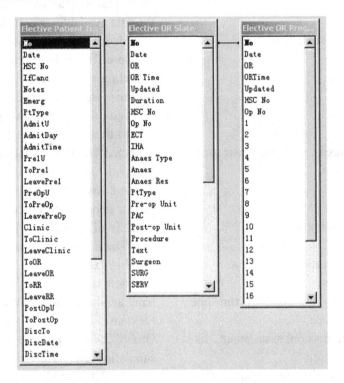

recording data of waiting time and total time that patients stay in the OR. Histograms are defined to display waiting time and total time of patients. A screenshot of the simulation model is shown in Figure 6. Figure 7 shows attributes and variables used in the simulation process.

The OR scheduling is modeled based on the definition of variables and data generated by the distribution functions as shown in Figure 8. Python programming (Python, 2008) is used for data operation and data analysis. Python is a dynamic object-oriented programming language. It offers a support for integration with other languages and tools. It comes with extensive standard libraries. Python is distributed under an OSI-approved open source license. The scheduling is generated using

Table 4. Variables used in the modeling

No	Item	Description
1	No	The number of the patient
2	ArrivalTime	The patient admitting time
3	MRBegings	The time when the patient arrives at the holding area
4	OPBegins	The time when the OR begins
5	OPEnds	The time when the OR ends
6	PACUBegins	The time when the patient arrives to PACU
7	LeaveTime	The time when the patient discharges
8	LOS	The length of stay
9	count	The count in the simulation model

Figure 4. The histogram of surgery processing time

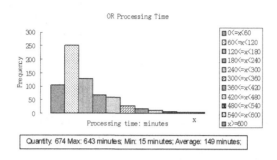

Figure 5. The length of Same Day (SD) patients

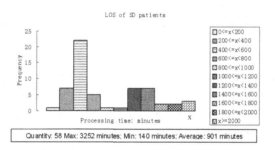

Table 5. Main distributions of processing time (unit: minutes)

Items	Time	Use
Patient arrival	PatientArrival (13)	Admitting
Admitting	UNIFORM (2,10,4)	Admitting
Interview	NEGEXP(10,10)	Holding area
Assessment	NEGEXP(10,11)	Holding area
Surgery	Duration (12)	Operating Room
Recovery	TRIANGLE (0,144,657,6)	PACU
OR cleaning	TRIANGLE (0,14,28,19)	Operating Room
OR setup	TRIANGLE (0,15,36,20)	Operating Room

Python to query the elective_patient_time table in the database. The input data are imported into the simulation model using text files. The processed data are written to output files. Python reads data from these files, and implements all functions needed in the processing. Python is also connected to a Microsoft Access database to record all patient information. Python retrieves data from the database to analyze data and to generate the distributions.

Table 6. Travel time between different units (minutes)

From- to	Distributions
Pre-op units to OR	TRIANGLE (0,21,41,1)
OR to PACU	TRIANGLE (0,4,10,20)
PACU to post-op unit	TRIANGLE (0,8,24,2)

The model testing is for the verification and validation of the simulation model. The verification and validation of the simulation model are important for ensuring that the model built is correct and right representation of the real system. The model validation is the key to guarantee the assumption of the conceptual model are right and close to the reality. Based on the simulation model built for the existing OR operations, the collected data are used to drive the simulation for the analysis of surgical patient flow and the operation performance in the OR department. The events from the five weeks data are counted to validate the model. The model performances are compared between the reality and model results by running 6 replications for five weeks of each

replication. The data in Table 7 show that the simulation results are very close the reality of the collected actual data.

The simulation model enables scenarios to analyze how observed variables in the OR will be affected by the data or resources change. By changing some of inputs, the model is able to show how the performance is automatically changed when resources and other pertinent data are revised. The alternatives are simulated after the verification and validation of the simulation model. The processing procedure and patients flow are simulated in the model. The model is used to simulate 'what-if' scenarios of the OR department in WHSC.

A series of experiments are simulated to iden-

Figure 6. A screen shot of the simulation model

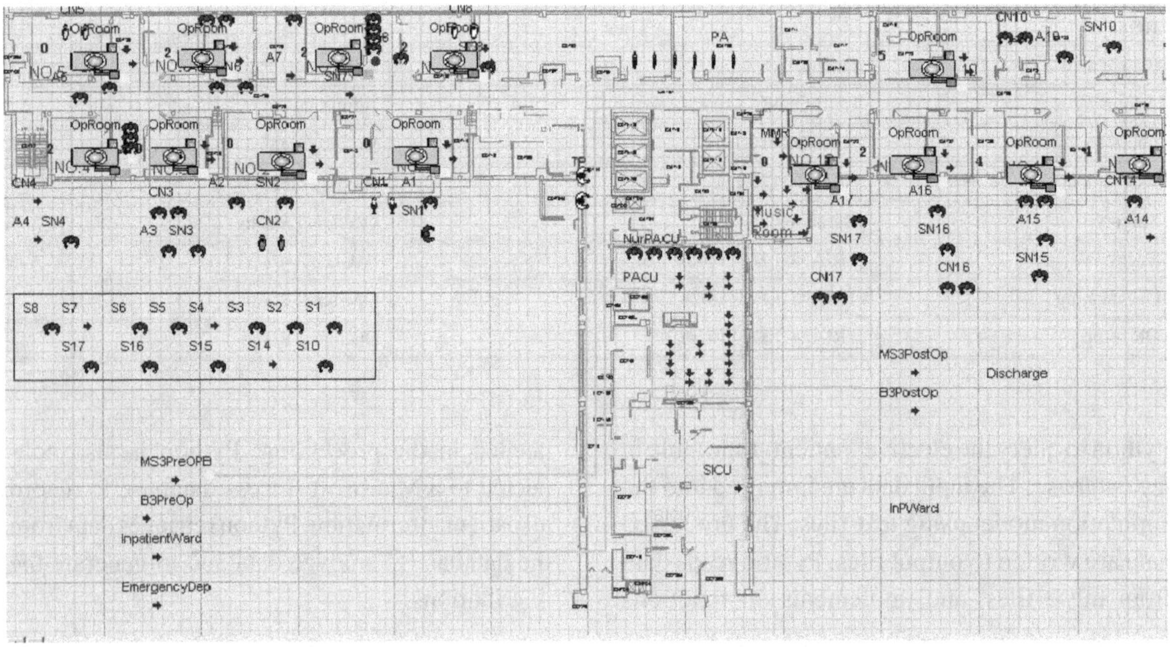

Figure 7. Attributes and variables in the simulation process

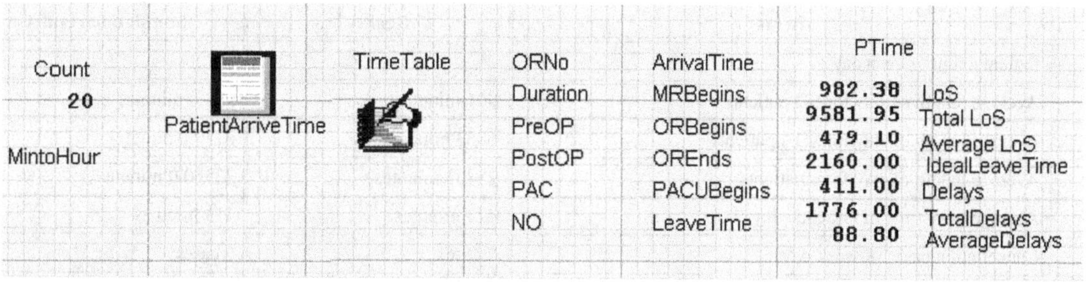

tify the bottleneck of the existing patient flow in the OR by changing different resources, such as numbers of nurses and beds. The patients' arrival schedule is based on the actual historical data. The OR number is assigned for the individual patient following the historical schedule. Based on the data collected from five weeks, the model running lengths and warm up periods of 25 days, and 3 days respectively are used for each replication to allow for the system to reach realistic operating conditions before collecting appropriate statistics. 6 replications of the simulation are undertaken.

Simulation is performed based on different scenarios. The overall utilization rate for each case is found for doctors, nurses and beds, respectively. The length of stay of patients in the OR is simulated. It is assumed that a fully loaded one week appointment booking is as input for the simulation. The simulation shows the detailed daily operation with patient arrivals and resource constraints.

Figure 8. The part of OR scheduling

<u>*Definition of attributes:*</u>
The first column is the patient type
The second column is the quantity of arrival patient
The third column is the time when the patient arrives
ORNo = The number of operating room
Duration = The surgery processing time
No =The No of the patient
PreOP = Pre-operative unit
PostOP = Post-operative unit
PAC = If patient went to PAC or not before surgery, 1 means that patient went to PAC before the surgery.

<u>*Part of scheduling file:*</u>

INP	*1*	*365*	*ORNo=8*	*Duration=241*	*NO=1*	*PreOP="D2"*
SDA	*1*	*373*	*ORNo=1*	*Duration=295*	*NO=2*	*PreOP="GMS3" PostOP="A3"*
	PAC=1					
SDA	*1*	*373*	*ORNo=2*	*Duration=296*	*NO=3*	*PreOP="GMS3" PostOP="A3"*
	PAC=1					
SD	*1*	*394*	*ORNo=16*	*Duration=124*	*NO=4*	*PreOP="GMS3"*
SDA	*1*	*410*	*ORNo=3*	*Duration=242*	*NO=5*	*PreOP="GMS3" PostOP="D2"*
	PAC=1					
SD	*1*	*428*	*ORNo=15*	*Duration=63*	*NO=6*	*PreOP="GB3"*

.
.

Table 7. The model validations

No	Items	Reality	Simulation results
1	Patient count of each day	26	27
2	Average length of stay for SD patients	901 minutes	923.0 minutes
3	Average length of stay for SDA patients	6063 minutes	6130.0 minutes
4	Average length of stay for inpatients	23401 minutes	23560.0 minutes
5	Average busy time of OR each day	421 minutes	413 minutes
6	Cancellation cases of week day	7 cases	6 cases

The experimental data include the arrival time of the patient and the category of the patient. Following two scenarios are experienced using the simulation model for the length of stays of elective patients.

Scenario 1: Four alternatives with the effect of changes in resources on:

- Number of operating rooms in the OR department;
- Number of beds in PACU;
- Number of chairs in the holding area.

Table 8 shows outcomes of the simulation for the average length of stay (LOS) of different patients and the reduced ratio of LOS under different resource conditions. Figure 9 shows the reduced LOS of SD patients with the resources of row No. 4 comparing with using the resources of row No. 1 in Table 8. It shows in Figure 8 that the frequency of short stay (0 < x <1400) is increased and the frequency of long stay is decreased (x> 1400).

Scenario 2: Four alternatives with the effects

of changing number of the transport personnel in the OR department.

The improvement is shown in Table 9 when increasing the number of transport personals (TPs). Patients are transported to operating rooms almost at the same time in the morning as all operating rooms are empty. Currently, there are only two TPs who move patients from the pre-op unit to the operating rooms.

Preliminary simulation experiments indicate that when more patients are expected to be processed at the OR, the patient waiting time becomes longer, unless the additional beds are allocated. Then, a stepwise procedure of operations planning is proposed to reduce the patient waiting time. Through a series of simulation experiments, the patient waiting time can be minimized, by adjust appropriate resources in the OR.

It seems obvious that an increase in resources would result in a reduced length of stay and increased patient flow. A feasible solution should improve the system efficiency without resources increase. Based on the system simulation and data

Table 8. The comparison of the resources change

No	Resources			SD		SDA		Inpatient	
	Beds in OR	Beds in PACU	Chairs in holding area	Average LOS	Change	Average LOS	Change	Average LOS	Change
1	13	12	6	923.0	0	6130.0	0	23560.0	0
2	13	12	10	865.0	6%	5993.0	2%	23298.0	4%
3	13	14	10	791.0	14%	5901.0	8%	23123.0	9%
4	14	14	10	717.0	22%	5843.0	14%	22986.0	17%

Figure 9. Reduced LOS of SD patients

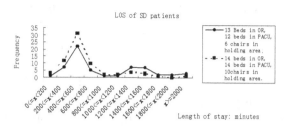

Table 9. Changing the number of TPs

No	Number of TPs	SD patients		SDA patients		Inpatients	
		Average LOS	Change	Average LOS	Change	Average LOS	Change
1	2	923.0	0	6130.0	0	23560.0	0
2	3	901.0	2.30%	6102.0	0.46%	23536.0	0.10%
3	5	853.0	7.60%	6062.0	3.20%	23494.0	2.01%
4	7	793.0	14.00%	5989.0	7.60%	23382.0	5.04%

analysis, it is identified that scheduling is one of the crucial tasks guaranteeing the efficiency of operating activities in the OR. One solution to improve the operation procedure without resources increase is to optimize the patient arrival schedule. The patient arrival schedule is an essential element of the model. Detailed information of an OR schedule includes admitting time, patient type, operation room number and the expected operation duration. Therefore, an agent-based method is introduced to extend the function of the simulation model to optimize the patient arrival schedule.

THE AGENT-BASED OPTIMIZATION FOR THE SYSTEM IMPROVEMENT

Healthcare systems consist of a large number of subsystems interacting with each other in a complex way. An *agent* in agent-based modeling systems for healthcare operations can make its own decision according to the resource available, patient types and operations. Each agent in the system could interact, communicate and collaborate with others to achieve a prospective aim. Each agent may also play the different role to solve a particular problem.

Operation scheduling plays an important role in planning daily routines of the OR department at WHSC. It is not easy to handle all types of scheduling problems efficiently using the existing process. It is difficult to plan an optimal OR operation using the simulation model only. The agent-based approach provides a good alternative for the scheduling flexibility. The agent-based technology can aid the simulation model to provide a solution for the problem. A multi-agent system can indicate possibly heterogeneous and computational entities with problem solving capabilities to reach the overall goal. The autonomous, distributed, and dynamic natures of the multi-agents fit the requirement for building a complex, flexible, robust, and dynamic operation scheduling (Wang, 2008). Therefore, a multi-agent approach is used as follows to model and optimize complex scenarios of the OR department.

Idea and Strategy:

- Using a dynamic schedule instead of the fixed schedule to make the system flexible. At the beginning, the system runs with the pre-assigned schedule. The system will then make its own decision depending on the actual situation to change or modify the schedule.
- Balancing the operation to increase the utilization of resources, and also balancing the personnel working time. When a patient stays in the holding area waiting for the operation, or the pre-assigned room is in use, the system will automatically assign one available OR room with max idle percentage.
- The priority and sequence will be set for nurses who have multi-missions during working.

Agent Definition

The multi-agent system is composed of different agents related to the OR operation. Each agent has its functions, goals, rules, and resources with following definitions.

Agent. Admitting

Function: Scheduling primary process including the patient arrival time and operation room number according to provided patient quantity and expected operation duration (EOD).

- Assigning patients to related pre-operation units.
- Recording the patient arrival time and assign the patient ID.
- Calculating each patient expected length of stay (ELOS).

- Calculating each patient expected Music Room leaving time (EMLT) and expected operating room leaving time (EOLT).
- Recording the LOS, MLT, OLT and discharge time for next day scheduling.

Rules: The schedule should balance the difference of ELOS and EOD for each patient or the ratio of ELOS/EOD for the high patient satisfaction level.

- The patient arrival time should avoid waiting in Pre-op units and Holding areas based on EMLT and EOLT to reduce average LOS.
- The schedule should also consider the earliest daily ending time for whole system.
- The operation room number arrangement should follow the rule to balance the OR percentage utilization, and EOD/available time.

Interaction: Delivering patients to Pre-OP units for waiting.

Agent.Pre-OP

Function: Accommodating patient waiting for transferring to holding areas.

- Recording the length of patient stay and patient entering and leaving time.
- Determining the patient expected leaving time.

Rules: Based on the patient assigned OR status. If available, the interview nurse should move to holding areas when the patient leaves Pre-OP to reduce LOS.

Interaction: Informing agent.TP to dispatch personnel to transfer patients.

- Informing agent.OR to dispatch nurses to Holding areas for ready to interview if possible.

Agent.Holidng

Function: Locating patient interview before the operation.

- Recording the length of patient stay, and patient entering and leaving time.
- Checking the patient assigned operation room status.
- Updating the patient schedule according to the OR status and OR utilization.

Rules: The patient waiting time should be reduced in holding areas.

- If there is waiting required, other suitable operation room will be assigned for the patient.
- If there is no operation room available, find out the earliest available operation room. Raising the priority of PACU nurses transferring task and cleaning task for such operation room.

Interaction: Informing the agent, OR to dispatch nurses for interview and transfer the patient to OR.

Agent.TP

Function: Transferring the patient from Pre-op to Holding areas and from PACU to Discharge.

- Assigning staff ID.
- Establishing the dynamic task and determining the task priority.

- Dispatching different staff for different tasks.

Rules: A task priority should be decided according to holding areas, OR and PACU current situation to reduce LOS. The different scenarios and related priorities are shown in Table 10. The staff dispatching will follow the rule of shortest distance moving.

Agent.OR

Function: The surgery operation.

- Recording each operation room status, patient entering and leaving time and cleaning finish time.
- Determining the operation time.
- Calculating the patient expected OR leaving time.
- Arranging doctors and nurses for each operation process.

Interaction: Accepting information from holding areas to assign patients for interview.

- Informing cleaning staff after each operation.
- Informing PACU nurse transferring patients to PACU unit.

Agent.PACU

Function: Accommodating patients waiting for discharge.

Table 10. The job priority

Holding Status	OR status	OR block	PACU status	Meaning	Priority
Not full	Not full	N/A	N/A	Patient will be treated immediately	3
Not full	full	N/A	N/A	Patient will be blocked in MMR	2
N/A	full	>=1	full	Should free OR as soon as possible	4
N/A	full	no	full	Patient will be blocked in OR	3
N/A	Not full		Not full	Working well	2
N/A	=0		>=1	Not so necessary	1

- Recording the length of patient stay and the patient entering and leaving time.
- Checking the patient LOS level status.
- Assigning staff ID.
- Establishing the dynamitic task and determining the task priority.
- Dispatching staff tasks.

Rules: The task priority should be decided according to the patient LOS level to reduce LOS. If the PACU bed is full or almost full, check the number of patients who stay in OR for waiting or based on the patient expected OR leaving time from agent.OR to arrange nurses transferring or nursing task. Beds are freed as much as possible to avoid PACU as bottleneck.

Interaction: Same as those in agent.OR.

Agent.Data and Analysis

Functions: Each agent builds its own data table to record the real-time information. The system builds a patient data table to record all the relevant information. The rules are modified as functions to be provided for agents to call.

Patients: Collecting the patient ID, expected unit time, each unit entering and leaving time,

operation room number and related information. Calculating the average, max and min LOS and analyzing the reason.

Units: Collecting each unit resource information, beds quantities, and percent utilization.

- Finding out the abnormal high or low percentage unit and analyze the reason.

Staff group: Collecting staff ID, busy time, and moving distance.

- Finding out the too busy or free staff and the reason.

The architecture of the proposed multi-agent based simulation system is depicted in Figure 10.

The capacity planning and schedule control are the two most important issues to determine the process setting and performance. A dynamitic schedule is built with following criteria.

- Customer satisfaction: with the reduced patient length of stay for the improved

Figure 10. The architecture of the agent-based simulation system

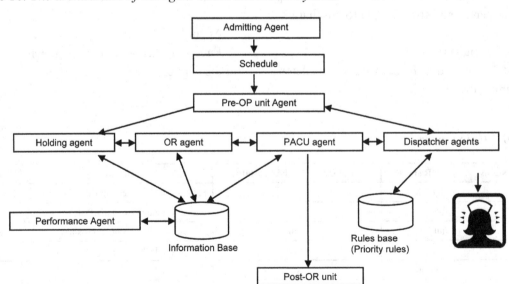

satisfaction level.

- Resource utilization: through balancing each unit work load and total time for the improved efficiency and utilization.
- Employee performance: by the measure of ratio of patients stay and staff working hours.

The capacity and schedule planning determine patients quantity, patients arrival time and operating room numbers assigned on each day. During the processing, the schedule is dynamically modified by each agent according to the environment achieved by following two steps:

Step 1: Patients quantity on each day is scheduled based on the historical data. The schedule is then modified with the arrival time and operating room number for each patient.

Step 2: the capacity of each day is determined according to the total expected operating time and staff working hours.

The agents coordinate operating iteratively to enable an optimal schedule to be carried out. The process also allows constraints of the system to be relaxed gradually during the agent interaction, so that scheduling is first carried out under existing constraints, but when solutions cannot be found, resources are regrouped to form alternative solutions.

The scheduling knowledge is integrated with agents in decision-making. The system performance is improved through dynamic interaction of agents for the reaction to an event and adjust existing schedule as shown in Figure 11. A self-interested activity agent can automatically cooperate with other agents in real-time to solve the problem of delay events through a decision-making process. For example, a longer stay may occur in the holding area (HA) when patients at the pre-operation unit are waiting for an assigned OR available. With the functions built for agents, the system can assign an available OR if the pre-assigned OR is in use. If there are more than one operation rooms are available, system will pick one OR number from available rooms according to the maximal idle percentage. Therefore, the system is able to modify the pre-assigned schedule according the operation room status dynamically.

Experiments are made based on the revised system with the same data in the simulation model. The comparison of the fixed schedule with the dynamic schedule is listed in Table 11. From Table 11, it can be found that the time from Arrival to ToOp is reduced, especially for the time between Holding areas and Operating rooms. However, there are slight increases of time from ToOpRoom to ToPostOp, and the stay in OR. The increased time after ORs probably is due to the bottleneck

Figure 11. Dynamic schedule solution

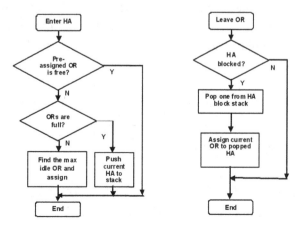

existed in PACU. The limited TPs also delay the delivery of patient to the Post Unites. This can be improved by the increase of TPs' number as shown in the previous simulation result. An ideal solution is to optimize the TP utilization that needs more data and strategy for the TP planning and scheduling. The agent-based system is still in the development when this chapter is written.

FUTURE TREND

Healthcare systems belong to typical service enterprises with a very personal, highly complex, and intangible outcome (Sibbel, 2001). The healthcare simulation is different from manufacturing simulation which mainly deals with material flows. Healthcare is a human-centered system including doctors, nurses, patients, and assistants. Human behaviors are different from those of machines. Human factor plays a central role in the integration of the operation, people and facilities to maximize patients' safety, systems' safety and productivity. Therefore, human behaviours and modeling levels of details should be integrated in the system modeling.

Because the healthcare system is dynamically changed, the fixed task priority cannot match the actual requirement. For example, the transport personnel transfer patients between departments. When they receive more than one task requirements, system will assign different priorities related different scenarios to decrease the patient stay time. The performance improvement of healthcare systems involves patient scheduling, patients'

safety, resource scheduling, physical resource requirements, and operating procedures.

The work described in this chapter is an initial step for the OR improvement. Further work will conduct in exploring the intelligence of an agent, such as learning from a scheduling history and making decision based on appropriate recorder or experience. Such learning ability will allow agents always to make favorable decisions that are best suited for the current situation.

Additional agents will also be added to separate the operation room agent to make the model more accurate. Dispatcher agents will also be created to dispatch each group of nurses to improve human resource utilization. More data will also be collected for the model. The emergency patients cases in the OR department will also be considered.

CONCLUSION

This research shows that simulation modeling and agent-based optimization are efficient tools for identifying problems and improving performance of healthcare systems. The simulation model is valuable to present the working flow and to predict the bottleneck of the healthcare systems. The model built is feasible to present the current patient flow of the OR department at WHSC to predict and improve the bottleneck of the healthcare system.

This research provides a reasonable assessment of the OR efficiency, resource utilizations and other performance measures. By using the simulation, a useful evaluation for the OR depart-

Table 11. The comparison of the fixed schedule and dynamic schedule

	Arrival to ToOpRoom	Arrival to ToPostOp	ToOpRoom to ToPostOp	ToHA to ToOP	Operation Room stay
Fixed schedule	149.82	434.99	285.17	89.06	279.58
Dynamic schedule	130.53	433.46	302.83	72,45	297.31
Difference (%)	-12.88	-0.35	6.23	-18.65	6.34

ment provides a chance to analyze and improve the current operation processing. The output of the simulation shows the analysis result with useful formation for the system improvement. The graphical user interface provides an effective tool for decision-making of the OR operation. Based on suggested actions for different scenarios to improve the system, the time from patient arrival to the operation is reduced. The resource utilization is also balanced.

ACKNOWLEDGMENT

This research is supported by the Winnipeg Regional Health Authority and Winnipeg Health Science Centre. Thanks for the support of staff members at WHSC for the data collection and comments for the simulation model.

REFERENCES

Abellán, J. J., Armero, C., Conesa, D., Pérez-Panadés, J., Martínez-Beneito, M. A., Zurriaga, O., et al. (2004). Predicting the Behavior of the Renal Transplant Waiting List in the Pais Valencia (Spain) Using Simulation Modeling. *Proceedings of Winter Simulation Conference* (pp. 1969-1974).

Baesler, F. F., Jahnsen, H. E., & DaCosta, M. (2003). The Use of Simulation and Design of Experiments for Estimating Maximum Capacity in an Emergency Room. *Proceedings of Winter Simulation Conference* (pp. 1903-1906).

Barnes, C. D., Quiason, J. L., Benson, C., & McGuiness, D. (1997). Success Stories in Simulation in Health Care. *Proceedings of the 1997 Winter Simulation Conference* (pp. 1280-1285).

Brailsford, S. C. (2007). Tutorial: Advances and Challenges in Healthcare Simulation Modeling. *Proceedings of Winter Simulation Conference* (pp. 1436-1448).

Centeno, M. A., Giachetti, R., Linn, R., & Ismail, A. M. (2003). A Simulation-ILP based Tools for Scheduling ER Staff. *Proceedings of the 2003 Winter Simulation Conference* (pp. 1930-1938).

Chen, Y., & Wang, S. (2007). Framework of agent-based intelligence system with two-stage decision-making process for distributed dynamic scheduling. *Applied Soft Computing*, 7, 229–245. doi:10.1016/j.asoc.2005.04.003

Ferrin, D. M., Miller, M. J., Wininger, S., & Neuendorf, M. S. (2004). Analyzing Incentives and Scheduling in a Major Metropolitan Hospital Operating Room Through Simulation. *Proceedings of Winter Simulation Conference* (pp. 1975-1981).

Flexsim Software Products, Inc. (2008). Retrieved Nov. 20, 2008, From http://www.flexsim.com/

Garcia, M. E., Valero, S., Argente, E., Giret, A., & Julian, V. (2008). A FAST Method to Achieve Flexible Production Programming Systems. *IEEE Transactions on Systems, Man and Cybernetics. Part C, Applications and Reviews*, 38(2), 242–252. doi:10.1109/TSMCC.2007.913921

Group, D. S. (2008). Retrieved Nov. 20, 2008, http://www.3ds.com/products/delmia/welcome/

Guo, M., Wagner, M., & West, C. (2004). Outpatient Clinic Scheduling – A Simulation Approach, *Proceedings of Winter Simulation Conference* (pp. 1981-1987).

Hassine, A. B., & Ho, T. B. (2007). An agent-based approach to solve dynamic meeting scheduling problems with preferences. *Engineering Applications of Artificial Intelligence*, 20, 857–873. doi:10.1016/j.engappai.2006.10.004

Lanner Group, Inc. (2008). Retrieved Nov. 20, 2008, From www.lanner.com.

Lowery, J. C., Hakes, B., Lilegdon, W. R., Keller, L., Mabrouk, K., & McGuire, F. (1994). Barriers to Implementing Simulation in Health Care. *Proceedings of Winter Simulation Conference* (pp. 868-875).

Mahapatra, S., Koelling, C. P., Patvivatsiri, L., Fraticelli, B., Eitel, D., & Grove, L. (2003). Pairing Emergency Severity Index 5-level Triage Data with Computer aided System Design to Improve Emergency Department Access and Throughput. *Proceedings of the 2003 Winter Simulation Conference* (pp. 1917-1925*).

Mes, M., Heijden, M., & Harten, A. (2007). Comparison of agent-based scheduling to look-ahead heuristics for real-time transportation problems. *European Journal of Operational Research, 181*, 59–75. doi:10.1016/j.ejor.2006.02.051

Miller, M. J., Ferrin, D. M., & Messer, M. G. (2004). Fixing the Emergency Department: A Transformational Journey with EDSIM. *Proceedings of Winter Simulation Conference* (pp. 1988-1993).

Mok, W. Y., Palvia, P., & Paper, D. (2006). On the computability of agent-based workflows. *Decision Support Systems, 42*, 1239–1253. doi:10.1016/j. dss.2005.10.010

Morrison, B. P., & Bird, B. C. (2003). A Methodology for Modeling Front Office and Patient Care Processes in Ambulatory Health Care. *Proceedings of Winter Simulation Conference* (pp.1882-1886).

CBC News (2006, December 1). *Public vs. private health care.*

Osidach, V. Z., & Fu, M. C. (2003). Computer Simulation of a Mobile Examination Centre. *Proceedings of Winter Simulation Conference* (pp. 1868-1875).

Python software foundation. (2008). Retrieved Nov. 20, 2008, From http://www.python.org/

Rodríguez, M. D., Favela, J., Preciado, A., & Vizcaíno, A. (2005). Agent-based ambient intelligence for healthcare. *AI Communications, 18*, 201–216.

Sibbel, R., & Christoph, U. (2001). *Agent-Based Modeling and Simulation for Hospital Management.* Retrieved Nov. 20, 2008, From http:// cuong.tgs.vn/ebook/Agent-Based.Modeling.and. Simulation.for. Hospital.Management.pdf.

Sinreich, D., & Marmor, Y. N. (2004). A Simple and Intuitive Simulation Tool for Analyzing Emergency Department Operations. *Proceedings of Winter Simulation Conference* (pp.1994-2002).

Takakuwa, S., & Shiozaki, H. (2004). Functional Analysis for Operating Emergency Department of a General Hospital. *Proceedings of Winter Simulation Conference* (pp. 2003-2011).

Wang, D., Nagalingam, S. V., & Lin, G. C. I. (2007). Development of an agent-based Virtual CIM architecture for small to medium manufacturers. *Robotics and Computer-integrated Manufacturing, 23*, 1–16. doi:10.1016/j.rcim.2005.09.001

Wang, S., Xi, L., & Zhou, B. (2008). FBS-enhanced agent-based dynamic scheduling in FMS. *Engineering Applications of Artificial Intelligence, 21*, 644–657. doi:10.1016/j.engappai.2007.05.012

Weng, M. X., Wu, Z., Qi, G., & Zheng, L. (2008). Multi-agent-based workload control for make-to-order manufacturing. *International Journal of Production Research, 46*(8), 2197–2213. doi:10.1080/00207540600969758

WHO. (2008). Primary Health Care – Now More Than Ever. The *World Health Report* (p. 82). Retrieved Nov. 20, 2008, from http://www.who. int/whr/2008/en/index.html

Xiang, W., & Lee, H. P. (2008). Ant colony intelligence in multi-agent dynamic manufacturing scheduling. *Engineering Applications of Artificial Intelligence*, *21*, 73–85. doi:10.1016/j.engappai.2007.03.008

Zhang, D. Z., Anosike, A., & Lim, M. K. (2007). Dynamically Integrated Manufacturing Systems (DIMS) - A Multiagent Approach. *IEEE Transactions on Systems, Man, and Cybernetics. Part A, Systems and Humans*, *37*(5), 824–850. doi:10.1109/TSMCA.2007.897710

Zhang, W. J., & Xie, S. Q. (2007). Agent technology for collaborative process planning: a review. *International Journal of Advanced Manufacturing Technology*, *32*, 315–325. doi:10.1007/s00170-005-0345-x

Chapter 6
Building a Health Care Multi-Agent Simulation System with Role-Based Modeling

Xiaoqin Zhang
University of Massachusetts Dartmouth, USA

Haiping Xu
University of Massachusetts Dartmouth, USA

Bhavesh Shrestha
University of Massachusetts Dartmouth, USA

ABSTRACT

Multi-Agent System (MAS) is a suitable programming paradigm for simulating and modeling health care systems and applications, where resources, data, control and services are widely distributed. We have developed a multi-agent software prototype to simulate the activities and roles inside a health care system. The prototype is developed using a framework called Role-based Agent Development Environment (RADE). In this chapter, the authors present an integrated approach for modeling, designing and implementing a multi-agent health care simulation system using RADE. They describe the definition of role classes and agent classes, as well as the automatic agent generation process. The authors illustrate the coordination problem and present a rule-based coordination approach. In the end, they present a runtime scenario of this health care simulation system, which demonstrates that dynamic task allocation can be achieved through the creation of role instances and the mapping from role instances to agents. This scenario also explains how agents coordinate their activities given their local constraints and interdependence among distributed tasks.

INTRODUCTION

Multi-Agent System (MAS) is a suitable programming paradigm for simulating and modeling health care systems and applications, where resources, data, control and services are widely distributed. We have developed multi-agent software to simulate the activities and roles inside a health care system. Such software can be used to assist the collaborative scheduling of complex tasks that involve multiple

DOI: 10.4018/978-1-60566-772-0.ch006

personals and resources. In addition, it can be used to study the efficiency of the health care system and the influence of different policies.

However, the application of multi-agent system has been limited by the difficulty of developing agent-based systems, and considerable amount of time and highly experienced programmers are required to develop a multi-agent system. After such system is built, it is also difficult to test and maintain the system because of its complexity. The reusability of such system is low; it is unlikely to use an existing system for another application domain with little or minor change. In this chapter, we will describe a role-based approach to building multi-agent systems for health care simulation and modeling. With this approach, we are able to separate the concern on domain knowledge and the concern on intelligent problem-solving capabilities. In this approach, conceptual roles, such as physicians, nurses and patients are defined with the domain related knowledge including goals, permissions, organizational relationship, and interaction protocols, etc; where an agent is a concrete entity equipped with motivations, resources and problem-solving capabilities, which can be used to represent a real person in a health care system. Each agent can be configured based on different specifications according to the real person's situation and needs. Then the agent instance is dynamically generated for the real person who enters the system.

In this chapter, we will also describe an automated agent generation process, which utilizes the existing tools and mechanisms as much as possible. We propose to create agents using a drag-and-drop mechanism where the user can select components to plug into the agent depending on application requirements. We adopt a utility-driven agent architecture with quantitative reasoning capabilities. Besides the logical reasoning on the matching of motivations and the conflicts among different roles, we adapt a quantitative model of motivation named MQ (motivation quantities) framework. Based on the MQ framework, an agent can perform

a quantitative reasoning on how important a role instance is, given its preference, its utility function and its current achievement. In the definition of a role, we introduce a formal language called RTÆMS (Role-based Task Analyzing, Environment Modeling, and Simulation) to represent the domain knowledge about how to achieve a goal. RTÆMS language is a hierarchical task network representation language with task interrelationships and quantitative descriptions of different alternatives to achieve a goal. The domain expert can specify how a complicated health service task should be performed with the collaboration of multiple roles inside the system. Each agent is also equipped with the capability for planning, scheduling and cooperation; hence, an agent can schedule its local activities with the consideration of the constraints from other agents. Meanwhile, a user of the system can choose different collaboration rules according to the organizational rules and the specific needs in the system.

In the rest of this chapter, we first discuss related work in several research areas. Afterwards, we describe how to construct a health care simulation system using the approach described above, and show how to define roles and their interrelationships, and how to define agent classes. Then, we present an automatic agent generation tool as well as a rule-based coordination approach. Finally, we use a runtime scenario to demonstrate how new role instances are created, how agents are taking new roles, planning and scheduling their tasks, and collaborating with each other to achieve a complex goal.

BACKGROUND

Researchers have studied a number of approaches for defining and developing autonomous agents and multi-agent system from different directions. Here we discuss related research work in four areas: agent development framework, role-based modeling of agent-based systems, specification of coordination rules, and model-driven development of multi-agent systems.

Agent Development Framework

DECAF (Graham, Decker & Mersic, 2003) and JADE (Bellifemine et. al, 2003) are examples of the frameworks that can be used to generate domain specific agents. DECAF (Distributed, Environment-Centered Agent Framework) developed in University of Delaware, is a toolkit to build multi-agent systems. The toolkit provides a stable platform to design, rapidly develop, and execute intelligent agents to achieve solutions in complex software systems. DECAF provides the necessary architectural services of an intelligent agent: communication, planning, scheduling, execution monitoring, coordination, and eventually learning and self-diagnosis. Plan editor is a GUI that provides the interface for control or programming of DECAF agents. In the Plan editor, executable actions are treated as basic building blocks, which can be chained together to achieve a larger and more complex goal in the style of a hierarchical task network. This provides a software component-style programming interface with desirable properties such as component reuse and some design-time error-checking. The chaining of activities can involve traditional looping and if-then-else constructs. This part of DECAF is an extension of the RETSINA (Williamson, Decker & Sycara, 1996) and TÆMS (Decker, 1996). task structure frameworks. Each action of an agent can also have a performance profile, which is used and updated internally by DECAF to provide real-time local scheduling services.

JADE (Java Agent Development Framework) (Bellifemine et. al, 2003) is a software framework fully implemented in Java language distributed by Telecom Italia. It simplifies the implementation of multi-agent systems through a middleware that complies with the FIPA specifications. The agent platform can be distributed across machines and the configuration can be controlled via a remote GUI. The configuration can be changed at runtime by moving agents from one machine to another, when required. The communication architecture offers flexible and efficient messaging, where JADE creates and manages a queue of incoming ACL messages, private to each agent; agents can access their queue via a combination of several modes: blocking, polling, timeout and pattern matching. JADE implements a full FIPA communication model, and its components have been clearly distinct and fully integrated: interaction protocols, envelope, ACL, content languages, encoding schemes, ontology, and finally, transport protocols. Most of the interaction protocols defined by FIPA are available and can be instantiated after defining the application-dependent behaviour of each state of the protocol. Agent management ontology has been implemented, as well as the support for user-defined content languages and ontology that can be implemented, registered with agents, and automatically used by the framework. JADE has also been integrated with JESS, a Java shell of CLIPS, in order to exploit its reasoning capabilities.

The goals of both these frameworks are to develop a modular platform to allow for rapid development of third-party domain agents, and provide a means to quickly develop complete multi-agent solutions using combinations of domain-specific agents and standard middle-agents. These frameworks specify agents in terms of roles they play, and assume that agents do not change their roles at run time. In contrast, we implemented an automated agent generation mechanism using the RADE framework. Using this framework, we can separate the domain knowledge and the intelligent problem solving capabilities. So an agent can be created with intelligent capabilities and motivations, and can take up different roles dynamically.

Role-Based Modeling

The related work in the second area is to propose role-based methodology for developing multi-agent systems. Approaches like Gaia (Wooldridge, Jenning, & Kinny, 2000; Zambonelli, Jennings & Wooldridge, 2003) and MaSE (DeLoach, Wood, & Sparkman, 2001) can be used to model multi-agent system societies in terms of organizations or groups composed of a collection of roles related to one another and participating in patterns of interactions with other roles. The agents are then specified in terms of a set of roles they play. These approaches explicitly assume that the inter-agent relationships and the abilities of agents do not change at run-time and that all the agents are explicitly designed to cooperatively achieve common goals.

The Gaia methodology can be used to model both the macro aspect and the micro aspect of a multi-agent system. It covers the analysis phase and the design phase. In the analysis phase, the role model and interaction model are constructed. Based on the analysis models, in the design phase, three models, the agent model, service model and acquaintance model are constructed during the initial design of the system, and then are refined during the detailed design phase using conventional object-oriented methodology. The later version of Gaia (Zambonelli, Jennings & Wooldridge, 2003) extends the former one in order to better suit to open multi-agent systems by introducing two new abstractions: (1) organizational rules (explicit identification of relationships and constraints between roles and protocols), and (2) organizational structures (explicit specification of organizations in terms of their topology and control regime).

The MaSE methodology is a specialization of more traditional software engineering methodologies (DeLoach, Wood, & Sparkman, 2001). During the analysis phase of the MaSE methodology, a set of roles are produced, which describes entities that perform some function within the system.

In MaSE, each role is responsible for achieving or helping to achieve specific system goals and sub-goals. During the design phase, agent classes are created according to the roles defined in the analysis phase.

In our approach, the components of role instances and agent instances are loosely coupled, where agents can take or release role instances at runtime without knowing the internal structure of role instances. Thus, role classes and agent classes can be designed and implemented independently.

Coordination Rules

The related work in the third area is definition of coordination rules. Projects such as AgenTalk (Kuwabara, Ishida, & Osato, 1995) use scripts and finite state machine to define coordination rules. AgenTalk is a language for describing coordination protocols for multi-agent systems co-developed by NTT Communication Science Laboratories and Ishida Laboratory, Department of Information Science, Kyoto University. It provides an explicit state representation of a protocol, and a finite state machine that allows variables to be used as a basis to describe coordination protocols, called a script. Using this model, states of a protocol are explicitly defined, and actions of an agent can be defined for each state. Protocols can be defined incrementally by extending existing scripts. It provides a programming interface that specifies the portion of a state transition rule that needs to be customized for each agent. The AgenTalk has been implemented in Common Lisp.

In ROPE project (Becht et. al., 1999), cooperation process is built as a separated component from the concrete agents; the ROPE engine provides execution of the cooperation process, which is described as a high-level Petri net class. However, the implementation of ROPE engine is based on shared memory, which is not always feasible for agents that are widely distributed on different machines. Additionally, the cooperation process in ROPE is based on token and transition firing, which is not feasible enough to support more proactive cooperation and collaboration, i.e. agents are able to consider the cooperation and coordination needs when they are planning their own activities.

A set of domain-independent general collaboration mechanisms, Generalized Partial Global Planning (GPGP) (Lesser, et. al. 2004), based on TÆMS language (Decker, 1996) has been developed. We have reused some of GPGP similar mechanisms in RADE (Zhang & Xu, 2006) framework based on RTÆMS language. In framework such as AgenTalk, the emphasis is on the flow of messages and how the dialog between agents is structured. Such framework combines finite state machines with enhancements. In contrast, GPGP focuses on a domain independent and quantitative evaluation of the interactions among tasks and the dynamic formation of temporal constraints to resolve and to exploit these interactions. Our implementation gives a user the freedom to choose the appropriate coordination rule according to the application domain.

Model-Driven Development

Previous work on model-driven development of multi-agent systems can be summarized as follows. Gracanina, Boher and Hincey proposed a model-driven architecture framework as an extension to Cognitive Agent Architecture (COUGAAR) (Gracanin, Bohner & Hinchey, 2004). The Cognitive Agent Architecture is a distributed agent architecture that has been developed primarily for very large-scale, distributed applications that are characterized by hierarchical task decompositions, and as such, it is well suited for autonomic systems. The framework consists of two main parts, General COUGAAR Application Model (GCAM) and General Domain Application Model (GDAM). The GCAM provides representation in its model of the COUGAAR basic constructs, and the GDAM defines the requirements and the detailed design.

Maria, Silva and Lucena (2005) proposed an MDA-based approach to developing multi-agent systems. They first use MAS modeling language (MAS-ML) to model MAS by creating the platform independent models (PIM). Then the MAS-ML models are transformed into UML models using the ASF framework, which defines a set of object-oriented models for MAS entities specified in MAS-ML. The UML models are then transformed into code.

We have proposed three levels of models for developing role-based open multi-agent systems (Xu, Zhang & Patel, 2007), namely AIPIM (Application Independent Platform Independent Model), ASPIM (Application Specific Platform Independent Model), and ASPSM (Application Specific Platform Specific Model), as a refinement process. In each level of the models, role components and agent components are always separated and designed independently. Role instances and agent instances interact with each other only at runtime through an A-R (Agent-Role) mapping mechanism.

ROLE-BASE MODELING APPROACH

The basic idea of the role-based agent development environment (RADE) is illustrated in *Figure 1*. The top level is the *role organization*, which defines the conceptual roles and their relationships such as inheritance, aggregation, association and incompatibility. In health care systems, conceptual roles represent all possible job titles in the system, such as *physician* and *nurse*. The relationships describe how these roles relate to each other. The second level is the *role space*, which consists of multiple role instances; each role instance is instantiated from a conceptual role dynamically. For example, whenever there is a need to cure a patient, a new physician role instance is created with the goal to cure a patient. A role instance represents the task that needs to be accomplished in the system. The bottom level is the *agent society*,

Figure 1. RADE Concept (© 2007, Journal of Computational Intelligence Theory and Practice. Used with permission.)

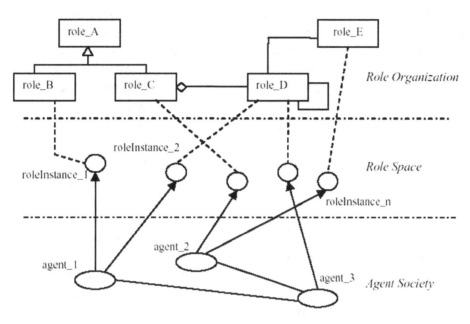

which consists of multiple agent entities. Agent can take or release role instances dynamically, where the mapping from role instances to agents is called A-R mapping, which represents that a real person takes a task in the system.

In an actual software system, agent instances are automatically generated based on the definition of agent classes. Each agent instance is a software entity that performs specific functions and also coordinates and communicates with other agent instances. On the contrary, role classes are defined to incorporate domain knowledge and organizational relationships. Each role class is associated with specific goals and detailed descriptions of how to achieve such goals. The relationships among different role classes also depict the organizational relationships among the real-world entities represented by these roles. Such information is expected to be provided by domain experts rather than software engineers. At system runtime, role instances are created dynamically either by a human user or by an agent when certain goals are needed to be realized. Those role instances mainly carry domain knowledge; however, they do not actually perform any actions like agents. When an agent takes a role instance, the agent uses the knowledge incorporated in the role instance in order to achieve the goals defined in it.

One major advantage of the RADE approach is that it supports the separation of domain knowledge and the agent framework for the simulation system. Any domain knowledge relates to the health care domain can be specified by domain experts through definition of roles and their interrelationships. On the other hand, software engineers are responsible to develop automatic agents that actually perform tasks in the simulation system.

DEFINING ROLES AND ROLE SPACE

The definition of a role class includes the following information:

1. A set of attributes, such as role name and identification.
2. A set of goals; each goal is associated with a plan tree, which is a hierarchal description of the alternatives to accomplish a goal.
3. A set of actions that can be performed by this role, i.e. a *Physician* role can perform an action of *Prescribe Medicine*.
4. Qualification: the requirement needed to take such a role.
5. The permission of this role, which specifies what information and resource are allowed to be access by this role. For instance, a *Physician* role has the permission to access the patient's medical record.
6. A set of protocols, which describe how this role should interact with other roles.

All above information is domain-dependent; hence an expert in health care domain who is familiar with all those rules and regulations can define those role classes. The formal definition of role class in Object-Z can be found in (Xu & Zhang 2005).

In the health care simulation system, we have defined the following role classes:

1. **Patient:** A person who seeks for health care.
2. **Physician:** A person who determines whether diagnostics are to be undertaken, provides prescriptions, performs medical and surgical interventions, has the ability to direct patient care and advance a patient to the next step of care.
3. **Medical Assistant:** A health care professional who performs a variety of clinical, clerical and administrative duties within a health care setting. There are two roles defined as subclasses of this role class:
   a. **Administrative Medical Assistant (MA Admin):** Medical assistant who performs the administrative job.
   b. **Clinical Medical Assistant (MA Clinical):** Medical assistant who performs the clinical job.
4. **Nurse:** There are two roles defined as subclasses of this role class:
   a. **Nurse Assistant:** a nurse who assesses the patient's medical problem, provides care and helps to set up laboratory specimen and medical instruments.
   b. **Nurse Practitioner:** a registered nurse who has completed an advanced training program in primary health care delivery, and may provide primary care for non-emergency patients, usually in an outpatient setting.

Figure 2 shows the RADE interface for a user to create role classes and define the interrelationships among role classes. In this example, the interrelationships include inheritance, association and incompatibility. An inheritance relationship describes the generalization/specification relationship between two role classes. For example, both *MA Admin* and *MA Clinical* inherit the *Medical Assistant* role class since they are specified medical assistants. Association is a very common relationship between role classes; it indicates that an instance of one role class may perform an action on an instance of another role class. Association relationships exist between *Physician* and *Nurse*, *Physician* and *Patient*, etc. Incompatibility relationship describes the constraints that the role instances of two role classes cannot be taken by the same agent in the same interaction scenario. For example, an agent cannot take a Physician role instance for treating a Patient role instance if the agent is already taking this Patient role instance; however, the agent can take another Physician role instance for treating another Patient role instance that is not taken by this agent. The definition of such relationships depends on the domain knowledge, so we feel that the domain experts are the best candidate to use this interface to define the role classes and their interrelationships.

Figure 2. RADE Interface for creating roles (© 2007, Journal of the Brazilian Computer Society. Used with permission)

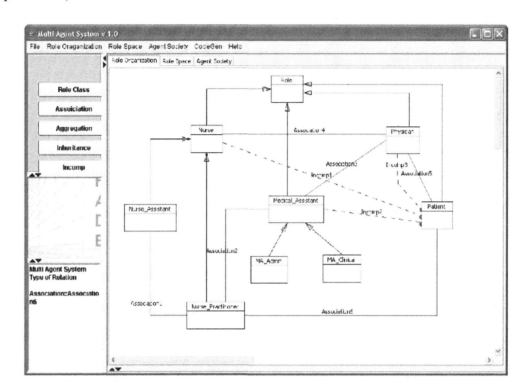

In this example, Physician role is defined with a goal to provide cure. The plan tree provides domain knowledge of how to accomplish this goal. To represent the domain knowledge, we introduce RTÆMS (Role-Based Task Analyzing, environment Modeling, and Simulation) language as an extension of the TÆMS language (Decker, 1996). TÆMS is a hierarchical task representation language, which supports representation of relationships among goals and sub-goals, the quantitative description of the atomic approaches and uncertainties, and resources. We extend the TÆMS language by introducing a role attribute for task nodes that represent goals and sub-goals. The attribute role specifies what roles are needed to carry out this goal or sub-goal. *Figure 3* shows the plan tree for the goal 'Provide Cure', which includes two sub-goals: 'Examine Patient' and 'Provide Treatment'. The goal 'Provide Cure'

is associated with a **min** quality accumulative function (**qaf**), which specifies the following relationship:

Quality(ProvideCure) = min(Quality(ExaminePatient), Quality(ProvideTreatment))

Each role is defined with a goal, a plan tree, a motivational quantity production set (MQPS), a certificate and other attributes. A goal represents a task that the role needs to accomplish, and the plan tree specifies the domain knowledge of how to accomplish the goal in terms of decomposing it as sub-goals. Consider the following role class.

ROLE: Physician

GOAL: Provide Cure

MQPS: (MQ_professional, p1), (MQ_moral, p2), (MQ_experience, p3)

CERTIFICATE: MD (Doctor of Medicine)

This min quality function associated with a

Figure 3. Plan tree for goal Provide Cure in RTÆMS representation (© 2007, Journal of the Brazilian Computer Society. Used with permission)

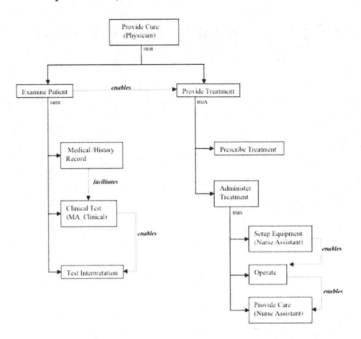

goal means that the success of this goal depends on the success of all of its sub-goals. Meanwhile, the use of max quality function specifies that there are several alternatives to achieve the goal. For instance, to 'Provide Treatment' for the patient, the Physician can choose either 'Prescribe Treatment' or 'Administer Treatment'. Other available quality accumulation functions in RTÆMS language are: *sum* and *seq_sum*.

Each sub-goal can be decomposed into smaller goals, i.e. 'Examine Patient' consists of three sub-goals: '(Read) Medical History Record', 'Clinical Test 'and 'Test Interpretation'. For those non-local goals, where the tasks need to be performed by other roles, the specification of other roles is included in the plan tree description. For example, 'Clinical Test' should be performed by a Clinical Medical Assistant (MA Clinical), and task 'Setup Equipment' and 'Provide Care' belongs to the Nurse Assistant role. The dash lines represent the interrelationship between goals/sub-goals. For example, 'Clinical Test', which enables 'Test

Interpretation,' means that the first goal 'Clinical Test' needs to be achieved successfully before it is possible to implement the second goal 'Test Interpretation'. In addition, '(Read) Medical History Record' facilitates the 'Clinical Test' process because it can provide some useful information about the patient. Other types of interrelationships defined in TÆMS include *disables* and *hinders*. The primitive goal (lowest-level goal) in the TÆMS representation can be specified with more details in another plan tree that is associated with another role. For example, the plan tree for the sub-goal 'Provide Care ' is described in ***Figure 3***, this information belongs to the role Nurse Assistant. The plan tree represented in RTÆMS shows all possibilities to achieve a goal and the interrelationship among goals/sub-goals. It provides fundamental knowledge for agents to plan and schedule its local activities, and it also supports the collaboration and cooperation among agents. More details about the plan tree will be discussed later in the Section of Coordination.

Each goal is associated with a motivational quantity production set (***MQPS***): MQPS = {(MQi, qi), (MQj, qj), (MQk, qk)...}, which represents the success accomplishment of the goal that generates qi amount of MQi, qj amount of MQj, qk amount of MQk, etc. The MQPS describes how this goal contributes quantitatively to some higher-level goals (abstract goals), which are built in an agent's motivation. For instance, when an agent fulfills a goal 'Provide Cure', it collects p1 units of MQ_professional, p2 units of MQ_moral and p3 units of MQ_experience. The agent uses the MQPS specification in the goal definition and its motivation to determine whether it is interested in a role instance, and how interested it is.

The *Qualification* defined in a role class describes the requirements for a particular role. Only an agent who has the specified certificate can take a role instance of that role class. For example, Physician role is defined with a certificate of MD (Medical Doctor); only an agent with a MD certificate can take a Physician role instance.

DEFINING AND DEVELOPING AGENT CLASSES

Agents are the real programmed entities running in the system. In the health care simulation system, each agent represents a personal assistant for a human user in the real world. The agent is responsible for scheduling a user's daily tasks according to the user's preference and constraints. The agent is also responsible for coordinating with other agents when coordination is needed between its own user and other users. A formal definition of agent class in Object-Z can be found in (Zhang, Xu & Shrestha 2007). An agent class definition includes: a set of attributes, motivations, utility function, sensor data, a set of reasoning mechanisms, and execution mechanisms.

Agent attributes include agent names, user, identification, and other descriptive characteristics. The values of these attributes are set when an agent instance is instantiated from the agent class. Different agent instances have different attribute values.

Motivation is defined as "any desire or preference that can lead to the generation and adoption of goals, and which affects the outcome of the reasoning or behavioral task intended to satisfy those goals" (Luck & d'Inverno, 1995). Motivation is the key for an agent to decide which goals it should pursue and how to pursue a goal. We adopt a quantitative view of motivation in our practice. Motivation is defined as a set of motivation quantities (MQs) (Wagner & Lesser 2002).) that the agent tracks and accumulates. Each MQ is associated with a preference function and represents progresses towards an abstract goal. An abstract goal is a long-term commitment to make progress toward certain direction but not a concrete task with a specified plan. For example, a user creates an assistant agent

named Adam. The user specifies his preference on choosing tasks by defining the motivation of this agent as:

Motivation: {MQ_Professional, 0, 0; MQ_Moral, 1, 1; MQ_Experience, 2, 2}

The motivation specifies three long-term goals the user has: professional achievement, moral achievement and experience achievement, which are represented by three types of MQs due to the user's Physician role. The two numbers following the MQ name is the function index and the initial amount of this type of MQ. The function index specifies a utility function that maps a certain number of units of MQ of this type into the agent's local utility. Since the function could be a non-linear function and is also context sensitive, the initial amount of this type MQ is also important. The user also provides this agent his qualification MD, so this agent can be qualified for a Physician role.

Each agent collects sensor data from the environment. For software agents built in this system, sensor data refers to the messages and information the agent receives from the environment including other agents. Based on the sensor data it collects and its motivation, the agent uses its reasoning mechanisms to make decisions. The decisions are made at different levels: selection of roles, selection of goals, and selection of the approach to fulfilling the goals. The first issue is resolved by A-R mapping mechanisms, and the later two issues are inter-related, which are solved by planning /scheduling mechanisms. Given the formal definition of motivations, goals and the detailed description of alternatives to achieve a goal, it is possible to build some general, domain-independent reasoning mechanisms/toolkits. The user can select appropriate components from such toolkits and add them to the agent; the user can also customize these general mechanisms and toolkits by setting up certain parameters. These general mechanisms and toolkits are reusable for agents in different application domains.

Each agent is equipped with some execution mechanisms that can be used to generate the output, which changes the environment. For software agents, the execution mechanisms are the primitive actions to change the environment state. Some of these execution mechanisms are domain-dependent. For example, in our health care simulation system, an agent representing a hospital worker is built with an execution mechanism to set up medical equipment, which is an action the person can perform in real world. Other execution mechanisms could be application-independent, such as sending a message to another agent.

AUTOMATIC AGENT GENERATION PROCESS

After the user has defined role classes and agent classes, agent can be automatically created using a tool we developed. The basic idea of automatic generation of agents is to use component-based agent architecture, where the user can select the components to be included in this agent, and specify a set of attributes of the agent.

The designer or the user of the agent needs to decide what reasoning tool should be built in and select the appropriate execution tools for the agent according to the design purpose of the agent. It is assumed that there are a set of reasoning and execution mechanisms available in the toolkit, which can be selected and plugged into the agent seamlessly.

Based on the general agent architecture, we developed a tool to support the automatic agent generation process. This tool is created by extending the JAF framework (Vincent, Horling & Lesser, 2001) developed by MAS lab at University of Massachusetts, Amherst. This tool includes a graphic user interface (GUI), which can be used to create new agents, modify existing agents, run agents and delete agents. A screen shot of the graphic user interface is shown in *Figure 4*.

The user also defines the agent's reasoning and execution mechanisms by selecting a number of ready-to-plug-in components such as: planning, scheduling, communication, etc. The user can select what coordination rule should be used by this agent. We will discuss more about the coordination rule in the next section. After an agent class is created, one or multiple agent instances (the executable programs) can be created from this class definition. Each agent instance is an independent program, and the agent is named after its class with a unique number ID. For example, when a user creates an agent class "X" and three agent instances of this class, the three agents are named as "X_1", "X_2" and "X_3," respectively. The user can run agents from this interface by clicking on the "RUN AGENT" menu box on the top, and selecting a number of agents to run from a list of agents that have already been created. Multiple agents can be created and run on difference machines. The user can choose to delete existing agents by clicking on the "DELETE AGENT" menu box. Finally, the user has an option to choose the coordination rules from three types of rules, namely simple rules, hard and soft relationships based rules, and priority based rules.

Figure 4. Automatic agent generation interface (© 2007, Journal of the Brazilian Computer Society. Used with permission

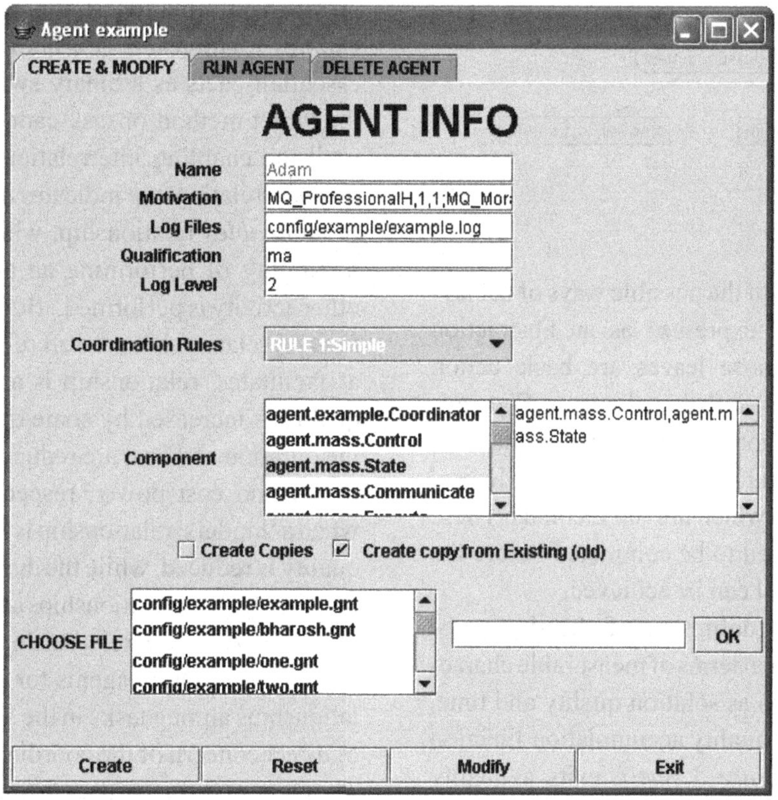

AGENT COORDINATION AND COOPERATION

In a health care simulation system with complex activities, distributed information and resources, agents need to coordinate and cooperate on their actions. Efficient coordination and cooperation mechanisms are important for the performance of the system. An agent should coordinate its own actions with those of other agents when there are constraints and interdependencies among their actions.

The RTÆMS language supports collaborations and cooperation by specifying interrelationship among goals and sub-goals, so agents know when and with whom they need to collaborate and cooperate. A set of domain-independent general collaboration mechanisms (GPGP) based on

TÆMS language (Lesser et. al., 2004), has been developed, where some of GPGP similar mechanisms are reused in RADE framework based on RTÆMS language. Agents can coordinate and cooperate with each other using the set of mechanisms according to the protocols defined in the role, which specify how the interaction between roles should proceed.

Figure 3 and *Figure 5* illustrate pictorially the information that are captured in a RTEAMS representation, which include:

1. Top-level goals that an agent intends to achieve including the deadline for their completion. In *Figure 3*, 'Provide Cure' is the top-level goal that needs to be completed and in *Figure 5*, 'Setup Equipment' is the top-level goal that needs to be completed.

Figure 5. Plan tree for 'Setup-Equipment' in RTÆMS representation

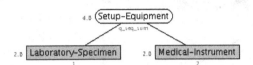

2. One or more of the possible ways of achieving goals is expressed as an abstraction hierarchy whose leaves are basic action instantiations, called methods. In ***Figure 5***, the top-level goal 'Setup Equipment' has sub-goals "Laboratory Specimen' and 'Medical Instrument', which are the methods. These sub-goals need to be completed before the top-level goal can be achieved.

3. Quantitative definition of the degree of achievement in terms of measurable characteristics, such as solution quality and time, is called the quality accumulation function (qaf). In ***Figure 5***, there exits a quality accumulation function *seq_sum* between the sub-goals "Laboratory Specimen' and 'Medical-Instrument'. The total quality of the goal "Setup Equipment" is the sum of the quality of its sub-goals "Laboratory Specimen' and 'Medical Instrument', and these two sub-goals need to be accomplished in a sequence order.

4. Task relationships indicate how basic actions or abstract task achievement affect task characteristics such as its quality and time, elsewhere in the task structure. In ***Figure 3***, there exits a "facilitates" relationship between the task 'Medical History Record' and 'Clinical Test'. A *facilitates* relationship indicates that if the task 'Medical History Record' is completed before the start of task 'Clinical Test', it will increase the quality, and reduce the cost and duration of task 'Clinical Test' by some value.

Task relationships represent a measure view of temporal constraints among activities as a result of information sharing relationships. An *enables* relationship is a hard relationship that essentially acts as a binary switch. In this case, the target method or task cannot accrue quality until the enabling interrelationship is active. A *disables* relationship indicates the exact converse of an *enables* relationship, which precludes the possibility of performing an activity when another activity is performed,. Both a *facilitates* and *hinders* relationship are soft relationships. When a 'facilitates' relationship is active, the targets' quality is increased by some quality power, and the duration and cost are reduced by the duration power and cost power, respectively. Similarly, when a 'hinders' relationship is active, the target's quality is reduced, while the duration and cost are increased. These relationships are called non-local effects if they are relationships between tasks situated in different agents for coordination. Relationships among tasks in the same agent are not of direct concern of the coordination component. The measured view of these relationships indicates how the quality of the information generated by an activity will affect the performance characteristics of the activity using this information, such as the length of its execution and the quality of its resulting solution.

There is a strong connection between the coordination module and a local scheduler module that is part of each agent's architecture. In our work, the agent's local optimization expert is the Design-to-Criteria Scheduler (DTC) (Wagner, Garvey & Lesser, 1998). During the coordination process, the coordination module queries the DTC scheduler repeatedly to explore the implications of constraints. The coordination and DTC module present in each agent can guide the agent's activities using knowledge of its own local situation and partial knowledge of the activities being carried by other agents. The coordination component in each agent also coordinates with that of other agents to generate constraints on local control that leads to

Figure 6. Agent A and Agent B's initial task view with enables relationship

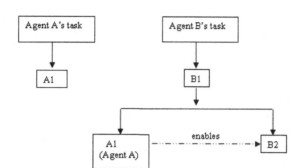

more coherent agent activities.

Each agent starts its coordination component by constructing its own local view of the activities that the agent intends to pursue, as well as the relationships among these activities (Lesser et. al., 2004). The RTÆMS representation is used by the problem solving, coordination and scheduling components as a common communication language. The coordination component helps to construct a global view for an agent, and to recognize and respond to particular inter-agent task structure relationships by making commitments to other agents. The commitments result in coordinated behavior by affecting the tasks an agent executes and the results transmitted. The DTC scheduler, based on commitments, agent's goal, the local and non-local values of tasks, and other agent activity constraints, creates a schedule of activities for the agent, which must meet the real-time deadlines. The coordination component coordinates the activities of an agent through modulating its local control as a result of placing commitments and constraints on the local scheduler.

The coordination component uses the RTÆMS task structure representation to add an extension of local and non-local commitments to task achievement. The coordination includes the goals that the agent is currently pursuing, the goals it will likely pursue in the near future, the characteristics of the abstract tasks and basic actions available to achieve these goals, their relationships to other tasks, and the degree of achievement necessary for each goal.

A user can choose a coordination rule from three types of coordination rules, namely Rule1 (simple), Rule 2 (hard and soft relation), and Rule 3 (priority based). The coordination mechanism between agents depends on selection of a specific rule.

Suppose we have two agents A and B shown in *Figure 6*. Agent B is performing task B1. Task B1 has subtask A1 and B2. Subtask A1 is performed by agent A and subtask B2 is performed by agent B itself. There is an 'enables' relationship from A1 to B2.

When a user selects Rule 1 (simple), the agents use a very simple coordination mechanism - they only consider the quality accumulation function but not the hard and soft relationships between the tasks. As shown in *Figure 6*, suppose there is a *seq_sum* quality accumulation function associated with task B1, agent B recognizes that the quality achievement of B1 depends on the accomplish of task A1 and it has to be performed before task B1, it then sends a message to agent A asking it to perform task A1 by a given deadline. Agent A replies with the start time and finish time for task A1 according to its local schedule. Upon receiving this message agent B reschedules the start time of its task B1 to the finish time of task A1. This is the Scenario 1 described in *Figure 7*.

Figure 7. Coordination scenarios using different rules

Scenario	Using Rule		Agent A - task A1				Agent B - task B2			
			Start time	Duration	Deadline	Priorty	Start time	Duration	Deadline	Priorty
1	Rule 1	Intial schedule	5	5	15	5	15	5	25	5
		After Coordination	5	5	15	5	10	5	25	5
2	Rule 2	Intial schedule	5	5	15	5	5	5	25	5
		After Coordination	0	5	15	5	5	5	25	5
3	Rule 2	Intial schedule	5	6	20	5	5	5	25	5
		After Coordination	0	6	20	5	6	5	25	5
			Agent A - task A1				Agent B - task B2			
			Start time	Duration	Deadline	Priorty	Start time	Duration	Deadline	Priorty
4	Rule 3	Intial schedule	5	5	25	3	5	6	15	5
		After Coordination	0	5	25	3	5	6	15	5
			Agent A - task A2							
		Intial schedule	0	5	25	7				
		After Coordination	5	5	25	7				

Rule 2 deals with both hard and soft relationships together with the quality accumulation functions and non-local tasks. Hard relationships include the *enables* and *disables* relationship, and soft relationships include *facilitates* and *hinders* relationships.

As shown in **Figure 6**, task A1 has *enables* relationship with task B2. Agent B sends a message to agent A saying that task B2 has an *enables* relationship with task A1 and should complete task A1 by a given deadline. Agent A checks the start time of task A1. If the start time of task A1 is less than or equal to the start time of task B2, then agent A makes a commitment to agent B that it can finish the task B2 by the given deadline. If the finish time of task A1 is greater than the start time of task B2, agent A then moves task A1's start time to task A1's earliest start time. Agent A sends the new start time and finish time of task A1 to agent B. If the finish time of task A1 proposed by agent A is less than or equal to the start time of task B2, agent B follows its normal schedule. Otherwise, agent B temporarily sets task B2's start time to the finish time of task A1 as proposed by agent A and calculates its new finish time for task B2. If the new finish time falls within the deadline of task B2, then agent B reschedules its task B2 with new values. Otherwise, task B2 is not performed.

Scenario 2 in *Figure 9* explains how agents coordinate with each other using Rule 2. In the initial schedule for task B2, the start time is 5. Agent A sets its start time to its earliest start time (0). Now the new finish time for task A1 is 5. Since the new finish time for task A1 is equal to the start time of task B2, the schedule for task B2 remains unchanged.

Scenario 3 shows a different case. In the initial schedule for task B2, the start time is 5. Agent A sets its start time to its earliest start time (0). Now the new finish time for task A1 is 6. Since the new finish time for task A1 is greater than the start time of task B2, rescheduling of task B2 is needed. Task B2 has a new start time as 6 after rescheduling.

Rule 3 is based upon priority of a task, which takes into consideration the hard and the soft relationships. Rule 3 is useful when an agent is performing more than one task. In the RTÆMS representation, each task has a new attribute called "priority", with its value ranging from 1 (i.e., the highest priority) to 10 (i.e., the lowest priority).

Let us assume that agent A has two tasks A2 and A1. Task A1 has *enables* relationship with task B2. Agent B sends a message to agent A saying that task A1 has an *enables* relationship with task B2 and requires task A1 to be completed by a given deadline. Agent A checks the start time of task A1. If the start time of task A1 is less than or equal to the start time of task B2, agent A makes a commitment to agent B that it can finish the task B2 by the given deadline. If the finish time of task A1 is greater than the start time of task B2, agent A then checks the start time and finish time of task A2. If task A2 is performed before task A1, agent A compares the priority of task A1 and A2. If the priority of task A1 is higher than that of task A2, agent A reschedules task A1 to be performed before task A2, and the new start time and finish time of task A1 is sent to agent B. Otherwise, agent A sets the start time to task A1 to its earliest start time. Agent A sends its new start time and finish time to agent B. If the finish time of task A1 proposed by Agent A is less than the start time of task B2, agent B follows its normal schedule. If the proposed finish time of task A1 is greater, agent B temporarily sets B2's start time to A1's finish time and calculates the new finish time for task B2. If the new finish time is no later than the deadline of task B2, agent B reschedules its task B2 with new values; otherwise, task B2 is not performed.

Figure 8. Plan tree for 'Get-Cure' in RTÆMS representation

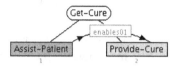

Scenario 4 in Figure 9 shows how Rule 3 works. The initial start time of task B2 is 5 and agent A cannot complete the task A1 before 5. Hence, agent A compares the priority of task A2 and A1. Since priority of task A1 is higher, A1 is performed before A2, and the new schedule is sent to agent B.

Similarly, these coordination rules can be used to support other non-local relationships, including disables, facilitates and hinders.

Figure 9. Task schedules

Agent		Intial schedule				New schedule			
Admin-MA	Task	Start time	Duration	Finish time	Priorty	Start time	Duration	Finish time	Priorty
	Clean	0	12	12	7	12	12	24	7
	Assist-Patient	12	12	24	3	0	12	12	3
	Answer-Telephone	12		15		0	3		
	Schedule-Appointment	15		18		3	6		
	Greet-Patient	18		21		6	9		
	Admit-Patient	21		24		9	12		
Physician	Task	Start time	Duration	Finish time	Priorty				
	Provide-Cure	12	67	79	3				
	Medical-History-Record	12		15					
	Clinical-Test	15		17					
	Test-Interpretation	17		20					
	Setup-Equipment	20		40					
	Operate	40		46					
	Provide-Care	46		79					
Nurse-Assistan	Task	Start time	Duration	Finish time	Priorty				
	Provide care	46	33	79	3				
	Walk-Patient	46		49					
	Clean-Room	49		52					
	Server-Meal	52		55					
	Dress-Patient	55		58					
	Check-Pulse	58		61					
	Check-Blood-Pressure	61		64					
	Check-Temperature	64		67					
	Check-Respiratory-Rate	67		70					
	Physical-Condition	70		73					
	Mental-Condition	73		76					
	Emotional-Condition	76		79					
Clinic MA	Task	Start time	Duration	Finish time	Priorty				
	setup-equipment	20	20	40	5				
	Laboratory-Specimen	20		30					
	Medical-Instrument	30		40					

RUNTIME SCENARIO

Now we present a runtime scenario for a hospital organization to describe how the health care simulation system works. The scenario demonstrates how the dynamic task allocation is accomplished through the A-R mapping mechanism, and how agents coordinate with each other in their activities. In this scenario, a special agent role space is first created. Role space agent is initially not taking any active role in the system; rather, it is mainly responsible for maintaining and managing the role instances in the system. The role space checks the plan tree of a role instance, when this role instance is taken by an agent, which recognizes the needs to create new role instances. The role space selects the appropriate agent for the role instance after verifying the qualification and consistency of the candidates.

When the system is initialized, the system administer creates several Patient role instances to express the expected service requirements from patients. The number of Patient role instances depends on the capability of the hospital. These patient role instances are posted in the role space and are not active until they are taken by some agents. When a (real) patient Bryan enters the hospital for services, a personal assistant agent named Bryan is created for this patient, and the agent takes one Patient role instance. In this case, Bryan uses the coordination Rule 3, which is specified when the user defines the Patient agent class.

When agent Bryan takes the Patient role instance, it has one goal to achieve: 'Get Cure'. The plan tree of this goal describes that two sub goals 'Assist Patient' and 'Provide Cure' must be achieved so that the goal 'Get Cure' can succeed. The goal 'Assist Patient' belongs to a MA Admin (Administrative Medical Assistant) role and the goal 'Provide Cure' belongs to a Physician role. Based on this information, a Physician role instance and an MA Admin role instance are created by the role space.

Four other agents, Adam, Cathy, Kevin and David that represent four medical professionals are also created and active in the system. Both agent Adam and the remaining agents are initialized with coordination Rule 3. They have been idle and sent requests to the role space for available role instances. When the MA Admin and Physician role instances are created in the role space, all three agents who are interested in taking any additional role instances receive a message for this update. After receiving the message, the agent checks the goal associated with the role instance, especially the MQPS, to see if it matches its own motivation. If the MQPS contains the same type of the agent's MQ in its motivation, the agent is said to be interested in taking that role instance.

For example, the Physician role instance has MQPS as: (MQ_professional, p1), (MQ_moral, p2), (MQ_experience, p3), all these three types MQ's belong to agent Adam's motivation. So Adam is interested in this role instance. How interested Adam is for this role instances depends on the actual values of p1, p2 and p3, the exact structures of the mapping functions with index 0, 1, and 2, and the current accumulation of these MQ's for agent Adam.

If agent Adam is interested in multiple role instance openings, it will compare the degree of interests in these role instances and select the most interested ones, and send requests to the role space. It is also possible that the role space receives requests from multiple agents for the same role instance. In this case, the role space verifies the qualification of each agent by matching the agent's qualification with the certificate requirement defined in the corresponding role class. For example, agent Adam is qualified for this role instance because it has a MD qualification that matches the certificate requirement of the Physician role class. The role space also checks if this role instance is compatible with other role instances the agent is taking right now. For instance, suppose agent Bryan has a MD qualification and it is also interested in this Physician role instance; however, according to the incompatibility relationship between the Physician role and the Patient role, agent Bryan cannot take this role instance because it takes the Patient role instance related to this Physician role instance.

After verifying the qualification and checking the consistency, the role space selects an appropriate agent (agent Cathy) for the MA Admin role instance, whose goal is to 'Assist Patient'. The role space then tells agent Cathy that the task 'Assist Patient' has an *enables* relationship with the task "Provide Cure'. The plan tree for the goal 'Assist Patient' consists of four sub goals: 'Greet Patient', 'Schedule Appointment', 'Admit Patient', and 'Answer Telephone'. All of these sub-goals can be performed by the same agent who takes the MA Admin role instance, so no new role instance has to be created.

After assigning the MA Admin role instance to agent Cathy, the role space assigns the Physician role instance to another appropriate agent - Adam, based on its qualification. The role space then tells agent Adam that task 'Assist Patient' enables its task 'Provide Cure'. The goal of taking the Physician role by agent Adam is to 'Provide Cure'. The role space reads the plan tree associated with the goal, and finds that in order to accomplish this goal, sub-goals 'Setup Equipment' and 'Provide Care' must be accomplished by other roles. In response to this need, new role instances Nurse Assistant and MA Clinical (Clinical Medical Assistant) are created. The role space then selects appropriate agents Kevin and David to take these role instances respectively. This process will continue until no more new role instance is needed, and all role instances have been taken. After a goal defined in a role instance is accomplished, the agent will collect the utility as defined in the MQPS of this role instance, and release the role instance, which will be further deleted by the role space.

After all role instances have been assigned to appropriate agents, the role space sends a table of roles to the agent who is performing that role, followed by a message to start the coordination. The agents can now begin the coordination pro-

cess. For example, as shown in *Figure 8*, Patient Bryan a goal to 'Get Cure", which has two non-local subtasks 'Assist Patient' and 'Provide Cure' performed by MA Admin Cathy and Physician Adam, respectively. Patient Bryan sends a message to both agents to ask them to complete the task within the deadline. Agents Cathy and Adam reply to Patient Bryan with their scheduled execution time. The Physician Adam coordinates with MA Admin Cathy using coordination Rule 3 to schedule the task 'Assist Patient' before 'Provide Cure'. There is a *facilitate*s relationship between task '(Read) Medical History Record' and task 'Clinical Test'. Since both tasks belong to the same agent, so the 'facilitates' relationship is taken care of by agent Cathy's local scheduler.

Since task 'Assist Patient' has an *enables* relationship with task 'Provide Cure', Physician Adam requests MA Admin Cathy to complete the task by 12. However, Cathy has another task 'Clean' that is scheduled for time 0 to 12, and the task 'Assist Patient' is scheduled for time 12 to 24. Cathy compares the priority of task 'Assist Patient' and task 'Clean': priority of task 'Assist Patient' is higher so this task is rescheduled before the task 'Clean'. Nurse Assistant Kevin can perform the task 'Provide Care' after task 'Operate' performed by Physician Adam. Similarly, Clinical MA David can perform the task 'Setup Equipment' before task 'Operate' and meet the deadline requested by Physician Adam. So no more rescheduling is necessary. The initial schedule for all tasks and new schedule for task 'Clean' are shown in *Figure 9*.

After the coordination is complete the agents can now begin execution, Patient Bryan can now begin executing its task 'Get Cure', which has subtasks 'Assist Patient' and 'Provide Cure'. The task 'Assist Patient' should be performed by MA Admin Cathy. Patient Bryan agent sends a message to MA Admin Cathy to begin the task 'Assist Patient'. MA Admin Cathy then begins executing the task 'Assist Patient', which has the subtasks 'Answer Telephone', 'Schedule Appointment',

Figure 10. Plan tree for 'Assist-Patient' in RTÆMS representation

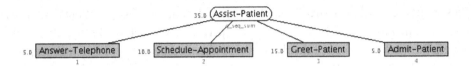

'Greet Patient' and 'Admit Patient'. The quality of the task 'Assist Patient' is defined by the quality accumulative function "seq_sum", which is the total quality of all of its sub-tasks performed in sequence. Since MA Admin Cathy itself can perform all of the subtasks, it starts the execution immediately. After Cathy completes the task 'Assist Patient', it collects the motivation quantities as defined in the MQPS of this role instance. (See Figures 10 and 11)

Upon receiving this message, patient Bryan updates its own task structure. MA Admin Cathy has rescheduled this task after the task 'Assist Patient'. So when Cathy completes the task 'Assist Patient', it begins executing the task 'Clean'. Now Patient Bryan can start executing the task 'Provide Cure'. Since the task 'Provide Cure' is performed by Physician Adam, so Patient Bryan sends a message to Physician Adam saying that it can start the execution. Physician Adam begins the execution of the task 'Provide Cure'. The task 'Provide Cure' has subtasks 'Examine Patient' and 'Provide Treatment' as shown in *Figure 3*.

Physician Adam begins executing 'Examine Patient', which has subtasks '(Read) Medical History Record', 'Clinical Test' and 'Test Interpretation', which can all be performed by Physician Adam. After completion of these subtasks, it then begins executing task 'Provide Treatment', which has subtasks 'Prescribe Treatment' and 'Administer Treatment' with the quality accumulative function "max", which means only one of these two subtask needs to be accomplished.

If Physician Adam decides to perform the task 'Administer Treatment', then the three subtasks

'Setup Equipment', 'Operate' and 'Provide Care' need to be accomplished. The task 'Setup Equipment' is performed by MA Clinical agent David. So Physician Adam sends a request to Clinical MA David to perform the task 'Setup Equipment'. David starts executing the task 'Setup Equipment', which has subtasks 'Laboratory Specimen' and 'Medical Instrument'. After the completion, David sends a message to Physician Adam, saying that the task has been completed, together with the quality accumulated, cost accrued and the time taken. Upon receiving this message, physician Adam updates its task structure and begins executing 'Operation', which is performed by itself.

Similarly, the task 'Provide Care' is performed by Nurse Assistant Kevin. Physician Adam sends a request to Kevin to execute the task. Kevin begins executing the task 'Provide Care', which has the subtasks 'Serve Patient', 'Provide Skin Care' and 'Observe Patient'. Nurse Assistant Kevin itself can perform all of these subtasks. (See Figure 12)

After the completion of the task, Kevin sends a message to Physician Adam, saying that the task has been completed, together with the quality accumulated, cost accrued and time taken. Upon

Figure 11. Plan tree for updated 'Get-Cure' in RTÆMS representation

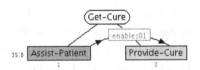

Figure 12. Plan tree for updated 'Provide Care' in RTÆMS representation.

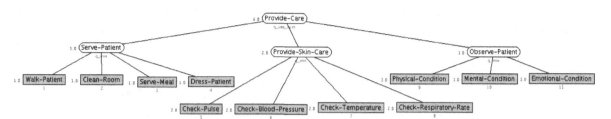

receiving this message, physician Adam updates its task structure. Since task 'Provide Cure' has now been completed, Adam sends a message to Patient Bryan that the task has been completed, together with the quality accumulated, cost accrued and time taken. Upon receiving this message, Patient Bryan updates its task structure.

FUTURE TRENDS

The future work includes further development of the system based on the current prototype. Especially, we are interested providing support for users to define interaction protocols in role classes, and integrating those domain-dependent protocols with domain-independent communication mechanisms in agents. We are also interested in experimenting with large systems, more complex scenario and analyzing the system performance.

CONCLUSION

In this chapter, we describe a multi-agent health care simulation system built using RADE framework. The integrated framework supports role-based design of multi-agent systems as well as implementation of utility-driven agents that can use a variety of existing agent reasoning and coordination mechanisms. We describe how the roles are defined, how agents are created, and how the role instances are mapped to agents. We also describe the rule-based coordination mechanisms

and present a runtime scenario that shows how the simulation system works and how agents coordinate with each other to schedule their local activities. This work verifies the feasibility of modeling health care system with multi-agent approach and demonstrates the strength of automatic coordination, planning and scheduling.

REFERENCES

Becht, M., Gurzki, T., Klarmann, J., & Muscholl, M. (1999). ROPE: Role-Oriented Programming Environment for Multi-Agent Systems. *Conference on Cooperative Information Systems* (pp. 325–333).

Bellifemine, F., Caire, G., Poggi, A., & Rimassa, G. (2003). JADE A White Paper. *EXP in search of innovation - Special Issue on JADE, TILAB Journal, 3*, 6-19.

Decker, K. (1996). TAEMS: A Framework for Environment Centered Analysis and Design of Coordination Mechanisms. In G. O'Hare & N. Jennings (Eds.), *Foundations of Distributed Artificial Intelligence* (pp. 429-448). Wiley Inter-Science.

DeLoach, S., Wood, M., & Sparkman, C. H. (2001). Multiagent Systems Engineering. *International Journal of Software Engineering and Knowledge Engineering, 11*, 231–258. doi:10.1142/S0218194001000542

Gracanin, D., Bohner, S. A., & Hinchey, M. (2004). Towards a Model-Driven Architecture for Autonomic Systems. *Proceeding of 11ᵗʰ IEEE International Conference and Workshop on the Engineering of Computer-Based Systems (ECBS'04)* (pp. 500-505).

Graham, J. R., Decker, K. S., & Mersic, M. (2003). DECAF – A Flexible Multi Agent System Architecture. *Autonomous Agents and Multi-Agent Systems*, 7(1-2), 7–27. doi:10.1023/A:1024120703127

Kuwabara, K., Ishida, T., & Osato, N. (1995). AgenTalk: Describing Multiagent Coordination Protocols with Inheritance. *Proc. 7th IEEE International Conference on Tools with Artificial Intelligence (ICTAI '95)* (pp. 460-465).

Lesser, V., Decker, K., Wagner, T., Carver, N., Garvey, A., Horling, B., Neiman, D., & Podorozhny, R., NagendraPrasad, M., Raja, A., Vincent, R., Xuan, P., & Zhang, X.Q. (2004). Evolution of the GPGP/TAEMS Domain- Independent Coordination Framework. *Autonomous Agents and Multi-Agent Systems*, 9(1), 87–143. doi:10.1023/B:AGNT.0000019690.28073.04

Luck, M., & d'Inverno, M. (1995). A Formal Framework for Agency and Autonomy. *Proceedings of the First International Conference on Multi-Agent Systems (ICMAS-95)* (pp. 254-260). AAAI Press/ MIT Press.

Maria, D. B. A., Silva, V. T., & Lucena, C. J. P. (2005). Developing Multi-Agent Systems Based on MDA. *Proceedings of the 17ᵗʰ Conference on Advanced Information Systems Engineering (CAiSE'05)*. Porto, Portugal.

Vincent, R., Horling, B., & Lesser, V. (2001). An Agent Infrastructure to Build and Evaluate Multi-Agent Systems: The Java Agent Framework and Multi-Agent System Simulator. *Lecture Notes in Artificial Intelligence: Infrastructure for Agents, Multi-Agent Systems and Scalable Multi-Agent Systems, 1887*.

Wagner, T., Garvey, A., & Lesser, V. R. (1997). Complex Goal Criteria and its Application in Design-to-Criteria Scheduling. *Proceedings of the Fourteenth National Conference on Artificial Intelligence*.

Wagner, T., & Lesser, V. (2002). Evolving Real-Time Local Agent Control for Large-Scale MAS. In J.J. Meyer & M. Tambe (Eds.), *Intelligent Agents VIII (Proceedings of ATAL-01), Lecture Notes in Artificial Intelligence*. Springer-Verlag, Berlin.

Williamson, M., Decker, K. S., & Sycara, K. (1996). Unified information and control flow in hierarchical task networks. *Proceeding of the AAAI-96 workshop on Theories of Planning, Action and Control*.

Wooldridge, M., Jennings, N., & Kinny, D. (2000). The Gaia Methodology for Agent-Oriented Analysis and Design. *Journal of Autonomous Agents and Multi-Agent Systems*, 3, 285–312. doi:10.1023/A:1010071910869

Xu, H., & Zhang, X. (2005). A Methodology for Role-Based Modeling of Open Multi-Agent Software Systems. *ICEIS, (3)*, 246–253.

Xu, H., Zhang, X., & Patel, R. J. (2007). Developing Role-Based Open Multi-Agent Software Systems. [IJCITP]. *International Journal of Computational Intelligence Theory and Practice*, 2(1), 39–56.

Zambonelli, F., Jennings, N., & Wooldridge, M. (2003). Developing Multiagent Systems: The Gaia Methodology. *ACM Transactions on Software Engineering and Methodology*, 12, 317–370. doi:10.1145/958961.958963

Zhang, X., & Xu, H. (2006) Towards Automated Development of Multi-Agent Systems Using RADE. *Proceedings of the 2006 International Conference on Artificial Intelligence (ICAI'06)* (pp. 44-50). Las Vegas, Nevada.

Zhang, X., Xu, H., & Shrestha, B. (2007). An Integrated Role-Based Approach for Modeling, Designing and Implementing Multi-Agent Systems. *Journal of the Brazilian Computer Society (JCBS) . Special Issue on Software Engineering for Multi-Agent Systems, 13*(2), 45–60.

Section 3
Physician/Patient Support Systems

Chapter 7
HeCaSe2:
A Multi-Agent System that Automates the Application of Clinical Guidelines

David Isern
University Rovira i Virgili, Spain

Antonio Moreno
University Rovira i Virgili, Spain

ABSTRACT

Clinical guidelines (CGs) contain a set of directions or principles to assist the healthcare practitioner with patient care decisions about appropriate diagnostic, therapeutic, or other clinical procedures for specific clinical circumstances. It is widely accepted that the adoption of guideline-execution engines in daily practice would improve the patient care, by standardising the care procedures. Guideline-based systems constitute part of a knowledge-based decision support system in order to deliver the right knowledge to the right people in the right form at the right time. The automation of the guideline execution process is a basic step towards its widespread use in medical centres. To achieve this general goal, different topics should be tackled, such as the acquisition of clinical guidelines, its formal verification, and finally its execution. This chapter focuses on the execution of CGs and describes the design and implementation of an agent-based platform in which the actors involved in health care coordinate their activities to perform the complex task of guideline enactment.

INTRODUCTION

In *electronic healthcare* (*e*-Health) it is increasingly necessary to develop computerised applications to support people involved in providing basic medical care, reducing costs and providing relevant patient information at the point of care (Lenz, et al., 2007; Wyatt & Sullivan, 2007). A *clinical guideline* (in

the following, CG) is a highly matured therapeutic plan that compiles optimum practices for treating patients in a well-defined medical syntax. Thus, the adoption of CGs is a promising way for standardising and improving health care practices (Field & Lohr, 1990; Mersmann & Dojat, 2004; Michie & Johnston, 2004).

More concretely, CGs are a set of directions or principles to assist the health care practitioner with patient care decisions about appropriate diagnostic,

DOI: 10.4018/978-1-60566-772-0.ch007

therapeutic, or other clinical procedures for specific clinical circumstances. CGs are developed by government agencies, institutions, organizations such as professional societies or governing boards, or by the convening of expert panels. They provide a foundation for assessing and evaluating the quality and effectiveness of health care in terms of measuring improved health, reduction of variation in services or procedures performed, and reduction of variation in outcomes of health care delivered (CancerWEB, 2008).

CGs are usually published as technical reports, papers and books, which are mainly disseminated through the Web. The data format includes natural language statements, tables, workflows of processes, and they report information about decisions to be made, drug therapies, diagnostic procedures, doses, etc. (*e.g.,* a CG can describe the screening, early detection, diagnostic and treatment of pre-eclampsia in pregnancy (Milne, et al., 2005)). From the creation of these documents, to their final use in daily care, several stages must be followed: representation, acquisition, verification and finally, execution. The first three tasks concern the authors of the guideline (e.g., governmental or professional organizations), whereas the latter is related to practitioners. Briefly, these steps can be described as follows:

a) *Choice of a representation language.* A CG contains several elements to be modelled, such as actions, required patient data, decisions to be made, constraints between tasks, temporal constraints in a global plan, etc. Different researchers have defined formal languages to model computer-interpretable clinical guidelines, such as PRO*forma*, EON, GLIF, GUIDE, SDA* or Asbru (Clercq, Blom, Korsten, & Hasman, 2004; Miksch, Shahar, & Johnson, 1997; Riaño, 2007; Wang, Peleg, Tu, Shortliffe, & Greenes, 2001). Some reviews of the main guideline representation languages can be found at (Peleg, et al., 2003) and (Mulyar, van der Aalst, & Peleg, 2007).

b) *Acquisition of CGs.* Clinical guidelines are based on the evidence collected from clinical trials and existing literature (Davis, Goldman, & Palda, 2007; Priori, Klein, & Bassand, 2003). Some authors are also currently working in the semi-automatic construction of computer-interpretable guidelines, by applying Machine Learning techniques from a corpus of clinical data collected in a medical centre (Riaño, 2004), directly from textual documents (Hrabak, Campbell, Tu, McClure, & Weida, 2007), or using mark-up techniques to guide the extraction of the main data structures and relations (Shahar, et al., 2004).

c) *Verification of CGs.* Verification includes two aspects: is a medical guideline well formed?, and, which of these two available CGs is the best? The first question seeks to verify the formal correctness of the guideline (Hommersom, Groot, Lucas, Balser, & Schmitt, 2007; ten Teije, et al., 2006). The second question is more difficult to answer since it is necessary to quantify how appropriate is a clinical guideline. To tackle this problem, some authors proposed an evaluation procedure called AGREE which calculates a set of parameters for a given guideline to evaluate its quality (AGREE, 2003). In addition a methodology to facilitate the whole development and evaluation of CGs can be found in (Ricci, Celani, & Righetti, 2006).

d) *Execution aspects.* As mentioned above, a CG contains a great amount of information to be considered (decisions to be made, constraints between tasks, temporal restrictions). Proper management and evaluation of heterogeneous data from different sources (*e.g.,* family doctor, nurses, and medical devices) during the enactment of CGs is a crucial task. In any case, these decision-support tools are used to assist the practitioner during a treatment in a supervised way. The patient, at the same time, receives the feedback from the system knowing his current status, outcomes, and remaining tests.

While representation, acquisition and verification stages are currently active research areas as shown in (Chesani, de Matteis, Mello, Montal, & Storari, 2006; Leong, Kaiser, & Miksch, 2007; Peleg, Keren, & Denekamp, 2008; Seyfang, et al., 2006), the execution of guidelines is a less developed field, and it is the main focus of this chapter. In addition, we study the use of the intelligent agent paradigm and its adoption to build a guideline-based execution system.

The rest of the chapter is organised as follows. First of all, a study of the application of agents to healthcare problems and a review of the available guideline-based execution engines are done. After that, the multi-agent system to execute CGs and its knowledge representation are explained in detail. The chapter finalises with some future lines of research and a set of concluding remarks of this application.

RELATED WORK

The main goal of this chapter is to describe the design and implementation of a guideline-based execution engine that improves the general performance with respect to similar systems by using a multi-agent system, which coordinates both the collection of data and their transmission to the correct point of care. The background is divided into two main issues: the use of agents in the healthcare domain, and the study of current guideline execution engines.

Agents Applied in the Healthcare Domain

The execution of CGs presents most of the general characteristics of the problems on the medical domain (Fox, Beveridge, & Glasspool, 2003;

Nealon & Moreno, 2003). Particularly, it is very usual that the knowledge required to solve a problem is spatially distributed among different locations, adding constraints in the planning of coordinated actions. Moreover, the solution of a problem involves the coordination of the effort of a set of individuals with different skills and functions. Finally there is a lot of knowledge spread around the Web and digital libraries that can be reused. Thus, the execution of CGs by using a multi-agent system (MAS) and the adequacy of this technology to healthcare problems can be argued as follows (Fox, et al., 2003; Nealon & Moreno, 2003):

- The components of a MAS may be running in different machines, and be located in many different places. Each of the agents may keep a part of the knowledge required to solve the problem, such as patient records held in different departments within a hospital. Therefore, a MAS offers a natural way of attacking inherently distributed problems.

- One of the main properties of an intelligent agent is sociability. Agents are able to communicate between themselves, using some kind of agent communication language, in order to exchange any kind of information. In that way they can engage in complex dialogues, in which they can negotiate, coordinate their actions and collaborate in the solution of a problem (*e.g.*, different units of a hospital may collaborate in the process of patient scheduling).

- When a problem is too complex to be solved by a single system, it is usual to decompose it in sub-problems (which will probably not be totally independent of each other). In multi-agent systems there are techniques of distributed problem solving, in which a group of agents may dynamically discuss how to partition a problem, how to distribute the different subtasks to be solved among them, how to exchange information to solve possible dependencies between partial solutions, and how to combine the partial results into the solution of the original problem. Thus, agent technology can handle the complexity of solutions through decomposing, modelling and organising the interrelationships between components.

- Another important property of agents is their pro-activity; their ability to perform tasks that may be beneficial for the user, even if he has not explicitly requested those tasks to be executed. Using this property, agents may find relevant information and show it to the user before he has to request it. For instance, if a personal agent knows that the user has had heart problems in the past and might need this information urgently, and it also knows that the user is about to travel abroad, it could look for information about the medical centres in the towns to be visited that have a cardiology department.

- The basic characteristic of an intelligent agent is its autonomy. Each agent takes its own decisions, based on its internal state and the information that it receives from the environment. Therefore, agents offer an ideal paradigm to implement systems in which each component models the behaviour of a separate entity, which wants to keep its autonomy and independence from the rest of the system (*e.g.,* each unit of the hospital may keep its private data).

- Agent technology offers advanced platforms for building expert systems to assist individual clinicians in their work.

- Distributed agent systems have the potential to improve the operation of healthcare organizations, where failures of communication and coordination are important sources of error.

Mainly, the most important characteristic that these systems offer their flexibility. This property is central in our approach, due to the heterogeneity of both roles and interactions of all care givers. Using a MAS (and not a centralised model) provides a great advantage to collect, monitor, and evaluate all the data required during the enactment of a CG.

Study of Guideline-Based Execution Engines

There are many approaches to the design and development of clinical guidelines execution engines, with different levels of coverage and facilities to include them into existing clinical management systems. The most prominent examples are Arezzo, DeGeL, GLARE, GLEE, NewGuide, and SAGE. Arezzo, DeGeL and NewGuide offer some level of distribution of elements, the first defining an agent-based model, and the rest, defining several client-server applications interconnected among them. The other tools (GLARE, GLEE and SAGE) were designed as centralised applications that work standalone. In the following sub-sections, a brief description and discussion of those tools is made (a more detailed analysis and comparison of those systems can be found at (Isern & Moreno, 2008)).

Arezzo

Arezzo is a commercial product to create, visualise and enact PRO*forma* guidelines (Fox, Alabassi, Patkar, Rose, & Black, 2006; Fox, et al., 2003). PRO*forma* is an executable process modelling language that has been successfully used to build and deploy a range of decision support systems, guidelines and other clinical applications (Fox, Patkar, & Thomson, 2006).

The tool is composed of three elements: a *Composer*, a *Tester* and a *Performer*. The *Composer* is a graphical tool used to create guidelines. The *Tester* is a tool created to test the guideline logic before deployment (it checks that all statements in decisions, tasks and enquiries are well written). The *Performer* inference engine allows running the guideline, taking into account data related to patients stored in an electronic medical record. The guideline is composed by different kinds of tasks (decisions, enquiries, actions and plans), which during the enactment change their internal state depending on whether a task is awaiting for data, suspended, finished or it cannot be accomplished taking into account the state of the patient. Arezzo uses the *Domino autonomous agent model* (Fox, et al., 2003). The model deals with a large class of medical problems and establishes a relationship between decision making and plan enactment procedures. The main goal of this model is to identify the basic elements required in any language to represent clinical guidelines that can be used for both decision making and plan management.

DeGeL

Digital electronic Guidelines Library (DeGeL) is a web-based, modular and distributed architecture, which facilitates the gradual conversion of clinical guidelines from text to a formal representation in Asbru (Miksch, et al., 1997; Shahar, et al., 2004; Young & Shahar, 2005).

The initial textual guidelines go through an intermediate layer between the textual and the final form, where experts add semantic information. The intermediate layer uses a meta-ontology that defines a hierarchy of basic concepts. Internally, Asbru organises a clinical guideline as a library of plans created during the decomposition process performed in the specification phase. These plans are interrelated in a hierarchical network of plans and sub-plans using a parent-child relationship which is encoded using control structures (*e.g.*, do in parallel).

The guideline execution module, Spock, incorporates an inference engine that can retrieve data stored in a patient's medical record. Spock is a modular client-server application that consists of:

(i) a set of classes, that allow to store any guideline, (ii) a parser, that interprets the content of a guideline, and (iii) a specialized module, the Controller, which synchronizes the communication between the system layers and external services (Young & Shahar, 2005; Young, et al., 2007).

GLARE

GuideLine Acquisition, Representation and Execution (GLARE) is a system to acquire and execute clinical guidelines (Anselma, Terenziani, Montani, & Bottrighi, 2007; Terenziani, Montani, Bottrighi, Molino, & Torchio, 2005; Terenziani, et al., 2004).

Guidelines use an *ad hoc* graph-based representation, where each action is represented by a node, while control relations are represented by arcs. This system is focused in the management of *temporal constraints* between different actions in the graph. An *execution module* allows executing/simulating a guideline using the appropriate data retrieved from a database. Each patient has his own medical record, which is updated continuously with the actions executed during the enactment. The architecture is complemented with a database of available resources in a given hospital, which allows making domain-dependent execution of guidelines. Moreover, GLARE allows the local adoption and update of guidelines to cope with both the need to apply them to new situations (countries, hospitals and/or departments), and with the need to manage updates (*e.g.*, authoring, recording the history of a guideline and learning from experience) (Terenziani, et al., 2005).

GLEE

GLEE is a tool for executing guidelines encoded in the 3rd version of GLIF (called GLIF3) (Wang, et al., 2004; Wang & Shortliffe, 2002). GLEE defines three levels of abstraction: *data, business logic*, and *user interface*. The data level contains the electronic medical record with a guideline repository and the *clinical event monitor*, that allows the execution (or simulation) of clinical guidelines through an event-driven model. The *business logic* level contains the GLEE execution engine, formed by a server and many clients. The server interacts with the data level, and clients interact with users (both through defined interfaces). At the bottom, there is the *user interface* level, where the clinical applications that exchange data with the upper levels are located (Wang & Shortliffe, 2002).

The execution model of GLEE takes the "system suggests, user controls" approach. A tracing system is used to record an individual patient's state when a guideline is being applied to him. It can also support an event-driven execution model once it is linked to the clinical event monitor in a local environment.

NewGuide

NewGuide is a framework for modelling and executing clinical practice guidelines (Ciccarese, Caffi, Boiocchi, Quaglini, & Stefanelli, 2004; Ciccarese, Caffi, Quaglini, & Stefanelli, 2005).

Guidelines are represented using the GUIDE representation language, which is based on Petri Nets (Quaglini, et al., 2000). It allows to model complex processes including temporal data. GUIDE is integrated into a workflow management system which proposes an infrastructure that enables inter- and intra-organizational communication through a *Careflow Management System* (CfMS) that, on the basis of the available best practice medical knowledge, is able to coordinate the care providers' activities.

The inference engine is composed of three main elements: a *general manager*, a *message manager*, and an *instance manager*. The inference engine is invoked by a clinician and automatically creates an instance of a guideline for the management of an individual patient. All the steps followed in the execution of a guideline are supervised by an *instance manager*. At the same time, all instances are controlled by a *general manager*. After loading the guideline, the *instance manager* needs to collect the entire patient's data stored in his patient record. The execution engine goes step-by-step recommending actions, such as drug prescription or laboratory tests and, at the same time, stores that information in a logs database. All log data is used to monitor the status of a patient in the CG in another module named *reporting system*. In addition, the communication between NewGuide and the external world is governed by the *message manager*, which delegates requests and responses to the web user interface or to an external entity (through a Web service interface) on the basis of the system configuration. The responsibility for maintaining the correct guideline flow and timing is left to the external CfMS (Ciccarese, et al., 2004).

SAGE

The SAGE project pursues two main goals. First of all, developing an infrastructure that allows medical experts to author and encode guidelines using a standard representation. The second goal is the use of this infrastructure to deploy those guidelines across heterogeneous clinical information systems (Berg, Ram, & Glasgow, 2004; Tu, et al., 2007; Tu, Campbell, & Musen, 2004; Tu & Glasgow, 2006).

The internal representation of guidelines in SAGE is made using the EON formalism which is comprised of a set of Protégé classes and plug-ins (Tu & Musen, 2001).

The execution engine, called *SAGEDesktop*, is implemented as a centralised element (Berg, et al., 2004). Given a guideline, it collects the required data from an internal repository and allows medical experts to emulate the real guideline behaviour. The execution engine interacts with the clinical information system (CIS) via an event listener and a set of services (terminology, patient record and general applications). The *terminology server* was added to customise the terms used in some specific local applications. Calls to/from the execution engine and the CIS are made through a set of defined APIs; the definition of an API provides interoperability with existing systems. Services related to the Electronic Medical Record (invoked using *medical record calls*) allow the engine to retrieve the appropriate patient data. After that, the *action service calls* allow the engine to initiate actions within the CIS.

Discussion

From the presented background in automated execution of CGs, several conclusions can be drawn:

- Most approaches define a set of interconnected modules that implement the main components of the guideline platform: an electronic medical record, a repository of guidelines, an interface with the (medical) expert user, a run-time engine to execute a guideline over a patient, and a structured language to represent CGs. Several of these elements act autonomously and are accessed as requested during the execution of a clinical guideline.
- These modules require defining appropriate interfaces and common understandable terminologies to exchange data.
- Representation languages define basic primitives to request the data, to represent logical conditions, and to describe actions to perform (diagnostic or treatment procedures). After its creation and verification, a CG can be deployed in different healthcare centres.
- In a real organization, some entities (human experts and resources) coordinate their activities in daily care. Systems in the healthcare domain should be able to exchange information and run continuously depending on the current status of the completed tasks and taking into account this information to

plan further pending tasks.
- The adoption of agents in the execution of CGs is a feasible approach due to the flexibility and communication skills that they provide.

AGENT-BASED EXECUTION OF CLINICAL GUIDELINES: HECASE2

The execution of a CG involves three main tasks: *a*) the definition of the (medical) data to handle, *b*) the interpretation of logical conditions in the decision points, and *c*) the description of the set of medical actions to be performed over the patient during a treatment. The proposed agent-based system aims to assist a practitioner during the enactment of a CG managing all those issues in a flexible way. Unlike a centralised system, our proposal allows to coordinate the daily activities of all actors of a healthcare organization that act autonomously according to their beliefs, desires, and intentions. Different kinds of agents have been modelled, such as doctors (representing a particular practitioner), patients, medical services (representing particular medical devices and nurses that provide different medical values into the system), and others that are required to model the structure of healthcare organizations such as medical centre agents or department agents. Later, the architecture will be explained in detail. In addition, the agents deal with data that must be represented appropriately to be exploited, including actions, predicates and concepts. The information contained in CGs contains sequences of actions to be performed in a procedural way (know-what), and they include data about enquiries, decisions and actions. The interpretation of these CGs by intelligent agents requires more information in order to know which actor is able to perform an action, or understand a criterion of a logical condition (know-how). This information is represented using declarative knowledge. Those execution-related elements could be included explicitly into the CG, but the same CG can be executed in a different way in two different medical centres or by different actors, and that option would suppose a loss of generality of CGs in front of versioning under particular circumstances. To tackle this problem a medico-organizational ontology was designed.

The rest of this section is structured as follows. First, it is explained how the agent-based architecture was designed following an agent-oriented software engineering methodology. After that, an explanation of the medico-organizational ontology is done. Finally, it is described how a clinical guideline is executed by the proposed agent-based system.

Development of the System using an Agent-Oriented Software Engineering Methodology

Nowadays, most developers of agent-based systems use an ad hoc approach. The use of an agent-oriented software engineering (AOSE) methodology in the preliminary stages of a MAS development (analysis and design) provides some advantages (*e.g.*, the possibility of reusing and sharing a common vocabulary and pieces of code in an easy way), and improves the quality of the software (Bernon, Cossentino, & Pavón, 2005; Cernuzzi, Juan, Sterling, & Zambonelli, 2004; Gómez-Sanz, Gervais, & Weiss, 2004; Henderson-Sellers & Giorgini, 2005).

One of the main problems to adopt a methodology in daily work is the wide range of available possibilities. Depending on the requirements of the project, several approaches can be applied, and the criteria for selecting one or another are difficult to evaluate. This section describes the procedure followed in order to apply a methodology to design the HeCaSe2 system. First of all, the selection of the methodology is described, and then, the steps followed in the construction of a prototype are detailed. Finally, the architecture of the system is presented.

AOSE Selection Process

Before analysing and comparing the existing AOSE methodologies, the system designer must define clearly the requirements to be accomplished. Several approaches to design a MAS are available, and a thorough review of these tools can be found at (Gómez-Alonso, Isern, & Moreno, 2007).

The criteria to select one or another methodology are very subjective because any of them covers all the requirements of HeCaSe2. A subset with the most well-known alternatives was selected considering their usability, the existence of CASE tools to facilitate the implementation, the coverage of the whole life-cycle (analysis, design and implementation), the agent-oriented programming language used during the codification, the level of formalisation and abstraction of the created documents, the expressiveness of agents and organizations, and the availability of documentation to ease learning. The approaches that could be used in a real implementation are: *Extended Gaia* (Zambonelli, Jennings, & Wooldridge, 2003), *INGENIAS* (Pavón, Gómez-Sanz, & Fuentes, 2005), *MaSE* (DeLoach, 2004), *Passi* (Cossentino, 2005), *Prometheus* (Padgham & Winikoff, 2004), and *Tropos* (Bresciani, Giorgini, Giunchiglia, Mylopoulos, & Perini, 2004). After analysing those methodologies, *Extended Gaia* was discarded because it only covers analysis and design, and the generated documents are difficult to translate into a programming language and to validate formally. The rest of tools offer a wide range of features and supportive elements, and it was difficult (and somewhat subjective) to select one of them. All the methodologies allow modelling agents (with formal representations), defining different roles of these agents, teams or groups of agents (organizations), and detailing communication issues (conversations and protocols). They also offer full life-cycle coverage, and provide some CASE tools. At the end, *INGENIAS* was selected. The most prominent features of this methodology, which have led to its selection in this work, are:

- It allows an agent developer to analyse and design a wide range of MAS.
- It permits to describe agents in different levels of abstraction, including social and organizational issues, goals and tasks.
- It is possible to detail the environment where the agents act.
- It allows the definition of conversations and messages to be exchanged.
- It allows the definition of an agent's mental state, which includes information about facts, beliefs, events and goals, and their changes depending on the agent's current role.
- It includes several examples that ease the learning of this methodology. Moreover, several research projects have adopted *INGENIAS* (Cuesta, Gómez Expósito, Rodríguez, & González, 2005; Soto, Vizcaino, Portillo, & Piattini, 2006).
- It provides an open source tool called *INGENIAS* Development Kit (IDK)1, which facilitates the implementation of projects as well as its learning.
- It also allows translating the designed models into a well-known agent-oriented programming language such as JADE (Bellifemine, Caire, & Greenwood, 2007).

Analysis-to-Implementation Steps

INGENIAS proposes the definition of different models in the analysis and design stages, and finally, a code-generator plug-in interprets these models in order to create a prototype using an agent programming language. The created prototype contains a general skeleton for all agents with the conversations patterns and the translation of all interaction models into communication protocols. In addition, it includes functional features applied to a particular organization (topology of agents),

internal roles of agents, and the sequences of general tasks included into workflows.

The created prototype does not cover the full functionalities of HeCaSe2, and other features such as the definition of ontology-related topics in the communications between agents or security issues were added *a posteriori*. However, the generated skeleton is very useful to organize a complex MAS and implement changes in the organization. Concretely, the identification of bottlenecks and reusing pieces of software are easy with this approach and, in addition, the generated models are used to document the functionalities of the final software in terms of agents, communication protocols, tasks and goals.

The first task to design the MAS is to define the set of requirements to be accomplished, which in our case are summarised as follows:

- The system should model a generic user (or patient) that wants to interact with a complex medical organization. The medical organization is inspired in the Catalan Health Service (CatSalut). From the user point of view, there is no direct communication with medical practitioners, and a representative of the organization is required. A broker allows the user to obtain a filtered collection of results from different medical centres.
- A medical organization includes medical services and doctors organized into departments. These medical services can be located in a particular department or shared by the whole medical centre. Some basic functions, such as booking a medical visit or searching a particular department, are offered to the user through the broker and the medical centre. An internal service used by doctors is the management of clinical guidelines. They are retrieved and executed by doctors, and can require the
- supervision of users to confirm pending activities. Internal tasks coded inside the

Figure 1. The organizational model of HeCaSe2

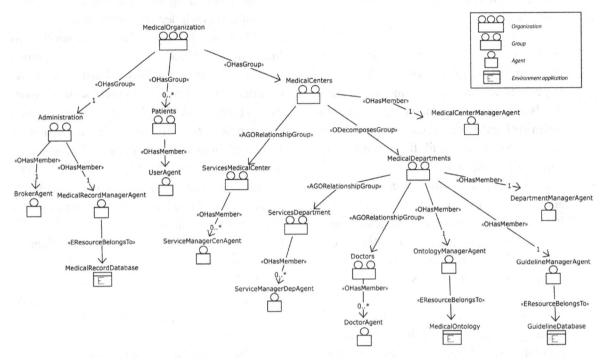

clinical guidelines require coordination among doctors and medical services in order to obtain a result.

- In addition, the medical knowledge used by doctors is represented in a medical ontology. Moreover, an electronic health record stores all results provided by services (tests results) or by doctors (results of medical visits).

The first step described in *INGENIAS* is the analysis of these requirements in order to extract the main entities and their relationships with the environment and between them. After that, the agent designer creates the *use cases diagram* (following the UML roles but replacing actors by agents), and the *environment* and *organization* models. The *environment model* describes the used resources such as external applications and databases. The *organizational model* is the most complex and interesting model of this stage (see Figure 1), and includes information about

organization's members (relations preceded with the letter O), agent operations (relations preceded with AGO), and environment resources (relations preceded with E). At the top of the model there is the root organization element, called Medical Organization.

It includes three different kinds of agents grouped by their basic functionalities: agents that compose a medical centre, administrative actors and patients. A deep analysis of the medical centre shows a hierarchical organization divided in departments. Each one includes doctors, a guideline manager and an ontology manager (linked with the corresponding database). In the case of medical services, they can be found at the level of the medical centre or in the department. The manager of the medical record and the broker are classified as administrative actors. Finally, patients are considered as another group of agents that are included into the medical organization.

All individual patients are instances of this group. Moreover, the medical organization has different workflows to manage the services, the guidelines, or the electronic medical record, which are identified in this stage. In addition, the agent designer should identify the main tasks and goals to be accomplished into the workflows and assign them to the actors (which may represent a particular agent or an organization).

The next step is the design stage. It includes the creation of more particular models that detail specific aspects of a MAS implementation (behaviours, patterns of communication, goals and tasks), which will be translated into the agent-based prototype. Basically, the results of this stage are the following: a collection of agent models, models of tasks and goals, decomposition of workflows, and mental states of the agents. This stage includes a refinement of the use cases diagram by grouping the common features and assigning interaction models to those cases. These models are defined using UML collaboration diagrams and other representations designed specifically for agent-based applications.

Each agent model describes single agents, their tasks, goals, and played roles. The *goals model* shows the relationships between the goals of the system. This model expresses the constraints and dependencies between goals, and the agent model links each goal to the agent who is able to perform it. After designing these two models, the *tasks model* defines all tasks in terms of goals, pre-conditions, post-conditions, required resources, and required external modules. Dependencies between tasks are expressed using the *workflow diagrams*. Workflow and goals models together describe how an agent acts.

Agents act autonomously in order to accomplish their goals, but they are achieved by executing tasks that can require exchanging data between several partners. This fact is represented using specification diagrams. *INGENIAS* supports two different representations: *UML collaboration diagrams* and *Grasia! diagrams*. The *UML collaboration diagrams* are used to represent sequences of messages. Figure 2 shows an example that

involves different partners during the execution of a clinical guideline from the doctor point-of-view. In this case, the first conversation allows getting a certain guideline from the guideline agent. Then, the doctor needs to know the details about the terms included in the guideline. Moreover, during the enactment, the doctor can require the interaction with services. This diagram allows expressing the receivers, the performative and the meaning of the message, but not the actions associated to each message; the model is just used to create the skeleton of the conversation. If the interaction is more complex, *INGENIAS* proposes the use of *Grasia! diagrams* that include all *UML collaboration diagrams* with new interaction features such as precedence or concurrence relations.

Finally, another of the interesting elements introduced in this methodology is the specification of the *mental states* of each agent. A *mental state diagram* allows building a plan for executing tasks in order to accomplish a goal. The *mental state* responds to events from the environment and infers something.

Architecture of HeCaSe2

The analysis and design stages are repeatedly revised, and when these stages are completed, the code generator of the IDK tool allows generating a prototype of the MAS. From the designed skeleton, the complete multi-agent architecture of HeCaSe2 is presented in Figure 3. This is an open architecture and, depending on the situation, there will be more or less instances running of each agent type, and more or less interaction between them. At the top, the patients are represented by User Agents (UA). All UAs can talk with the Broker Agent (BA).

The BA is the bridge between users and the medical centres, and it is used to discover information. The user can even check personal information about his medical record through his medical centre. The BA knows about the medical centres located in a city or in an area. A

Figure 2. The Collaboration diagram in UML that shows a clinical guideline execution

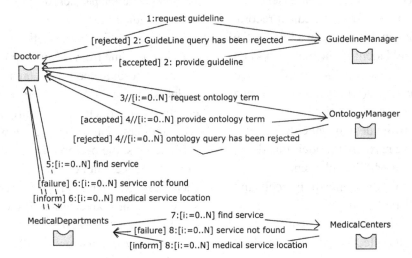

Medical Centre Agent (MCA) monitors all of its departments, represented by Department Agents (DAs), and a set of general services (represented by Service Agents (SAs)). Each department is formed by several doctors (represented by Doctor Agents (DRAs)) and more specific services (also modelled as SAs). Moreover, in each department there is a Guideline Agent (GA) that performs all

Figure 3. Complete architecture of HeCaSe2

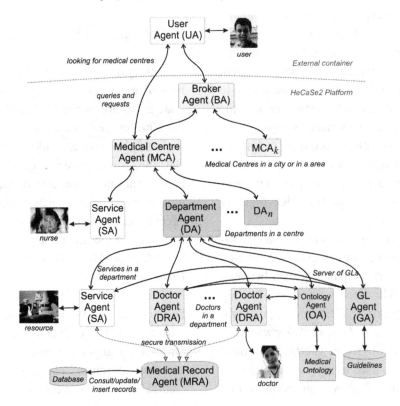

actions related to guidelines, such as looking for a desired CG, storing and/or changing a CG made by a doctor, etc. This GA manages only CGs related to the department where it is located but, if it is necessary to use another guideline (*e.g.*, when treating a patient with multiple pathologies), the GA could request it from other GAs.

Each department also contains an Ontology Agent (OA) that provides access to the designed medical ontology (to be described later) and complements the information provided by the GA.

At the bottom of the architecture there is the Medical Record Agent (MRA), which controls the access to a database that stores all patient health records in the medical centre. This agent provides a secure transmission of sensitive data (Moreno, Sánchez, & Isern, 2003).

A Medico-Organizational Ontology

The previous section has described the architecture of the system, including the roles of all agents and their relationships. Now, a more precise description of how the information contained into CGs is used by the appropriate agents in the appropriate way is explained. For instance, a practitioner is able to perform some basic activities, monitor the current state of the patient, and refer the patient to specialized procedures, such as a venography, which is performed by a surgeon. This basic example shows how an agent should combine medical information (*e.g.*, venography) with other related with the healthcare organization (*e.g.*, refer the patient to another department). The interpretation of a CG by intelligent agents requires specifying the actions allowed to each particular actor, understanding the parameters contained in a logical condition, and interpreting all internal relations between medical terms. This information is implemented through a medico-organizational ontology. The scope of the ontology presented in this section covers all the relations established in the multi-agent system associated to a healthcare organization (Isern, Sánchez, & Moreno, 2007). The ontology is divided in three main groups of concepts: (*a*) description of all health care entities with their relations, (*b*) linkage of semantic categories to the medical concepts, and (*c*) representation of all medical terms shared among all partners.

The ontology, developed using Protégé as editor, has been coded using OWL-DL, which allows the maximum level of expressiveness and, at the same time, permits to perform inference of facts (McGuinness & van Harmelen, 2004).

Description of the Healthcare Entities

The *Agent* hierarchy of classes includes all main concepts related with the internal organization of the multi-agent system. In this hierarchy there are *Departments*, *Patients*, *Practitioners*, *Medical centres* and *Services*. All these elements have internal relations, such as *Cardiology* is-a *Department* that belongsTo *Medical-center*. More complex relations between doctors and services are also mapped, such as *Nurse* belongsTo *Department* because a nurse can be located in any department, or *Family-doctor* belongsTo (*General medicine* $\cup$ *Emergency* $\cup$ *Paediatrics*) that means that an instance of family doctor could belong to any instance of these three departments. Relations between *Agent* subclasses are inspired in usual healthcare organizations.

The inverse relations are also available to know which kinds of doctors compose a department or which kinds of services are located in a department or medical centre. Although most of the departments are similar in the majority of medical centres, it is possible to represent different variations. In those cases, a specialisation of the ontology could be made. For instance, the oncology department is different in a hospital or in a primary attention centre that covers a part of a city or a set of villages. In these cases, two subclasses of the oncology department would be created. The parent class would keep all common features and the two siblings would contain the features or resources for each one.

Description of Semantic Types of Medical Concepts

The next set of classes concerns the different semantic types of the medical concepts. There are two main hierarchies, named *Entity* and *Event*, which were picked from UMLS Metathesaurus (Humphreys, Lindberg, Schoolman, & Barnett, 1998). Currently, UMLS defines 135 different semantic types divided in two groups: meanings concerned with healthcare organizations or entities, and meanings related with events or activities in a daily care flow. Both hierarchies are organized as a taxonomy with is-a relations between concepts, such as *Disease or Syndrome* is-a *Pathologic* function.

All this information is used by agents to know exactly the function of any required concept and further connections with others. For instance, if a concept is a *Finding* and a *Finding* isResponsibilityOf a *Practitioner*, the agent knows that a patient's finding should be given by a practitioner.

Medical Domain Terminology

The last part of the ontology represents the specific vocabulary used in clinical guidelines. It systematises all specific knowledge required in any guideline execution engine, divided in *Diseases*, *Procedures* and *Personal data*. It is necessary to define a set of relations between each concept and its identifier (Code Unique Identifier or CUI), its semantic type, which entity of the system is responsible of its accomplishment, and the produced result type (*i.e.*, if it as number, a boolean, an enumerate or a complex object). Relations are bidirectional because it is interesting to know that the finding *Active cancer* isResponsibilityOf a *Family Doctor*, and the family doctor's responsibilities. Each agent can access the concepts related to its own domain and

be aware of the consequences of the application of an action. The medical expert must update the ontology with the concepts, relations, actions, and effects included in the CG, before adding a new CG to the system.

If there is no information about a concept, the agent requests the doctor to make a decision. If a concept has more than one semantic type, the agent cannot follow an option because both directions are correct. For instance, the term *smoke* has two semantic types as *Environmental Effect of Humans* and *Hazardous or Poisonous Substance*, but the action *smoking* is only an *Individual Behaviour*. In this case, it is recommended to create another term, by searching the UMLS repository, which fits better with the ontology; the percentage of terms with more than one semantic meaning in UMLS is very low because the creators of this repository tried to avoid these kinds of problems and facilitate its use by decision support systems.

Combination of Medical and Organizational Knowledge

As explained above, three main groups of concepts are defined in the medical ontology: agent-based health care concepts, semantic types of entities and events, and medical concepts (Figure 4 shows the whole ontology with the relations). All the defined concepts have taxonomic and non-taxonomic interrelations. The former are based on *is-a* relations and are established by generalisation-specialisation of concepts. Some are picked from UMLS and others are picked from healthcare organizations. The second kind of relations is more difficult to establish, due to its semantic dependency. In fact, they are usually omitted in standard repositories.

By analysing the information required in the execution of a clinical guideline, a set of relations were defined. They are shown below with their type and description. When a new CG is added, all new concepts should be added and all required relationships between concepts should be estab-

Figure 4. Medico-organizational ontology with main relations

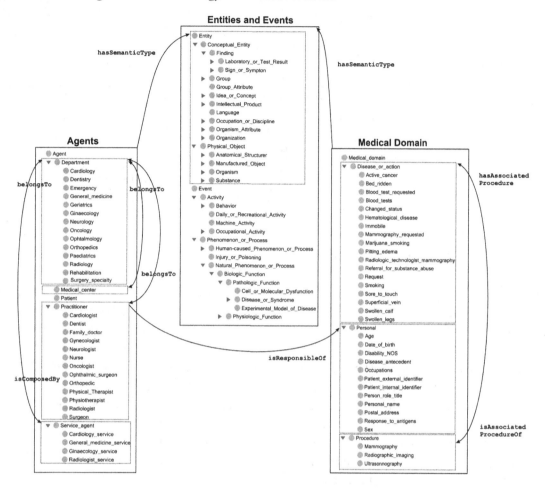

lished. *Object properties* establish relationships between pairs of individuals and allow performing ontological inference (see Table 1). In addition, there are other particular relations called data type properties that relate an individual to a data value (string, integer, float, etc.); they can be considered attributes (see Table 2).

Applying a Clinical Guideline

The procedural knowledge embedded within clinical guidelines should be complemented with a representation of declarative knowledge that allows to know exactly the semantic meaning of all elements, and hence, to implement a guideline execution engine to follow step-by-step all the stages of the CG.

The basic pieces to consider in any guideline are decisions, actions, and inputs of data. The CG consists in a combination of these elements with labeled transitions between them: temporal constraints. The execution of a CG involves different kinds of actors, with different skills and constraints. In the case of HeCaSe2 the execution of a CG is a semi-supervised procedure handled by the doctor. In the following subsections, all the procedures followed by agents, the decisions made by the system, and the information requested to the users (patients and practitioners) is explained.

Table 1. Object properties defined in the medical ontology

Object properties	Description
belongsTo	Any instance of a class that belongs to another.
hasAssociatedProcedure	A medical concept has an associated procedure. It is used by doctors to simplify a search (from UMLS).
hasResponsible	Establish the responsibility of any medical concept that has to be performed by a healthcare party.
hasSemanticType	Functional property to specify the semantic type of a concept.
isAssociatedProcedureOf	Inverse of hasAssociatedProcedure.
isComposedBy	If an instance $a \in A$ belongsTo $b \in B$ then, $b \in B$ isComposedBy $a \in A$. It is not just the the inverse because the first relation is $1 - N$ and the second is $M - N$.
isResponsibleOf	Inverse of hasResponsible.

Retrieving the Appropriate Guideline

The first task to accomplish during the enactment is sending the requested CG to the practitioner when required. HeCaSe2 has a particular agent called guideline agent (GA) that stores a collection of CGs of a medical centre. These CGs are annotated with information about the department where they belong, the author, the version, the date of inclusion into the repository, and the names of the owner medical centre as well as of the clinical guideline itself. These attributes are used to filter the requested CGs and, at the same time, maintain a versioning of guidelines.

When the doctor begins a medical visit with a patient, his DRA proactively performs a set of tasks, such as getting the patient's medical record, getting the information of the medical visit, and getting the list of available CGs. The patient's data are collected through the medical record agent (MRA) and the list of available CGs from the GA. If there is no previous information about the patient, the doctor receives an empty medical record. Otherwise, he receives the personal details of the patient (*e.g.*, name, address, date of birth, phone, and allergies), the collection of results of past medical visits, and the information of current ongoing CGs. If the patient is currently following a CG, the name of this guideline is highlighted in the list of guidelines, but the doctor can decide to

Table 2. Data type properties defined in the medical ontology

Object properties	Description
hasCUI	Value of the CUI (Code Unique Identifier) (from UMLS).
hasDescription	Concept definition provided from UMLS (when it is available).
hasResult	Type of output of an element (action or data concept).
hasResultBoolean	Sub class of hasResult that sets a Boolean as output.
hasResultInteger	Sub class of hasResult that sets an Integer as output.
hasResultString	Sub class of hasResult that sets a String as output.
hasResultEnumerate	Sub class of hasResult that sets an enumerate as output.
hasResultComplex	Sub class of hasResult that sets a complex element formed by one or more simple results (concepts) as output.
hasTUI	In UMLS, semantic types are labelled with a Type Unique Identifier.

change it. After selecting the CG to follow, the DRA requests the content of this CG to the GA. The DRA receives the CG, and establishes the current status of the patient.

Enactment of a Clinical Guideline

As shown in previous sections, the combination of a knowledge base and an agent-based system that exploits that knowledge can be interesting to achieve flexibility and re-usability. In order to illustrate how these elements have been integrated, in this section we explain the procedure followed in a CG adopted from the National Guideline Clearinghouse and coded in PRO*forma* (Sutton & Fox, 2003), which is intended to diagnose and treat Gastrointestinal Cancer (GC).

First of all, the doctor selects the GC guideline from the repository (following the procedure explained above). The DRA receives the CG which is graphically presented to the doctor.

The DRA indicates to its guideline execution module that this guideline must be loaded to be executed, and the DRA is ready to receive events from this module. First of all, the DRA needs to determine the exact entry point within the CG to begin the execution (usually, there is only one entry point), and gets the required data to begin the enactment. When the DRA receives these data, it collects all past values from the patient's health record, and puts these values automatically.

The guideline execution module is able to load and follow step-by-step a requested guideline. The DRA delegates execution aspects to this module and observes the events related with the execution. Particularly, two important methods need an especial mention those that are triggered when a decision or an action are reached. In the first case, the module informs to its listener (DRA) that a decision has been reached. The agent can check the information related to this decision, such as the attached logical condition. The DRA informs to the medical expert through his graphical interface and it does not need any other step. In the second

case, the method informs that an action should be performed. First, the DRA must search the entity able to execute this action. This information is collected through the medical ontology, and after inferring this information, the agent knows which kind of actor is required to perform a task. Then, the DRA finds this actor whitin the department, inside the centre, or outside the centre. In the case that the current state is an enquiry of data, these data are collected in the same way than the actions explained previously. Each item to be collected is searched in the medical ontology, and the entity able to perform or to provide this item is contacted.

Going back to the execution of the GC guideline, the first step is to assess the importance of the disease. The DRA analyses the CG and observes that the first enquiry is composed by six parameters. For each one, the DRA asks the Ontology Agent (OA) to know more details. The OA replies with the information found in the Medical Ontology. In this case, the parameter *Age* is included in the category of *Personal* that can be found in the medical record. The DRA requests to the MRA that value. Other required parameters like *Pain site*, *Weight loss*, *Pain time* and *Smoking*, are *Findings* that the doctor can evaluate and set if the record is not found in the patient's history. The ontology also contains information about each element, like the resulting format output and the allowed values, which are stored using data type properties (see Table 2). For instance, in the case of *Pain time*, due to its nature, the allowed data values are *short*, *moderate*, and *long*. Finally, the last value to consider is the result of the *Biopsy*.

A *Biopsy* is an invasive *Diagnostic Procedure* that isResponsibleOf a *Surgery specialty*. In that case, if the biopsy has not been performed previously, the DRA is able to look for a surgeon (*Practitioner* that belongsTo a *Surgery specialty* department) and book a meeting for the patient (at first, it looks for available surgeons, and then, it begins a contract net negotiation with them). If agreed, the enactment is stopped until that result is received. In a future medical visit, the doctor will have the result of the biopsy and he will be able to perform a first diagnosis: if the biopsy is negative, the patient will follow a plan for gastro-intestinal treatment of a *Peptic ulcer*. Otherwise, the patient suffers from cancer and should be treated for that disease.

In the case of cancer, there is a final step to be performed before referring the patient to a surgeon: to check if the patient is elderly or not. In the former case, the patient cannot be hospitalised and should be treated with symptomatic treatments. In the latter case, there are two possible plans to follow, a chemical treatment such as *Chemotherapy*, or a *Surgery*. The decision is taken by the surgeon in a further medical visit.

As shown through the example, the CG provides the general care flow to follow (declarative and explicit knowledge) and the ontology provides semantic information about all concepts or actions to be performed. Detailed information allows to represent relations between all entities and to collect all required data by agents in order to know which decision to take. When the doctor agent considers the term *Biopsy* it does not know if that concept is a procedure or a finding or any other kind of element, and it does not know the existing relations of that concept either. The ontology allows to correlate all elements present in the CG and know exactly all the details. This information is not included in CGs because it depends on the specific scenario or organization where the CG should run.

FUTURE WORK

In this section we describe several future lines of research and present some preliminary ideas on how they can be tackled.

- Monitoring the use of a guideline execution engine may be useful to evaluate the adherence indicators during the enactment of CGs over patients. These measures will show if the CGs are being followed exactly as they are defined or some steps are repeatedly avoided by practitioners. All this information can be used to refine and improve the use of CGs in daily practice.

- The retrieval of the CG that has to be applied over a patient may be improved if additional recommendation processes are considered. As (Shahar, et al., 2003) propose, the use of information stored in the patient's health record and the annotation of available CGs can allow to collect the most appropriate CGs according to the current circumstances of the patient, using case-based reasoning or other learning methods. This improvement, to be added in the guideline agent, can produce a rated and sorted list of appropriate guidelines and ease the selection process of the practitioner.

- There is the possibility to connect different guideline agents belonging to different medical centres creating a network of guideline agents. This group of agents may be used to share and adapt other CGs in a particular medical centre.

- The execution of a CG is a complex task that involves several actors during a treatment. An improvement can be the delegation of execution during a treatment. This fact is done when a patient is referred from a department to another to perform a clinical procedure. In this case, the patient can begin another CG to perform the referred procedure and, at the end, establish some result or diagnostic, required during the main treatment. This improvement will require updating the medical record to allow the execution of different CGs at the same time (with its control) and to update the current management of CGs in the doctor agent.

CONCLUSION

The main aim of the present work has been to develop a distributed platform that allows executing clinical guidelines in an efficient way. The most important and novel point is the complete integration of different actors, allowing a coordination of their daily activities, and representing all the used knowledge in an effective way.

Several guideline-based execution engines, which provide functionalities similar to those of HeCaSe2, have been developed in the past, but it is not until now that researchers are starting to focus their efforts to exploit the benefits of the inclusion of CGs in the daily practice. This inclusion requires building open and easy-to-deploy systems to allow a customisation to diverse medical centres that usually have proprietary and local clinical management systems. Although this platform has been designed with a particular purpose and provides a concrete set of services, the novel point-of-view is to represent the active actors of health care organizations (*e.g.,* practitioners, nurses, patients) as autonomous entities with different goals to achieve and acting with different roles and permissions. This permits to implement flexible systems and, at the same time, tackle some barriers that limit or restrict the adherence to CGs. Representing all participants separately allows adding special features for particular actors, or groups of them, in a scalable way.

Regarding the design of the MAS, an accurate analysis, design and implementation have been done, following the *INGENIAS* agent-oriented software engineering methodology. This point is not usually done by developers of MAS and allowed us to structure, document and improve the quality of the final product.

In addition, the use of ontologies to represent all the knowledge has proved to be an appropriate approach. This work proposes the combination of application ontologies (*e.g.,* medical terms and relations included for each clinical guideline) designed to cover particular issues, with some domain ontologies (*e.g.,* classification of the semantic types of medical terms) designed for general purposes, used to automate the enactment of clinical guidelines.

Finally, the evaluation of several ideas of this work is currently ongoing in two research projects called *HYGIA* (Alonso, et al., 2008) and *K4Care* (Campana, Moreno, Riaño, & Varga, 2008). They provide encouraging results on the suitability of our approach for executing clinical guidelines in two well distinguished domains. The appropriate execution of CGs between different actors or the collection of the patient's data will be thoroughly tested. In addition, the medical partners of these projects are providing several CGs (*e.g.,* chronic obstructive pulmonary disease, hypertension, post-stroke, heart failure), real patient's data for testing them, and finally, they will verify and use the final implemented prototypes (Hospital Clínic in the case of *HYGIA*, and Amministrazione Comunale di Pollenza in the case of *K4Care*). Taking all of these characteristics into consideration, we believe that our proposal represents a new and interesting addition over the current state-of-the-art of agent technology applied in medical informatics.

REFERENCES

AGREE, C. (2003). Development and validation of an international appraisal instrument for assessing the quality of clinical practice guidelines: the AGREE project. *Quality & Safety in Health Care, 12*(1), 18–23. doi:10.1136/qhc.12.1.18

Alonso, A., Marcos, M., Alonso, J. R., Gelabert, G., Martínez-Salvador, B., & Riaño, D. (2008). (in press). A Knowledge-Acquisition Framework to Facilitate the Development and Reengineering of Care Plans in Electronic Format. *Journal of Telemedicine and Telecare*.

Anselma, L., Terenziani, P., Montani, S., & Bottrighi, A. (2007). Automatic Checking of the Correctness of Clinical Guidelines in GLARE. In K. A. Kuhn, J. R. Warren & T.-Y. Leong (Eds.), *Proc. of the 12th World Congress on Health (Medical) Informatics, MEDINFO 2007* (pp. 807-811). Brisbane, AUS.

Bellifemine, F., Caire, G., & Greenwood, D. (2007). *Developing multi-agent systems with JADE*. Chichester, England: John Wiley and Sons.

Berg, D., Ram, P., & Glasgow, J. (2004). SAGEDesktop: An Environment for Testing Clinical Practice Guidelines. In Z.-P. Liang (Ed.), *Proc. of the 26th Annual Conference of the IEEE Engineering in Medicine and Biology Society, IEEE-IEBMS 2004* (pp. 3217-3220). San Francisco, US.

Bernon, C., Cossentino, M., & Pavón, J. (2005). Agent-oriented software engineering. *The Knowledge Engineering Review, 20*(2), 99–116. doi:10.1017/S0269888905000421

Bresciani, P., Giorgini, P., Giunchiglia, F., Mylopoulos, J., & Perini, A. (2004). TROPOS: An Agent-Oriented Software Development Methodology. *Autonomous Agents and Multi-Agent Systems, 8*(3), 203–236. doi:10.1023/B:AGNT.0000018806.20944.ef

Campana, F., Moreno, A., Riaño, D., & Varga, L. (2008). K4Care: Knowledge-Based Homecare e-Services for an Ageing Europe. In R. Annicchiarico, U. Cortés, & C. Urdiales (Eds.), *Agent Technology and e-Health* (pp. 95-115). Basel, Switzerland: Birkhäuser Basel.

Cancer, W. E. B. (2008). *CancerWEB Project.* Retrieved July 29, 2008, from http://cancerweb.ncl.ac.uk/.

Cernuzzi, L., Juan, T., Sterling, L., & Zambonelli, F. (2004). The Gaia Methodology: Basic Concepts and Extensions. In F. Bergenti, M. P. Gleizes, & F. Zambonelli (Eds.), *Methodologies and Software Engineering for Agent Systems* (pp. 69-88). Springer US.

Chesani, F., de Matteis, P., Mello, P., Montal, M., & Storari, S. (2006). A Framework for Defining and Verifying Clinical Guidelines: A Case Study on Cancer Screening. In F. Esposito, Z. W. Ras, D. Malerba, & G. Semeraro (Eds.), *Proc. of the Proceedings of 16th International Symposium on Methodologies for Intelligent Systems, ISMIS 2006* (pp. 338-343). Bari, Italy.

Ciccarese, P., Caffi, E., Boiocchi, L., Quaglini, S., & Stefanelli, M. (2004). A Guideline Management System. In M. Fieschi, E. Coiera, & J. X. Li (Eds.), *Proc. of the 11th World Congress on Medical Informatics, MEDINFO 2004* (pp. 28-32). San Francisco, USA.

Ciccarese, P., Caffi, E., Quaglini, S., & Stefanelli, M. (2005). Architectures and Tools for innovative Health Information Systems: the Guide Project. *International Journal of Medical Informatics, 74*(7-8), 553–562. doi:10.1016/j.ijmedinf.2005.02.001

Clercq, P. A. d., Blom, J. A., Korsten, H. H. M., & Hasman, A. (2004). Approaches for creating computer-interpretable guidelines that facilitate decision support. *Artificial Intelligence in Medicine, 31*(1), 1–27. doi:10.1016/j.artmed.2004.02.003

Cossentino, M. (2005). From Requirements to Code with the PASSI Methodology. In B. Henderson-Sellers & P. Giorgini (Eds.), *Agent-Oriented Methodologies* (pp. 79-106). Idea Group.

Cuesta, P., Gómez Expósito, A., Rodríguez, F. J., & González, J. (2005). Developing a Multiagent System for Mobile Devices. *Revista Iberoamericana de Inteligencia Artificial, 25,* 49–57.

Davis, D., Goldman, J., & Palda, V. A. (2007). *Handbook on Clinical Practice Guidelines*. Ottawa, CA: Canadian Medical Association.

DeLoach, S. A. (2004). The MaSE Methodology. In F. Bergenti, M. P. Gleizes, & F. Zambonelli (Eds.), *Methodologies and Software Engineering for Agent Systems: The Agent-Oriented Software Engineering Handbook* (pp. 107-125). Kluwer Academic Publishers.

Field, M. J., & Lohr, K. N. (Eds.). (1990). *Clinical Practice Guidelines: Directions for a New Program*. Washington, DC: National Academy Press.

Fox, J., Alabassi, A., Patkar, V., Rose, T., & Black, E. (2006). An ontological approach to modelling tasks and goals. *Computers in Biology and Medicine, 36*(7-8), 837–856. doi:10.1016/j.compbiomed.2005.04.011

Fox, J., Beveridge, M., & Glasspool, D. (2003). Understanding intelligent agents: analysis and synthesis. *AI Communications, 16*(3), 139–152.

Fox, J., Patkar, V., & Thomson, R. (2006). Decision Support for Healthcare: the PROforma evidence base. *Informatics in Primary Care, 14*, 49–54.

Gómez-Alonso, C., Isern, D., & Moreno, A. (2007). *Software Engineering Methodologies to Develop Multi-Agent Systems: State-of-the-art* (Research Report No. DEIM-RR-07-003). Tarragona, Catalonia: University Rovira i Virgili.

Gómez-Sanz, J., Gervais, M. P., & Weiss, G. (2004). A Survey on Agent-Oriented Software Engineering Research. In F. Bergenti, M. P. Gleizes, & F. Zambonelli (Eds.), *Methodologies and Software Engineering for Agent Systems* (Vol. 11, pp. 33-64): Springer US.

Henderson-Sellers, B., & Giorgini, P. (2005). Agent-Oriented Methodologies: An Introduction. In B. Henderson-Sellers & P. Giorgini (Eds.), *Agent-Oriented Methodologies* (pp. 1-19). Idea Group.

Hommersom, A., Groot, P., Lucas, P. J., Balser, M., & Schmitt, J. (2007). Verification of the Medical Guidelines using background knowledge in Task Networks. *IEEE Transactions on Knowledge and Data Engineering, 19*(4), 281–316.

Hrabak, K. M., Campbell, J. R., Tu, S. W., McClure, R., & Weida, R. (2007). Creating Interoperable Guidelines: Requirements of Vocabulary Standards in Immunization Decision Support. In K. A. Kuhn, J. R. Warren, & T.-Y. Leong (Eds.), *Proc. of the Proceedings of the 12th World Congress on Health (Medical) Informatics, MEDINFO 2007* (pp. 930-934). Brisbaine, AU.

Humphreys, B. L., Lindberg, D. A. B., Schoolman, H. M., & Barnett, G. O. (1998). The Unified Medical Language System: An Informatics Research Collaboration. *Journal of the American Medical Informatics Association, 5*(1), 1–11.

Isern, D., & Moreno, A. (2008). Computer-Based Execution of Clinical Guidelines: A Review. *International Journal of Medical Informatics, 77*(12), 787–808. doi:10.1016/j.ijmedinf.2008.05.010

Isern, D., Sánchez, D., & Moreno, A. (2007). An ontology-driven agent-based clinical guideline execution engine. In R. Bellazzi, A. Abu-Hanna, & J. Hunter (Eds.), *Proc. of the 11th Conference on Artificial Intelligence in Medicine, AIME 2007* (pp. 49-53). Amsterdam, The Netherlands.

Lenz, R., Blaser, R., Beyer, M., Heger, O., Biber, C., & Bäumlein, M. (2007). IT support for clinical pathways - Lessons learned. *International Journal of Medical Informatics, 76*(S3), 397–402. doi:10.1016/j.ijmedinf.2007.04.012

Leong, T.-Y., Kaiser, K., & Miksch, S. (2007). Free and Open Source Enabling Technologies for Patient-Centric, Guideline-Based Clinical Decision Support: A Survey. *IMIA Yearbook of Medical Informatics . Methods of Information in Medicine, 46*(Suppl. 1), 74–86.

McGuinness, D., & van Harmelen, F. (2004). *OWL Web Ontology Language.* Retrieved August 24, 2008, from http://www.w3.org/TR/owl-features/.

Mersmann, S., & Dojat, M. (2004). SmartCareTM - Automated Clinical Guidelines in Critical Care. In R. L. de Mántaras & L. Saitta (Eds.), *Proc. of the 16th European Conference on Artificial Intelligence, ECAI 2004* (pp. 745-749). València, Spain.

Michie, S., & Johnston, M. (2004). Changing clinical behaviour by making guidelines specific. *British Medical Journal, 328,* 343–345. doi:10.1136/bmj.328.7435.343

Miksch, S., Shahar, Y., & Johnson, P. (1997). Asbru: A Task-Specific, Intention-Based, and Time-Oriented Language for Representing Skeletal Plans. In E. Motta, F. V. Harmelen, C. Pierret-Golbreich, I. Filby & N. Wijngaards (Eds.), *Proc. of the 7th Workshop on Knowledge Engineering: Methods & Languages, KEML-97* (pp. 1-20). Milton Keynes, UK.

Milne, F., Redman, C., Walker, J., Baker, P., Bradley, J., & Cooper, C. (2005). The pre-eclampsia community guideline (PRECOG): how to screen for and detect onset of pre-eclampsia in the community. *British Medical Journal, 330,* 576–580. doi:10.1136/bmj.330.7491.576

Moreno, A., Sánchez, D., & Isern, D. (2003). Security Measures in a Medical Multi-Agent System. In I. Aguiló, L. Valverde & M. T. Escrig (Eds.), *Proc. of the Artificial Intelligence Research and Development. Proceedings of 6th Catalan Conference in Artificial Intelligence, CCIA 2003* (pp. 244-255). Palma de Mallorca, Spain.

Mulyar, N., van der Aalst, W. M. P., & Peleg, M. (2007). A Pattern-based Analysis of Clinical Computer-interpretable Guideline Modeling Languages. *Journal of the American Medical Informatics Association, 14*(6), 781–787. doi:10.1197/jamia.M2389

Nealon, J. L., & Moreno, A. (2003). Agent-Based Applications in Health Care. In J. L. Nealon & A. Moreno (Eds.), *Applications of Software Agent Technology in the Health Care Domain* (pp. 3-18). Basel, Switzerland: Birkhäuser Verlag.

Padgham, L., & Winikoff, M. (2004). *Developing Intelligent Agent Systems: A Practical Guide*: John Wiley and Sons.

Pavón, J., Gómez-Sanz, J. J., & Fuentes, R. (2005). The INGENIAS Methodology and Tools. In B. Henderson-Sellers & P. Giorgini (Eds.), *Agent-Oriented Methodologies* (pp. 236-276). Idea Group.

Peleg, M., Keren, S., & Denekamp, Y. (2008). Mapping computerized clinical guidelines to electronic medical records: Knowledge-data ontological mapper (KDOM). *Journal of Biomedical Informatics, 41*(1), 180–201. doi:10.1016/j.jbi.2007.05.003

Peleg, M., Tu, S. W., Bury, J., Ciccarese, P., Fox, J., & Greenes, R. A. (2003). Comparing Computer-Interpretable Guideline Models: A Case-Study Approach. *Journal of the American Medical Informatics Association, 10*(1), 52–68. doi:10.1197/jamia.M1135

Priori, S. G., Klein, W., & Bassand, J.-P. (2003). Medical Practice Guidelines: Separating science from economics. *European Heart Journal, 24*(21), 1962–1964. doi:10.1016/S0195-668X(03)00438-X

Quaglini, S., Stefanelli, M., Cavallini, A., Micieli, G., Fassino, C., & Mossa, C. (2000). Guideline-based Careflow Systems. *Artificial Intelligence in Medicine, 20*(1), 5–22. doi:10.1016/S0933-3657(00)00050-6

Riaño, D. (2004). Time-Independent Rule-Based Guideline Execution. In R. L. de Mántaras & L. Saitta (Eds.), *Proc. of the 16th European Conference on Artificial Intelligence, ECAI 2004* (pp. 535-538). Valencia, Spain.

Riaño, D. (2007). The SDA* Model: A Set Theory Approach In P. Kokol, V. Podgorelec, M. Dušanka, M. Zorman, & M. Verlic (Eds.), *Proc. of the 20th IEEE International Symposium on Computer-Based Medical Systems, CBMS 2007* (pp. 563-568). Maribor, Slovenia.

Ricci, S., Celani, M. G., & Righetti, E. (2006). Development of clinical guidelines: methodological and practical issues. *Neurological Sciences, 27*(S3), 228–230. doi:10.1007/s10072-006-0623-x

Seyfang, A., Miksch, S., Marcos, M., Wittenberg, J., Polo-Conde, C., & Rosenbrand, K. (2006). Bridging the Gap between Informal and Formal Guideline Representations. In G. Brewka, S. Coradeschi, A. Perini & P. Traverso (Eds.), *Proc. of the 17th European Conference on Artificial Intelligence* (pp. 447–451). Riva del Garda, Italy.

Shahar, Y., Young, O., Shalom, E., Galperin, M., Mayaffit, A., & Moskovitch, R. (2004). A Framework for a Distributed, Hybrid, Multiple-Ontology Clinical-Guideline Library and Automated Guideline-Support Tools. *Journal of Biomedical Informatics, 37*(5), 325–344. doi:10.1016/j.jbi.2004.07.001

Shahar, Y., Young, O., Shalon, E., Mayaffit, A., Moskovitch, R., Hessing, A., et al. (2003). DEGEL: A Hybrid, Multiple-Ontology Framework for Specification and Retrieval of Clinical Guidelines. In M. Dojat, E. Keravnou & P. Barahona (Eds.), *Proc. of the 9th Conference on Artificial Intelligence in Medicine in Europe, AIME 2003* (pp. 122-131). Protaras, Cyprus.

Soto, J. P., Vizcaino, A., Portillo, J., & Piattini, M. (2006). Modelling a Knowledge Management System Architecture with INGENIAS Methodology *of the 15th International Conference on Computing (CIC 2006)* (pp. 167-173). Mexico City, Mexico.

Sutton, D. R., & Fox, J. (2003). The syntax and semantics of the PROforma guideline modeling language. *Journal of the American Medical Informatics Association, 10*(5), 433–443. doi:10.1197/jamia.M1264

ten Teije, A., Marcos, M., Balser, M., van Croonenborg, J., Duelli, C., & van Harmelen, F. (2006). Improving medical protocols by formal methods. *Artificial Intelligence in Medicine, 36*(3), 193–272. doi:10.1016/j.artmed.2005.10.006

Terenziani, P., Montani, S., Bottrighi, A., Molino, G., & Torchio, M. (2005). Clinical Guidelines Adaptation: Managing Authoring and Versioning Issues. In S. Miksch, J. Hunter, & E. Keravnou (Eds.), *Proc. of the 10th Conference on Artificial Intelligence in Medicine, AIME 2005* (pp. 151-155). Aberdeen, Scotland.

Terenziani, P., Montani, S., Bottrighi, A., Torchio, M., Molino, G., & Correndo, G. (2004). The GLARE Approach to Clinical Guidelines: Main Features. In K. Kaiser, S. Miksch, & S. W. Tu (Eds.), *Proc. of the Symposium on Computerized Guidelines and Protocols, CGP 2004* (pp. 162-166). Viena, AU.

Tu, S. W., Campbell, J. R., Glasgow, J., Nyman, M. A., McClure, R., & McClay, J. (2007). The SAGE Guideline Model: Achievements and Overview. *Journal of the American Medical Informatics Association, 14*(5), 589–598. doi:10.1197/jamia.M2399

Tu, S. W., Campbell, J. R., & Musen, M. A. (2004). SAGE Guideline Modeling: Motivation and Methodology. In K. Kaiser, S. Miksch & S. W. Tu (Eds.), *Proc. of the Symposium on Computerized Guidelines and Protocols, CGP 2004* (pp. 167-171). Prague, Czech Republic.

Tu, S. W., & Glasgow, J. (2006). *The SAGE Guideline Model Technical Specification* (Research report No. SMI-2006-1243). Stanford, CA: Stanford Medical Informatics.

Tu, S. W., & Musen, M. A. (2001). Modeling Data and Knowledge in the EON Guideline Architecture. In V. Patel, R. Rogers & R. Haux (Eds.), *Proc. of the 10th Triennial Congress of the International Medical Informatics Association, MEDINFO 2001* (pp. 280-284). London, UK.

Wang, D., Peleg, M., Tu, S. W., Boxwala, A. A., Ogunyemi, O., & Zeng, Q. (2004). Design and Implementation of the GLIF3 Guideline Execution Engine. *Journal of Biomedical Informatics, 37*(5), 305–318. doi:10.1016/j.jbi.2004.06.002

Wang, D., Peleg, M., Tu, S. W., Shortliffe, E., & Greenes, R. A. (2001). Representation of Clinical Practice Guidelines for Computer-Based Implementations. In V. Patel, R. Rogers & R. Haux (Eds.), *Proc. of the 10th Triennial Congress of the International Medical Informatics Association, MEDINFO 2001* (pp. 285-289). London, UK.

Wang, D., & Shortliffe, E. H. (2002). GLEE – A Model-Driven Execution System for Computer-Based Implementation of Clinical Practice Guidelines. In AMIA (Ed.), *Proc. of the American Medical Informatics Association Annual Symposium, AMIA 2002* (pp. 855-859). San Antonio, TX, USA.

Wyatt, J. C., & Sullivan, F. (2007). eHealth and the future: promise or peril? *British Medical Journal, 331*, 1391–1393. doi:10.1136/bmj.331.7529.1391

Young, O., & Shahar, Y. (2005). The Spock System: Developing a Runtime Application Engine for Hybrid-Asbru Guidelines. In S. Miksch, J. Hunter, & E. Keravnou (Eds.), *Proc. of the 10th Conference on Artificial Intelligence in Medicine, AIME 2005* (pp. 166-170). Aberdeen, Scotland.

Young, O., Shahar, Y., Liel, Y., Lunenfeld, E., Bar, G., & Shalom, E. (2007). Runtime application of Hybrid-Asbru clinical guidelines. *Journal of Biomedical Informatics, 40*, 507–526. doi:10.1016/j.jbi.2006.12.004

Zambonelli, F., Jennings, N. R., & Wooldridge, M. (2003). Developing Multiagent Systems: The Gaia Methodology. *ACM Transactions on Software Engineering and Methodology, 12*(3), 317–370. doi:10.1145/958961.958963

ENDNOTE

[1]	Free to download at http://ingenias.sourceforge.net [last visit: 08/08/2008]

Chapter 8
An Agent–Based Modeling System for Wellness

Luigi Benedicenti
University of Regina, Canada

Chitsutha Soomlek
University of Regina, Canada

ABSTRACT

This chapter introduces an agent-based wellness visualization system. The visualization system integrates and analyzes health information collected from existing portable health monitoring devices, users, and other existing health information resources (e.g. hospital's databases). It can be used as a single wellness indicator for an individual and a one-station examination for health care professionals. The single wellness indicator provides a simplified view of health information of an individual. Thus, the individual will have a better understanding in personal wellness and will be encouraged to be aware of both personal and public's health. The one-station examination assists healthcare professional to have rapid evaluation and boosts healthcare services. Initial result indicates that the proof of concept of the research will provide direct benefits to the public, research communities, and enterprises.

INTRODUCTION

Health is a major public issue: a healthy life is desired by everyone. Unfortunately, we do not have a sufficient number of doctors, nurses, and medical practitioners compared to the size of human population at the present (*Core Health Indicators*, 2007). Therefore, we need mechanisms that assist health care professionals to work faster with efficiency to serve the public needs. One possible solution is to integrate health information on one single station, providing correlations and patterns of clinical data of a patient, and then identify anomalous situation. This would make it faster for medical professionals to access, interpret, and analyse the clinical data. In turn, this leads to better care and services for more people.

Another potential solution is to offer triage training, disease protection and prevention training, and health monitoring devices directly to the public. Triage addresses the seriousness of a condition or injury for people in an emergency but it does not

DOI: 10.4018/978-1-60566-772-0.ch008

protect people from diseases and chronic health conditions. Disease protection and prevention training gives people a better understanding of the factors affecting the onset of a disease and of how to reduce the risk of contracting diseases; however, it is hard for people to do so when their health conditions are unknown. Portable health monitoring devices provide primitive health information, e.g. heart rate; blood pressure; and blood sugar content. The information is meaningful, useful, and interpretable by health care professionals; but the information is not readily understandable for people without training or specific knowledge. To let people be on the watch for their own health conditions, health information should be displayed in a way that is easy to understand with simple explanations and suggestions for general users.

The research described in this chapter aims to develop an agent-based visualization system that provides a comprehensive display of primitive health information for both health care professionals and non-professional users. The visualization system will show primitive health information, relevant information, history, wellness indicator, profile, and significant change of patient condition or anomaly for rapid evaluation by medical practitioners. The system will also provide a simple explanation and a set of suggestions that are understandable for general users. The objectives of the research are described in the following section. The research plan is given in Section III. The description of analysis and approaches is provided in section IV. The architecture of the system is introduced in section V. The system design, results, conclusions and future work are provided in section VI, VII and VIII respectively.

OBJECTIVES

The agent-based visualization system cannot replace any health care professional. It cannot diagnose a symptom. Instead, it assists the health care professionals to work faster with high efficiency and encourages an individual to be aware of his/ her own health. The objective of this research is to develop an agent-based visualization system that can:

1. Help an individual to follow up and maintain his/her own health; and can assist a health care professional to provide better services to each patient.
2. Be used as a one-station examination for health care professionals and a single wellness indicator for patients.
3. Aggregate and integrate primitive health information collected from users.
4. Analyze correlations among parameters and display all relevant information in a comprehensive way to users.
5. Analyze patterns from primitive health information collected from a user and can identify anomaly from the patterns.
6. Has expandability and modularity characteristics.

RESEARCH PROGRESS AND PLAN

This section explains the research plan and main contributions by the team members. This research involves four main tasks spanning over three years. Details about each task are as follows:

Task 1: Literature Reviews and Data Collection

The first task allows the research team to gain knowledge from existing methods and technologies; and be able to conduct the research in the right direction. This task is accomplished by searching through existing research papers, books, products, and other existing resources. All relevant information are gathered and studied by the team members. This task can be performed in parallel with the other tasks because we may need more information and knowledge when we perform the other tasks. As a result, this task is still ongoing.

So far, we have studied existing visual display techniques for quantitative information, commonly used statistical methods in medical research and diagnosis, well-known data clustering and classification algorithms, database systems and design, and existing portable health monitoring devices. Some free clinical datasets, which will be employed in this research, have been collected; see (Keogh, Lin, & Fu) as an example. However, we do need more datasets for this research. If available datasets from public sources are not enough for the research validation, we will request datasets from health research communities. Simulation data suffices for conceptual validation, but the final validation will be based on real data annotated with diagnostic information. This will also be used to derive the final set of rules for the inference system employed in the wellness visualization system.

Currently, techniques and models for integrating data from various sources and Ajax are being studied. We are using these techniques to integrate users' information from various sources for the agent-based visualization system and to be able to implement Ajax as part of a distributed Java application (Java is the programming language adopted by our agent system). However, we need to refine the selection of a pattern analysis mechanism, allowing us to create the most effective measure of wellness from available information, and the rules for detecting data anomalies.

Task 2: System Analysis and Design

This began by defining research objectives and requirements. The initial design introduced in section V is developed based on the objectives, requirements, and knowledge from the first task. The initial design gives us a big picture of what is needed and what is developed in this research. Moreover, more details of each components and communication protocols among components will be clarified and developed in Section VI.

The detailed design of the statistical tools component has been already developed by the team members. There are many statistical methods used in medical research and diagnosis at the time of writing. However, we are not going to implement all the statistical methods; besides, the agent-based wellness visualization is designed to be expandable. Thus, more methods can be added in the future. Currently, only statistical methods that are perceived to be useful for our research and the commonly used statistical methods for medical research and diagnosis will be developed. As a result, twelve methods have been selected based on information from (Harris & Taylor, 2003; *Introduction to Medical Statistics*, 2001; Walker, 2002). The selected methods are the followings: Descriptive statistics (i.e. percentage, mean, median, mode, standard deviation, and confidential intervals), P-value, Two samples t-test, Mann-Whitney U test, Risk ratio, Odd ratio, Spearman rank correlation, Pearson's correlation, Sensitivity value, Specificity value, Positive predictive value, and Negative predictive value.

Other parts of the system have been integrated from previous work: for example, the agent-based inference system was the result of previous research from the group (Asadachatreekul, 2004). In this case, the research plan calls for an integration effort, with very little rework, as a result of the architectural choice of agents, which presents inherent extensibility.

Task 3: System Implementation

This task relates to the development of each component of the visualization system and unit testing. Unit testing has been performed frequently to ensure that the developed functions meet our requirements and work correctly. In addition, there continues to be some interactions among Task 1, 2, and 3 as needed because the literature review could return additional design and more information.

Task 4: System Integration and Testing

System integration is continuously performed throughout the research, even at this stage, as additional components of the wellness visualization system are developed. Continuous integration activities allow us to synchronize the components in the system and to find unexpected errors faster than with conventional integration phases. Testing activities in this research are divided into three subtasks: unit testing, system verification, and system evaluation. Unit testing is done together with system implementation activities to verify the correctness of every part of the visualization system. System verification occurs after the visualization system is successfully developed. System verification activities verify whether the agent-based visualization system complies with the research objectives and requirements. The activities also measure whether the system works correctly based on the design. Final system evaluation will be performed by one or more health care professionals in the region. Since health care professionals will be one of the end users, we need their feedback and opinions to ensure that the wellness visualization system can be useful for health services, and can assist them and the public. Therefore, although it is not necessary to use a clinical trial specifically for this system, it is nonetheless crucial to access an annotated dataset for the final part of the verification and validation operations.

As planned, the GUI will be the last part to be developed; system evaluation will be possible through a temporary GUI depicted in this chapter to start to receive feedback and opinions from experts. If more functions are needed, there will be the need for additional design. After the agent-based wellness visualization system is fully developed, a final acceptance test will be run for both categories of users: patients and health care practitioners. All demonstration and questionnaires needed for the system evaluation will be developed in accordance with scientific protocol.

ANALYSIS AND APPROACHES

The word "wellness" was introduced for the first time in 1959 by Halbert L. Dunn (Dunn, 1959). Then, wellness was defined as good health; where "health is a state of complete physical, mental, and social well-being and not merely the absence of disease and infirmity" (Dunn, 1959). Since then, many definitions of wellness have been introduced; examples can be found in (*Health Promotion Glossary Update*, ; *The six dimensional wellness model*, ; *What is wellness?*). Most of the definitions indicate that wellness comprises many dimensions. However, existing portable health monitoring devices cannot measure all dimensions of wellness, such as the dimensions of social, mental, spiritual, and emotional health. Therefore, we need to identify the term "wellness" that will be visualized by this research.

Since the research employs the benefits of primitive health information collected from existing portable health monitoring devices and resources, the agent-based visualization system is an indicator of wellness for the physical condition of an individual. However, when information of other wellness dimensions is available, it is possible to expand the visualization system to cover those dimensions of wellness in the future. The physical condition of an individual can be described by the results of clinical measurement. For instance, in an extremely simplified case, if the blood sugar content of a patient is in the normal range but the blood pressure is high, then we can tell that the physical condition of the patient is good in terms of the blood sugar content but it is not good in terms of the blood pressure. Thus, the level of wellness of the patient can be calculated from these two factors, based on the information available.

The definition of wellness is not the only thing that we need to consider in building a visualization system. There are other issues that we need to take into consideration. For example, we cannot tell that the level of wellness of a person is high or low from specific factors at all time. The wellness of the person in a period of time is changed by a group of factors. In other periods of time, the wellness of the patient could be changed by other factors. Thus, the agent-based visualization system must provide a mechanism that allows users to change the most appropriate weights for the factors to be used at a period of time. More issues that must be considered are described in the following subsections.

The Level of Wellness

A scale of wellness is designed to be used as a wellness indicator or a representation of the level of wellness of each user in the agent-based wellness visualization system because the scale is easy to interpret and understandable by everyone. Users can tell their wellness condition by looking through the scale of wellness. If the highlighted part of the scale is close to the "good" end, then the wellness of the user is potentially in good condition. On the other hand, if the highlighted part of the scale is closed to the "bad" end, then the wellness of the user is potentially in an unhealthy condition. The scale of wellness should encourage a user to maintain his/her wellness and avoid seeing his/her wellness move toward the "bad" end of the scale. Thus, it is possible that the user would maintain a high level of wellness and try to make it better (i.e. the user tries to improve the highlighted contributing factors to wellness by improving his/her health condition).

The level of wellness is calculated based on existing health information and adjustable weights because each patient is affected by different factors (or variables in the visualization system). For example, heart rate and blood pressure could be the main factors for a patient who has a heart disease. Therefore, variables should have different weights for different users. The wellness indicator or scale of wellness will be calculated based on the variables and their weights. If we allow the wellness indicator to be configurable,

the visualization system could potentially provide more accurate and effective results. Thus, it is a good idea to allow a health care professional to assign the weights of the variables that are used to calculate of the level of wellness of a patient.

The caregiver will assign weights for each variable relative to existing clinical data in the configuration page of the visualization system. This can only be done by a trained medical professional, who also has knowledge of the patient's history. As part of the support system for the caregiver, the system makes an educated guess on the weights to be used for the calculation of wellness, and gives the caregiver the option to use the suggested weights with an explanation of the guessing process. The variables and their weights are used to calculate the level of wellness. The level of wellness will be visualized on the scale of wellness displayed by the GUI (Graphic User Interface). Since modularity and expandability are two of the major goals of this research, if more types of clinical data become available, they will be added into the visualization system in the future. When new health monitoring devices or new types of clinical data of a patient become available for the system, the health care professional can assign weights for any new factors to calculate the level of wellness for each patient. Moreover, when the patient's condition changes, the weight of the factors that affect the patient's wellness will be changed as well. The caregiver can decide to adjust the weight of each variable as needed. If the weight of each factor is not assigned, the default value will be used.

Agent Technology and Platform

Since expandability and modularity are parts of the research objectives, agent technology is applied in this research. An agent can be added or removed from its platform and a software system easily. Thus, an agent-based system is inherently modular and easy to expand. Agent technology does not only provide modularity and expandability but also provides flexibility and distributed architecture for the visualization system. A distributed architecture allows one to distribute computational resources and process tasks on multiple processing units.

There are many choices of the agent execution platform available for the visualization system, such as TEEMA (TRLabs Execution Environment for Mobile Agents), Aglets, and Concordia (*Aglets*, 2002; *Concordia*, 2004; Martens et al., 2001). We choose TEEMA because TEEMA has been successfully employed in many previous research problems. In addition, there are benefits stemming a great deal of local experience and the resources of TEEMA are immediately available for this research.

Portable Health Monitoring Devices

Currently, portable health monitoring devices are easy to find at, say, local stores; and new products are introduced frequently. The devices can be classified in many ways. In this research, we wish to employ the benefits and results from the existing portable health monitoring devices. Thus, we must take the data provided by existing devices into consideration. As a result, the existing portable health monitoring device is divided into two categories:

1. **A portable heath monitoring device without data record:** the device shows measurement results to its users but it does not record any of these measurements. Therefore, if users want to keep track on their health information, they have to record the measurement results by themselves. Moreover, we cannot obtain health information from the device through network systems because most of the devices cannot connect to a computer or a network device. To solve this problem, the visualization system should allow patients and care givers to enter the results from the measurement together with the time

of measuring into the system. The time of measuring is necessary because results can be entered into the system at different time from the measurement occurs. In addition, it allows us to have more accurate health information, create history charts, and generate any other forms of graphical information. Examples of such a device can be found in (Bellin, Fellner, & Tchorbajian, 1985; *Heart Rate Monitor*, ; *Monitoring asthma symptoms*).

2. **A portable health monitoring device with data record:** the collected data is kept in data storage or in a database. The device may provide health information history, analysis trend, graphical display, and data management. Often, it is possible to obtain health information from the records on the device. In addition, some devices can be connected to a computer or to a local area network (in which case they are called telemonitoring devices). This type of device can be further classified in two categories. The first category is a device designed for monitoring specific parameters. The device provides only specified parameters and generates alarms when the monitored parameters reach a preset point. Another category is a device designed for general purpose. The device in the second category measures all basic parameters but it might not generate alarms when patient's condition changes. Most portable health monitoring devices with data recording capabilities adopt proprietary data structures for recording the measurement results. Therefore, there should be a mechanism that can identify the type of retrieved data and cluster the same type of data that come from different sources together. We need a method that can determine the relationships among the retrieved data as well. Examples of the portable health monitoring devices with data record can be found in (*Blood Pressure Monitor*, ; Brown,

2007; *Omron HJ-720ITC Pocket Pedometer with Advanced Omron Health Management Software*, ; Raymond, Gordon, & Singer, 1998).

User Interface

The agent-based wellness visualization system is designed for both health care professional and non-professional users. Therefore, there will be two types of users in the visualization system: health care professional (e.g. doctor, nurse, caregiver, etc.) and general user (e.g. patient). In the case of health care professionals, the users already have knowledge about health care and ability to evaluate clinical data. Therefore, the user interface should include the entirety of the data collected from a patient. The visualization system should allow the users to customize information to be displayed on the screen to meet their needs. This wellness visualization system has two types of users: general users and health professional users. For general users, the user interface should provide the information that is easy to understand for them. The user interface must be user-friendly for both types of users. The data presented by the visualization system must be visual, intuitive, and active to be of interest to the users.

The user interface will be divided into two modes: regular and advanced. The regular mode shows information to the general user. In the regular mode, general information; profile; alarm list; and summary are provided. The advanced mode displays information for the health care professional. In the advanced mode, more detailed information on a patient and options are provided to the users. Both modes can be accessed by all types of users, but general users default to the regular mode whereas health care professionals default to the advanced mode. Thus, the health care professional can see the screen that is shown to each of a patient. In addition, the general user can see what is viewed by the health care professional as well. To verify that the user interface

will be satisfactory by end users, both general users and available health care professionals in the region will be asked to evaluate the wellness visualization system.

Security

We must respect the privacy of every user. Dealing with health care information is a very sensitive issue. All health information and user information must be confidential. In addition, the data must not be accessible by unauthorized users. Thus, users will have to login to the wellness visualization system before they can obtain any information provided by the system. In the agent-based visualization system, health information is transferred among software agents and other system's components. Therefore, any sensitive data must be encrypted before the data transfer is performed. Moreover, we must not allow all health care professionals to view all patients' information. A health care professional is allowed to view only information of a patient who is under his/her care. As a result, a list of authorized users must be created to control the access to information. Additional security measures, such as the use of RFIDs and/or Bluetooth appliances, are other possibilities to provide identity certificates and authorizations to the system.

Moreover, the security control in the wellness visualization system must comply with standards and frameworks relative to health information system that are accepted by medical communities such as Health Level 7 (HL7) (*Health Level 7*, 1997). Thus, we can ensure that the visualization system will meet with the health community satisfaction and will be compatible with other health information systems.

ARCHITECTURE

Figure 1 illustrates the main components of the agent-based wellness visualization system and

Figure 1. Block diagram of the agent-based wellness visualization system

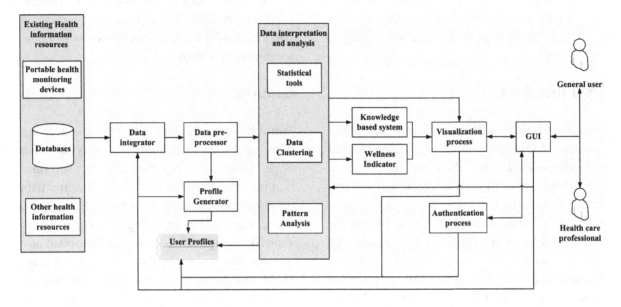

the relationships among the components. Each component in the system has its own responsibility. A component may contain more than one software agent and other pieces of software. More details about the components are described in the following subsections.

Existing Health Information Resources

This component provides health care information to the visualization system. Existing health care information can be gathered from portable health monitoring devices, hospital's databases, health care service providers, etc.

Data Integrator

The data integrator is responsible for collecting health care information of a user from various existing health information resources and from the users. The component also maintains the locations of the resources. This component may contain passwords to access existing health information resources, compatibly with security requirements and access protection protocols.

Data Pre-Processor

This component transforms retrieved health care information into a format that can be used by other components in the visualization system. If the information does not need to be transformed, then the component will forward the information to other parts of the system.

Profile Generator

This component is responsible for generating a profile for each user of the visualization system. The profile generator also updates the profile when changes occur. The profile generator is the only one component in the visualization system that can change any information in the user's profile to avoid errors, such as latest information is replaced by older information. Thus, if any other components want to update a profile, they have to send their requests to the profile generator.

Data Interpretation and Analysis

The data interpretation and analysis component is responsible for interpreting and analysing the health care information. It comprises of three sub-components:

1. **Statistical tools:** this sub-component comprises various statistical methods. It calculates commonly used statistical information of the health care information received from the data pre-processor. Examples of commonly used statistical methods provided by the sub-component are mean, median, mode, standard deviation, etc. More advanced statistical methods can be added to the sub-component in the future.
2. **Data clustering:** this sub-component clusters similar data together to reveal the structure of the health care information to the users. There are many data clustering algorithms at present. In this research, k-means is one of the most likely candidate algorithms to be used because it provides effective results to many research problems with low computational cost (Mirkin, 2005).
3. **Pattern analysis:** this sub-component identifies patterns from received health information collected from a user. Once a pattern is discovered, we can employ the pattern to identify anomalies.

Knowledge-Based System

This component generates an alarm based on received information from other components. It also provides simple suggestion to the users.

Wellness Indicator

The wellness indicator evaluates the level of wellness of a user of the agent-based visualization system. The level of wellness is calculated based on the health care professional's setting (i.e. weights of the variables) and available information from other components in the system.

Visualization Process

This component translates all received information to graphical formats. The component decides which format is the most appropriate to visualize the data. This component is the only one component that can access to the GUI to avoid other components to change any display by themselves.

Authentication Process

This component verifies that only authorized users can access to the visualization system. Thus, all users have to login before they can access to the system.

GUI

GUI or Graphic User Interface allows users to interact with the visualization system. The component is also responsible for showing information and results of the agent-based wellness visualization system to its users. Moreover, users can view, change, modify their profiles; information; and setting through the GUI.

SYSTEM DESIGN

Figure 1 illustrates what have been developed. The "agent-based rule-based system" and the "agent-based statistical tools" components work together to provide support information to the users. When new information of a user is added into the system, the FactorEvaluator agent will evaluate the information to update the good/bad factor list of the user; and the agent-based rule-based system will identify if the values of received information is normal or not. The rule-based system also

Figure 2. System design overview

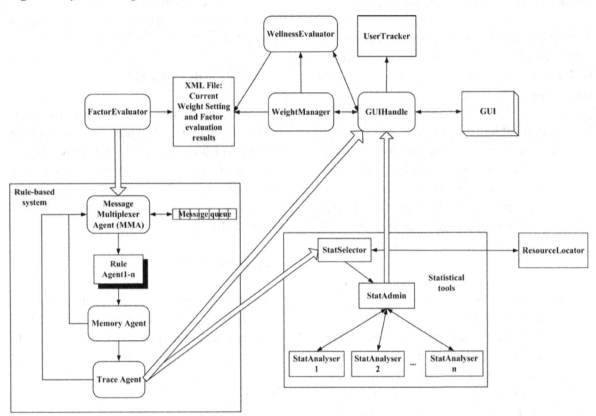

provides description and suggestion for the user. If the rule-based system detects anomaly, it will tell the agent-based statistical tools to give statistical information relative to the anomaly to the user. Moreover, the WellnessEvaluator will update the wellness level of the user based on information in the good/bad factor evaluation results and weight setting.

The Statistical tools component needs assistances from the ResourceLocator agent to obtain user's information. The StatSelector agent selects statistical methods that are appropriate to the retrieved information. For example, if multiple variables are retrieved, statistical methods

Table 1. Communication protocol

Host agent name	Message kind	Message content	Destination agent name
StatAnalyser	SIGNIN	STAT + method name	StatAdmin
StatAnalyser	SIGNOUT	-	StatAdmin
StatAdmin	ANALYSEDATA	Username + number of datasets + number of data entry in each dataset + initial data from each dataset e.g. "Alice 1 5 data1 1 2 3 4 5" "Alice 2 4 6 data1 1 2 3 4 data2 1 2 3 4 5 6" Note: maximum number of datasets = 2	StatAnalyser
StatAnalyser	ANALYSERESULT	Username + method name + result	StatAdmin

Table 2. Agent developed

Agent name	Method name	Approach and Usage (Broyles, 2006; Daly & Bourke, 2000; Fowler, Jarvis, & Chevannes, 2002; Jantachume, 1999; Munro, 2005)	Conditions and Results
StatAnalyser1	Mean	**Arithmetic mean** 1. Describing and summarizing the structure of quantitative data 2. Can be used for examining associations among two or more variables 3. Measure the average of data	**Results:** Mean of a single variable **Conditions:** -
StatAnalyser2	Median	**Median** 1. Describing and summarizing the structure of quantitative data 2. Can be used for examining associations among two or more variables 3. Measure an average and a frequency of distribution	**Results:** Median of a single variable **Conditions:** -
StatAnalyser3	Trend Analysis	**Average rate of periodic change** 1. Estimating the trend of time series data 2. Summarizing the movement or the average rate of periodic change	**Results:** Approximate trend of time series data (+ increase/- decrease) **Conditions:** -
StatAnalyser4	Mode	**Mode** 1. Describing and summarizing the structure of quantitative data 2. Can be used for examining associations among two or more variables 3. Measure an average in ordinal scale and a frequency of distribution	**Results:** Modal class of a single variable **Conditions:** -
StatAnalyser5	STD	**Root mean square deviation** 1. Describing and summarizing the structure of quantitative data 2. Describing variability/spread within quantitative data	**Results:** Standard deviation of a single variable **Conditions:** -
StatAnalyser6	Range	**Range** 1. Describing and summarizing the structure of quantitative data 2. Describing variability/spread within quantitative data 3. Measures the highest observation, lowest observation, and range of a sample.	**Results:** Range, lowest data value, and highest data value **Conditions:** -
StatAnalyser7	t-test1	**t-test for two independent samples:** t-value is calculated by using pooled variance estimate Comparing means or geometric means of two independent samples	**Results:** t value and degree of freedom **Conditions:** 1. Standard deviations of the populations of both samples are unknown. 2. Standard deviations of the populations of both samples are equal. 3. The sample sizes are not equal.
StatAnalyser8	t-test2	**t-test for two independent samples:** t-value is calculated by using separated variance estimate Comparing means or geometric means of two independent samples	**Results:** t value and degree of freedom **Conditions:** 1. Standard deviations of the populations of both samples are unknown. 2. Standard deviations of the populations of both samples are not equal. 3. The sample sizes are not equal.

Table 2. continued

Agent name	Method name	Approach and Usage (Broyles, 2006; Daly & Bourke, 2000; Fowler, Jarvis, & Chevannes, 2002; Jantachume, 1999; Munro, 2005)	Conditions and Results
StatAnalyser9	t-test3	**t-test for two independent samples:** t-value is calculated by assuming that the two distributions have the same variance Comparing means or geometric means of two independent samples	**Results:** t value and degree of freedom **Conditions:** 1. Standard deviations of the populations of both samples are unknown. 2. Standard deviations of the populations of both samples are equal. 3. The sample sizes are equal.
StatAnalyser10	t-test4	**t-test for testing correlation coefficient** To test if any two samples have linear relationship to each other **Note:** This t-test will be used with the four correlation coefficients to find if any two variables have linear correlation.	**Results:** t value and degree of freedom **Conditions:** Can test the following coefficients only 1. Pearson product-moment correlation coefficient 2. Spearman rank correlation coefficient 3. Point biserial correlation coefficient 4. Kendall rank correlation coefficient
StatAnalyser11	t-test5	**t-test for two dependent samples** Comparing means or geometric means of two dependent/paired samples, i.e. Pre-test vs. Post-test	**Results:** t value and degree of freedom **Conditions:** -
StatAnalyser12	Variance	**Variance (square of the standard deviation)** 1. Describing and summarizing the structure of quantitative data 2. Describing variability/spread within quantitative data	**Results:** Variance of a single variable **Conditions:** -
StatAnalyser13	Pearson1	**Pearson product-moment correlation coefficient** Measuring the degree of linear relationship between two variables	**Results:** correlation coefficient $(-1 < r < 1)$ **Condition:** calculated for n samples
StatAnalyser14	Pearson2	**Pearson product-moment correlation coefficient** Measuring the degree of linear relationship between two variables	**Results:** correlation coefficient $(-1 < r < 1)$ **Condition:** calculated for the population
StatAnalyser15	CoeffDetermin	**Coefficient of determination** 1. Measuring the association between two variables 2. Measuring the proportion of the change in one variable that is accounted for by change in another variable	**Results:** The square of r **Conditions:** work with Pearson product-moment correlation coefficient

designed for multiple variables are selected (e.g. finding correlation coefficients among pairs of variables). If a single variable is retrieved, statistical methods designed for single variables are selected (e.g. finding mean of the variable). Results of the agent-based system are given in the next section.

Agent Development

Fifteen StatAnalyser agents have been developed. The detail about each agent and its corresponding statistical method is described in Table 2. The communication protocol is explained in Table 1.

Figure 3. The architecture of the agent-based rule-based system

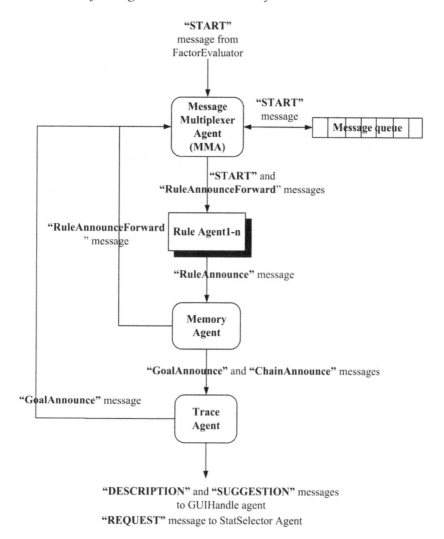

Agent-Based Rule-Based System

The agent-based rule-based system is modified from (Asadachatreekul, 2004). It is responsible for making inference to the knowledge base obtaining from humans to find a solution to a problem. In this research, the problem is to find the wellness level of a person, any anomaly in the health of a person, descriptions, and suggestions for a user. The problem is solved by employing the forward chaining method. Currently, there is no backtracking in the rule-based system, but it is planned to be added in the future. This rule-based system

comprises the following:

1. **MMA (Message Multiplexer Agent):** an agent that is responsible for registering/tracking Rule Agents in the system and sharing information to all Rule Agents.
2. **Rule Agents:** a group of agents. Each rule agent contains a set of rules; where each rule is a part of the knowledge base.
3. **Memory Agent:** an agent that selects the best rule to be used from all fired rules.
4. **Trace Agent:** an agent that is responsible for keeping the chain of fired rules and finding

Table 3. Communication messages developed for the agent-based rule-based system

Host agent name	Message kind	Message content	Destination agent name
Rule Agents	"SIGNIN"	"RULE"	MMA
	Example messages from a log file: 30/08/08 11:10:51 AM: Platform.sendAgentMessage(): msg.sendAgentName = Rule2@192.168.1.107:10010 msg.destHost.name = 192.168.1.107 msg.destAgentName = Multiplexer@192.168.1.107:10010 this.platformAddress.name = 192.168.1.107 messageType = SIGNIN messageContent= RULE		
Rule Agents	"SIGNOUT"	-	MMA
MMA	"START"	Username + Initial data	Rule Agents
	Example messages from a log file: 30/08/08 11:13:12 AM: Platform.sendAgentMessage(): msg.sendAgentName = Multiplexer@192.168.1.107:10010 msg.destHost.name = 192.168.1.107 msg.destAgentName = Rule3@192.168.1.107:10010 this.platformAddress.name = 192.168.1.107 messageType = START messageContent= Alice Female 25 HeartRate 110 BLANK		
MMA	"RuleAnnounceForward"	Username + Data after firing rule actions	Rule Agents
Rule Agents	"RuleAnnounce"	Username + Data before firing rule actions + firing rule name & priority + Data after firing rule actions	Memory Agent
	Example messages from a log file: 30/08/08 11:13:12 AM: Platform.sendAgentMessage(): msg.sendAgentName = Rule1@192.168.1.107:10010 msg.destHost.name = 192.168.1.107 msg.destAgentName = MemoryAgent@192.168.1.107:10010 this.platformAddress.name = 192.168.1.107 messageType = RuleAnnounce messageContent= Alice Female 25 HeartRate 110 BLANK Rule1@192.168.1.107:10010 1 Alice Female 25 HeartRate 110.0 LOWER 117-166[beat/min.]		
Memory Agent	"GoalAnnounce"	Username + Data before firing rule actions + firing rule name & priority + Data after firing rule actions	Trace Agent
	Example messages from a log file: 30/08/08 11:13:14 AM: Platform.sendAgentMessage(): msg.sendAgentName = MemoryAgent@192.168.1.107:10010 msg.destHost.name = 192.168.1.107 msg.destAgentName = TraceAgent@192.168.1.107:10010 this.platformAddress.name = 192.168.1.107 messageType = GoalAnnounce messageContent= Alice Female 25 HeartRate 110.0 BLANK Rule1@192.168.1.107:10010 1 Alice Female 25 HeartRate 110.0 LOWER 117-166[beat/min.]		
Memory Agent	"ChainAnnounce"	Username + Data before firing rule actions + firing rule name & priority + Data after firing rule actions	Trace Agent
Memory Agent	"RuleAnnounceForward"	Username + Data after firing rule	MMA
Trace Agent	"GoalAnnounce"	-	MMA
	Example messages from a log file: 30/08/08 11:13:15 AM: Platform.sendAgentMessage(): msg.sendAgentName = TraceAgent@192.168.1.107:10010 msg.destHost.name = 192.168.1.107 msg.destAgentName = Multiplexer@192.168.1.107:10010 this.platformAddress.name = 192.168.1.107 messageType = GoalAnnounce messageContent=		
Trace Agent	"DESCRIPTION"	Username+ Description about the goal	GUIHandle Agent
	Example messages from a log file: 30/08/08 11:13:14 AM: Platform.sendAgentMessage(): msg.sendAgentName = TraceAgent@192.168.1.107:10010 msg.destHost.name = 192.168.1.107 msg.destAgentName = GUIHandle@192.168.1.107:10010 this.platformAddress.name = 192.168.1.107 messageType = DESCRIPTION messageContent= Alice Your heart rate(110.0 beat/min.) is lower than the nomal range: 117-166[beat/min.]		

Table 3. continued

Host agent name	Message kind	Message content	Destination agent name
Trace Agent	"SUGGESTION"	Username + Suggestion information relative to the goal	GUIHandle Agent
	Example messages from a log file: 30/08/08 11:13:14 AM: Platform.sendAgentMessage(): msg.sendAgentName = Trace-Agent@192.168.1.107:10010 msg.destHost.name = 192.168.1.107 msg.destAgentName = GUIHandle@192.168.1.107:10010 this.platformAddress.name = 192.168.1.107 messageType = SUGGESTION messageContent= Alice Low heart rate is caused by many causes such as drug usage, metabolic issues, unbalance electrolyte, etc. If you are a trained athlete, your heart rate can be considered as normal. Please consult with your doctor for more information.		
Trace Agent	"REQUEST"	Username + parameter name	StatSelector Agent
	Example messages from a log file: 30/08/08 11:13:14 AM: Platform.sendAgentMessage(): msg.sendAgentName = Trace-Agent@192.168.1.107:10010 msg.destHost.name = 192.168.1.107 msg.destAgentName = StatSelector@192.168.1.107:10010 this.platformAddress.name = 192.168.1.107 messageType = REQUEST messageContent= Alice HeartRate		

the best description and suggestion for the goal.

Agent-Based Statistical Tools

The "agent-based statistical tools" is a component that provides statistical information to other components of the wellness visualization system. The statistical information is considered as support information to a user, especially for a health care professional. For example, finding a trend in a single parameter and finding linear correlation among parameters. There are three main components in the agent-based statistical tools:

1. **StatSelector Agent:** an agent that selects statistical methods that are appropriated to retrieved data.
2. **StatAdmin Agent:** an agent that is responsible for registering/tracking StatAnalyser Agents in the system. It also distributes information to the selected StatAnalyser

Figure 4. The architecture of agent-based statistical tools

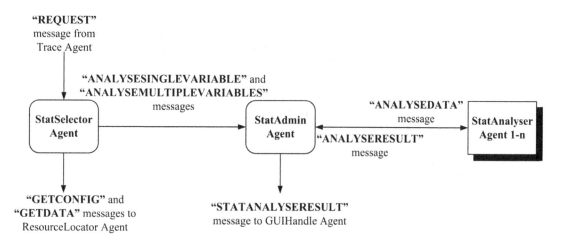

Table 4. Communication messages developed for the agent-based statistical tools

Host agent name	Message kind	Message content	Destination agent name
StatAnalyser Agents	"SIGNIN"	"STAT" + statistical method's name	StatAdmin Agent
	Example messages from a log file: 30/08/08 11:11:17 AM: Platform.sendAgentMessage(): msg.sendAgentName = StatAnalyser1@192.168.1.107:10010 msg.destHost.name = 192.168.1.107 msg.destAgentName = StatAdmin@192.168.1.107:10010 this.platformAddress.name = 192.168.1.107 messageType = SIGNIN messageContent= STAT Mean		
StatAnalyser Agents	"SIGNOUT"	-	StatAdmin Agent
StatSelector Agent	"ANALYSE SINGLE VARIABLE"	Username + no. of parameter type + no. of data entry + dataset	StatAdmin Agent
	Example messages from a log file: 30/08/08 11:13:15 AM: Platform.sendAgentMessage(): msg.sendAgentName = StatSelector@192.168.1.107:10010 msg.destHost.name = 192.168.1.107 msg.destAgentName = StatAdmin@192.168.1.107:10010 this.platformAddress.name = 192.168.1.107 messageType = ANALYSESINGLEVARIABLE messageContent= Alice 1 10 HeartRate 110 112 115 113 110 105 102 99 101 90		
StatSelector Agent	"ANALYSE MULTIPLE VARIABLES"	Username + no. of parameter type + no. of data entry + "data" + parameter's name + data set+ ...	StatAdmin Agent
	Example messages from a log file: 30/08/08 11:13:15 AM: Platform.sendAgentMessage(): msg.sendAgentName = StatSelector@192.168.1.107:10010 msg.destHost.name = 192.168.1.107 msg.destAgentName = StatAdmin@192.168.1.107:10010 this.platformAddress.name = 192.168.1.107 messageType = ANALYSEMULTIPLEVARIABLES messageContent= Alice 4 10 data HeartRate 110 112 115 113 110 105 102 99 101 90 data Temperature 36.7 37.4 37.7 37.5 37.8 37.3 37.1 37.0 37.1 37.2 data SystolicPressure 112 115 117 111 110 108 105 104 102 102 data DiastolicPressure 71 75 77 76 74 75 77 72 74 70		
StatAdmin Agent	"ANALYSE DATA"	Username + no. of parameter type + no. of data entry + dataset	StatAnalyser Agents
	Example messages from a log file: 30/08/08 11:13:15 AM: Platform.sendAgentMessage(): msg.sendAgentName = StatAdmin@192.168.1.107:10010 msg.destHost.name = 192.168.1.107 msg.destAgentName = StatAnalyser1@192.168.1.107:10010 this.platformAddress.name = 192.168.1.107 messageType = ANALYSEDATA messageContent= Alice 1 10 HeartRate 110 112 115 113 110 105 102 99 101 90		
StatAdmin Agent	"ANALYSE DATA"	Username + no. of parameter type + no. of data entry + "data" + parameter's name + dataset + ...	StatAnalyser Agents
	Example messages from a log file: 30/08/08 11:13:16 AM: Platform.sendAgentMessage(): msg.sendAgentName = StatAdmin@192.168.1.107:10010 msg.destHost.name = 192.168.1.107 msg.destAgentName = StatAnalyser13@192.168.1.107:10010 this.platformAddress.name = 192.168.1.107 messageType = ANALYSEDATA messageContent= Alice 4 10 data HeartRate 110 112 115 113 110 105 102 99 101 90 data Temperature 36.7 37.4 37.7 37.5 37.8 37.3 37.1 37.0 37.1 37.2 data SystolicPressure 112 115 117 111 110 108 105 104 102 102 data DiastolicPressure 71 75 77 76 74 75 77 72 74 70		
StatAnalyser Agents	"ANALYSE RESULT"	Username + statistical method's name + result	StatAdmin Agent
	Example messages from a log file: 30/08/08 11:13:15 AM: Platform.sendAgentMessage(): msg.sendAgentName = StatAnalyser1@192.168.1.107:10010 msg.destHost.name = 192.168.1.107 msg.destAgentName = StatAdmin@192.168.1.107:10010 this.platformAddress.name = 192.168.1.107 messageType = ANALYSERESULT messageContent= Alice Mean 105.7		

Table 4. continued

Host agent name	Message kind	Message content	Destination agent name
StatSelector Agent	"GETCONFIG"	Username + configured data type	ResourceLocator Agent
	Example messages from a log file: 30/08/08 11:13:14 AM: Platform.sendAgentMessage(): msg.sendAgentName = StatSelector@192.168.1.107:10010 msg.destHost.name = 192.168.1.107 msg.destAgentName = ResourceLocator@192.168.1.107:10010 this.platformAddress.name = 192.168.1.107 messageType = GETCONFIG messageContent= Alice CONFIGDATAENTRY		
StatSelector	"GETDATA"	"SINGLE" + Username + parameter's name **Note:** get data for single parameter	ResourceLocator
	Example messages from a log file: 30/08/08 11:13:15 AM: Platform.sendAgentMessage(): msg.sendAgentName = StatSelector@192.168.1.107:10010 msg.destHost.name = 192.168.1.107 msg.destAgentName = ResourceLocator@192.168.1.107:10010 this.platformAddress.name = 192.168.1.107 messageType = GETDATA messageContent= SINGLE Alice HeartRate		
StatSelector	"GETDATA"	"ALL" + Username + no. of data entry from configuration file of the user **Note:** Get specific number of data entries from all parameter for the user. It is suggested that the system should not allow anyone to process all data in the system at a time especially when the database is huge. The reason is to avoid the system to blow up or take forever to process the data.	ResourceLocator
	Example messages from a log file: 30/08/08 11:13:15 AM: Platform.sendAgentMessage(): msg.sendAgentName = StatSelector@192.168.1.107:10010 msg.destHost.name = 192.168.1.107 msg.destAgentName = ResourceLocator@192.168.1.107:10010 this.platformAddress.name = 192.168.1.107 messageType = GETDATA messageContent= ALL Alice 10		
StatSelector	"GETDATA"	"PERIOD" + Username + parameter's name + First period of time + Second period of time **Note:** Get data from a single parameter for two period of time	ResourceLocator
StatAdmin Agent	"STAT ANALYSE RESULT"	Username + statistical method's name + result	GUIHandle Agent
	Example messages from a log file: 30/08/08 11:13:16 AM: Platform.sendAgentMessage(): msg.sendAgentName = StatAdmin@192.168.1.107:10010 msg.destHost.name = 192.168.1.107 msg.destAgentName = GUIHandle@192.168.1.107:10010 this.platformAddress.name = 192.168.1.107 messageType = STATANALYSERESULT messageContent= Alice Mean 105.7		

Agents.

3. **StatAnalyser Agents:** a group of agents containing statistical methods. Some StatAnalyser Agents have to work together to get the final results. For example, the agent containing "coefficient of determination" method has to work with the agent containing "Pear product-moment correlation coefficient" method to find a result.

Wellness Indicator

The agent-based wellness indicator is an implementation of the wellness evaluation model. The wellness evaluation model gives wellness level of a person and level of wellness will be shown on the wellness scale of the visualization system. The wellness level of a person is calculated from available objective data and weight setting of the

Figure 5. The architecture of agent-based wellness indicator

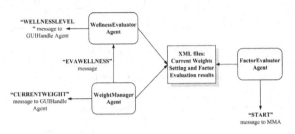

person. Figure 6 illustrates the wellness evaluation model.

The wellness indicator contains the following agents:

1. **FactorEvaluator Agent:** an agent that contains comparison and mapping functions. The comparison function compares all available objective data with its normal value. Then, the mapping function will assign each parameter as a good or bad factor based on the comparison result.

2. **WeightManager Agent:** an agent that manages the weights to be used in the wellness evaluation model.

3. **WellnessEvaluator Agent:** an agent that evaluates the wellness level of a person based on the wellness evaluation model.

Other Agents

Agents in this group support and provide services to other agents in the wellness visualization system. Agents in this group could be discarded from the system or developed to be a part of other components of the system when the wellness visualization system is complete. ResourceLocator agent is designed to be an agent that has the location of user's information and retrieves information from the sources. GUIHandle agent is the only one agent that can modify the GUI. Thus, any agent, that wants to show its results to the user, must submit the results to the GUIHandle agent. UserTracker agent is designed for tracking logged-in user. The agent will assist the wellness visualization system to support multiple users at a time in the future. Test agent is created for testing purposes. With test agent, we can assume that an event occurs or the system received expected messages from other components of the agent-based systems.

INITIAL RESULTS

A proof of concept is the major expected result of this research. The proof of concept must fulfil the objectives of the research and can be

Figure 6. Model for measuring the wellness of a person based on available objective data and weight setting

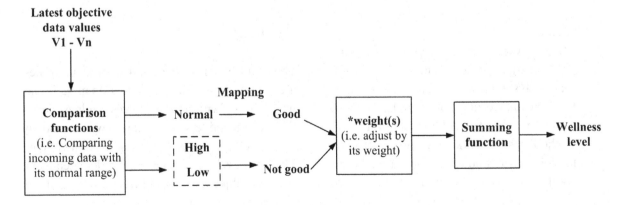

Table 5. Communication messages developed for the agent-based wellness indicator

Host agent name	Message kind	Message content	Destination agent name
FactorEvaluator Agent	"START"	Initial data	MMA
Example messages from a log file: 30/08/08 11:13:12 AM: Platform.sendAgentMessage(): msg.sendAgentName = FactorEvaluator@192.168.1.107:10010 msg.destHost.name = 192.168.1.107 msg.destAgentName = Multiplexer@192.168.1.107:10010 this.platformAddress.name = 192.168.1.107 messageType = START messageContent= Alice Female 25 HeartRate 110 BLANK			
WellnessEvaluator Agent	"WELLNESSLEVEL"	Username + wellness level	GUIHandle Agent
Example messages from a log file: 30/08/08 11:13:03 AM: Platform.sendAgentMessage(): msg.sendAgentName = WellnessEvaluator@192.168.1.107:10010 msg.destHost.name = 192.168.1.107 msg.destAgentName = GUIHandle@192.168.1.107:10010 this.platformAddress.name = 192.168.1.107 messageType = WELLNESSLEVEL messageContent= Alice 75.0			
WeightManager Agent	"CURRENTWEIGHT"	Username + parameter's name + corresponding weight +...	GUIHandle Agent
Example messages from a log file: 30/08/08 11:13:03 AM: Platform.sendAgentMessage(): msg.sendAgentName = WeightManager@192.168.1.107:10010 msg.destHost.name = 192.168.1.107 msg.destAgentName = GUIHandle@192.168.1.107:10010 this.platformAddress.name = 192.168.1.107 messageType = CURRENTWEIGHT messageContent= HeartRate 1.0 Temperature 1.0 SystolicPressure 1.0 DiastolicPressure 1.0			
WeightManager Agent	"EVAWELLNESS"	Username	WellnessEvaluator

improved to become a standard. This research also encourages people to have self-awareness of personal wellness and public health. If the research is successfully developed, the agent-based visualization system will provide benefits to the public, research communities, and commercial enterprises. The visualization system will be used as a single indicator of an individual's wellness and will generate a simplified view of the health information collected from existing resources and the user. The wellness of an individual is measured by using health information collected from each person. Moreover, the visualization system can be used as a one-station examination for health care professionals as well. The collected health information of each user with analysed information will be provided. In addition, the agent-based system potentially boosts up the health services. Therefore, the research has high potential in giving direct benefits to the public.

In case of the research communities, the agent-based system can be used as framework for health information integration, data analysis, visualization, and software agent research areas. All finding in this research can be used as a fundamental in developing more sophisticated systems. Furthermore, all knowledge, findings, and experiences of the research are expected to be transferrable to develop a product that will benefit all end users.

The results in this chapter are still preliminary, and are based on synthesized data patterned around the literature available on the subject. The results have been generated according to a number of test cases, the most relevant of which are reported below. Since the initial evaluation is intended to align the wellness indicator with a patient's health, this approach is acceptable, but requires a thorough validation with annotated data. All test cases succeed and provide the expected results with no discrepancies.

Table 6. Communication messages developed for the agents that provide services to other agents in the agent-based wellness visualization system

Host agent name	Message kind	Message content	Destination agent name
ResourceLocator Agent	"RETURN CONFIG"	Username + configuration information	StatSelector Agent
	Example messages from a log file: 30/08/08 11:13:14 AM: Platform.sendAgentMessage(): msg.sendAgentName = ResourceLocator@192.168.1.107:10010 msg.destHost.name = 192.168.1.107 msg.destAgentName = StatSelector@192.168.1.107:10010 this.platformAddress.name = 192.168.1.107 messageType = RETURNCONFIG messageContent= Alice 10		
ResourceLocator Agent	"RETURN USERDATA"	"SINGLE" + Username + no. of parameter + no. of data entries + parameter's name + dataset	StatSelector Agent
	Example messages from a log file: 30/08/08 11:13:15 AM: Platform.sendAgentMessage(): msg.sendAgentName = ResourceLocator@192.168.1.107:10010 msg.destHost.name = 192.168.1.107 msg.destAgentName = StatSelector@192.168.1.107:10010 this.platformAddress.name = 192.168.1.107 messageType = RETURNUSERDATA messageContent= SINGLE Alice 1 10 HeartRate 110 112 115 113 110 105 102 99 101 90		
ResourceLocator Agent	"RETURN USERDATA"	"All" + Username + no. of parameter + no. of data entries for a parameter + "data" + parameter's name + dataset +...	StatSelector Agent
	Example messages from a log file: 30/08/08 11:13:15 AM: Platform.sendAgentMessage(): msg.sendAgentName = ResourceLocator@192.168.1.107:10010 msg.destHost.name = 192.168.1.107 msg.destAgentName = StatSelector@192.168.1.107:10010 this.platformAddress.name = 192.168.1.107 messageType = RETURNUSERDATA messageContent= ALL Alice 4 10 data HeartRate 110 112 115 113 110 105 102 99 101 90 data Temperature 36.7 37.4 37.7 37.5 37.8 37.3 37.1 37.0 37.1 37.2 data SystolicPressure 112 115 117 111 110 108 105 104 102 102 data DiastolicPressure 71 75 77 76 74 75 77 72 74 70		
ResourceLocator Agent	"RETURN USERDATA"	"PERIOD" + Username + parameter's name + no. of data entries for the first period + no. of data entries for the second period + "data" + dataset1 + "data" + dataset2	StatSelector Agent
GUIHandle Agent	"SIGNIN"	Username	UserTracker Agent
	Example messages from a log file: 30/08/08 11:13:03 AM: Platform.sendAgentMessage(): msg.sendAgentName = GUIHandle@192.168.1.107:10010 msg.destHost.name = 192.168.1.107 msg.destAgentName = UserTracker@192.168.1.107:10010 this.platformAddress.name = 192.168.1.107 messageType = SIGNIN messageContent= Alice		
GUIHandle Agent	"EVAWELLNESS LEVEL"	Username	WellnessEvaluator Agent
	Example messages from a log file: 30/08/08 11:13:03 AM: Platform.sendAgentMessage(): msg.sendAgentName = GUIHandle@192.168.1.107:10010 msg.destHost.name = 192.168.1.107 msg.destAgentName = WellnessEvaluator@192.168.1.107:10010 this.platformAddress.name = 192.168.1.107 messageType = EVAWELLNESSLEVEL messageContent= Alice		

Table 6. continued

Host agent name	Message kind	Message content	Destination agent name
GUIHandle Agent	"GETWEIGHT"	Username	WeightManager Agent
	Example messages from a log file: 30/08/08 11:13:03 AM: Platform.sendAgentMessage(): msg.sendAgentName = GUIHandle@192.168.1.107:10010 msg.destHost.name = 192.168.1.107 msg.destAgentName = WeightManager@192.168.1.107:10010 this.platformAddress.name = 192.168.1.107 messageType = GETWEIGHT messageContent= Alice		
GUIHandle Agent	"CHANGEWEIGHT"	Username + weight setting mode (+ parameter's name + weight value) **Note:** if weight setting mode = "DEFAULT", the system will automatically set up default weight value for all parameter. Otherwise, the system will set weight value for each parameter as given by the user.	WeightManager Agent
Test Agent	"EVAFACTOR"	Username + new arrival data **Note:** Test Agent is designed for testing purposes. Message type and message content can be different in different test cases.	FactorEvaluator Agent
	Example messages from a log file: 30/08/08 11:13:12 AM: Platform.sendAgentMessage(): msg.sendAgentName = TestAgent@192.168.1.107:10010 msg.destHost.name = 192.168.1.107 msg.destAgentName = FactorEvaluator@192.168.1.107:10010 this.platformAddress.name = 192.168.1.107 messageType = EVAFACTOR messageContent= Alice Female 25 HeartRate 110 Temperature 36.7 SystolicPressure 112 DiastolicPressure 71		

Test Case 1: Factor Evaluation

Requirement

This test case verifies that the agent-based system can evaluate good/bad factors, which will be employed to calculate the wellness level of a person, by using latest parameter values.

Method

This test case is performed by simulating two different datasets of parameter values with the default weight setting. Each dataset is injected into the system by using an agent. It is assumed that each parameter value in a dataset is the latest information of the corresponding parameter.

Results

The system can update an XML file (i.e. WeightContainer_username.xml) to have current factor types for all parameter values submitted into the system.

Test Case 2: The Effects of Weight Setting Toward the Wellness Level of a Person

Requirement

This test case verifies that the agent-based system can produce the result of wellness evaluation model correctly (i.e. the wellness level). The test case also demonstrates the affects of weight setting used in the wellness evaluation model toward the wellness level of a person.

Method

This test case is performed by simulating one user's condition with various weight settings. There are seven datasets with different weight settings but the same parameter values. The data is injected into the system by developing an agent to submit the data into the system. The results will be compared with manually calculated results.

Results

Different weight settings for the same parameter values will enforce the system to produce different wellness levels for a person.

Test Case 3: The Affects of Parameter Values toward the Wellness Level of a Person

Requirement

This test case verifies that the agent-based system can produce the result of wellness evaluation model correctly (i.e. the wellness level). The test

case also demonstrates that the wellness level is not only affected by the weight setting but also the parameter values.

Method

This test case is performed by simulating different user conditions with the same weight setting. The data is injected into the system by developing an agent to submit the data into the system.

Results

The agent-based system produces different wellness levels for different sets of parameter values with the same weight setting.

Test Case 4: The Agent-Based Rule-Based System

Requirement

This test case verifies that the agent-based rule-based system can evaluate a user's condition based on available information and can provide suggestion to the user.

Table 7. Stored data for Alice

Heart Rate (beat/minute)	Body Temperature (degree Celsius)	Systolic Pressure (mmHg)	Diastolic Pressure (mmHg)
110	36.7	112	71
112	37.4	115	75
115	37.7	117	77
113	37.5	111	76
110	37.8	110	74
105	37.3	108	75
102	37.1	105	77
99	37.0	104	72
101	37.1	102	74
90	37.2	102	70

Figure 7. Result showing on the GUI of the agent-based system

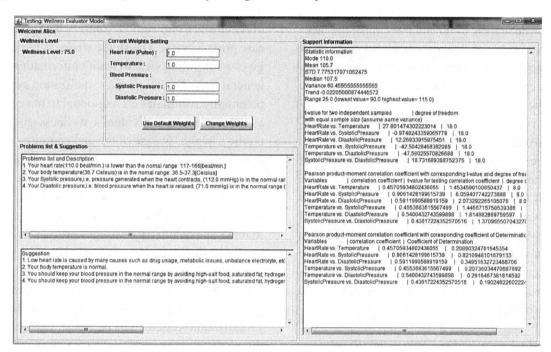

Method

This test case is performed by simulating different user conditions; then injecting the data into the system by developing an agent to submit the data into the system.

Results

The agent-based system produces a short description of received information with suggestion on the GUI.

Test Case 5: System Test

The following results obtained by using a Test agent to submit new arrival data into the agent-based system. In other words, we assume that the Test agent is a component that detects new arrival data and is responsible for notifying other components in the system when new information is added. The following data is injected into the agent-based system by the Test agent:

"Alice Female 25 HeartRate 110 Temperature 36.7 SystolicPressure 112 DiastolicPressure 71"

The information above indicates that the updated data belongs to Alice; Alice is a 25-year-old female; following by her new arrival data. The stored data (including new arrival data) of Alice are shown in Table 7.

Figure 7 shows the current wellness level and current weight setting for Alice when she logs into the system, and the results produced by the agent-based system when the new data comes while user is logging in. The Problem list and Description Textarea tells Alice about normal and abnormal in her new arrival health information with description. The Suggestion Textarea gives Alice simple suggestion corresponding to the list in the Problem list and Description Textarea. In this case, there is an anomaly in Alice's heart rate (i.e. lower than normal range). Thus, the agent-based system provides statistical information relatives to the heart rate parameter to her as well. With the statistical information, the user obtains descriptive statistical information about the heart rate parameter from the past to present. The system also evaluates the trend and how much the heart rate parameter is linearly correlated with other parameters of the users. In this case, the heart rate parameter has highest linear-correlation with the systolic pressure parameter (i.e. Pearson's correlation coefficient = 0.9061428199615739, Coefficient of Determination = 0.8210948101679133, t-value =6.059407742273888 and degree of freedom = 8.0)

All test cases submitted to the system have been validated and confirm the correctness of the system. However, the use of simulated data can only be acceptable for preliminary results. To validate the system and improve the effectiveness of its rules, the system needs to be tested with real data with full diagnostic information.

CONCLUSION AND FUTURE WORK

This paper presents an agent-based visualization system that will provide direct benefits to the public. The visualization system is designed to be used as a single wellness indicator for an individual and a one-station examination for health care professionals. The single wellness indicator gives a simplified view of health information to a general user. Therefore, the visualization system potentially stimulates an individual to have self-awareness in an individual's wellness and the public's health. In case of the one-station examination, the visualization system assists the health care professionals by providing comprehensive health information with analyse information. That information can be used for rapid evaluation and to make the health care services process faster.

The major expected result of this research is a proof of concept that meets the objectives highlighted in Section II. All findings and experience gained in developing the agent-based wellness visualization system will be made available to the medical community and to the public. Since modularity and expandability is pursued in this research, it is possible for the wellness visualization system to be expanded to develop more sophisticated systems in the future.

Figure 8. Data management component

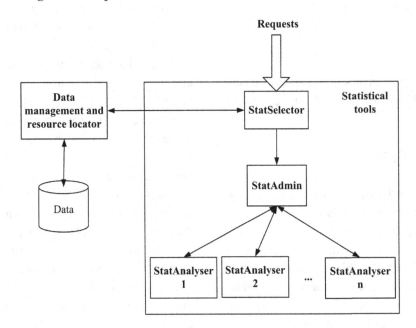

Figure 9. Multi user concurrent system

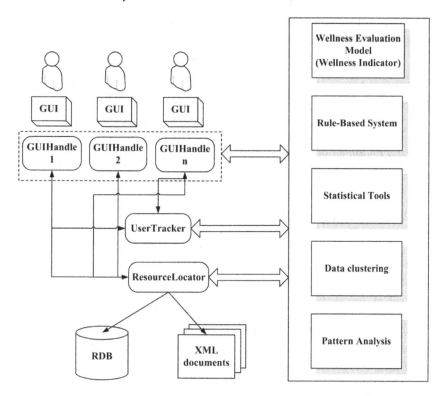

The next step of development is to add StatAnalyser agents that can calculate other statistical methods, as directed by the results. Currently, the StatAdmin agent can only receive initial data from simulated messages, and then, forward the data to all StatAnalyser agents registered to it. In reality, we need a mechanism that selects statistical methods matching with all requests from the outsiders and retrieves corresponding information from the data sources. This idea will be developed in the next step as well, for better efficiency and scalability.

This research also has not yet been validated with a full-scale trial. As this system is not a diagnostic system, there is no need for a double blind clinical trial, and instead we can make use of existing annotated data to refine the rules and the behaviour of the complete system. However, such annotated datasets are not readily available,

and currently the research team is in the process of obtaining one.

Figure 9 shows a multi-user concurrent access system, the final objective of this research.

REFERENCES

Aglets (2002). Retrieved July 27, 2006, from http://www.trl.ibm.com/aglets/

Asadachatreekul, S. (2004). *An Agent-based Distributed Inference Engine for Expert System Construction.* University of Regina, Regina.

Bellin, H. T., Fellner, D., & Tchorbajian, N. (1985). *Portable EKG monitoring device for ST deviation.* Retrieved July 4, 2007, from http://www.freepatentsonlines.com/4546776.html

Blood Pressure Monitor. Retrieved December 20, 2007, from http://www.omronhealthcare.com/enTouchCMS/app/viewCategory?catgId=23

Brown, M. (2007). *U of A contributes to all-in-one health device*. Retrieved December 20, 2007, from http://www.expressnews.ualberta.ca/article.cfm?id=8955

Broyles, R. W. (2006). *Fundamentals of statistics in health administration* (1st ed.). Sudbury, Massachusetts: Jones & Bartlett Publishers.

Concordia (2004). Retrieved July 27, 2006, from http://www.merl.com/projects/concordia/

Core Health Indicators. (2007). Retrieved December 24, 2007, from http://www.who.int/whosis/database/core/core_select_process.cfm

Daly, L. E., & Bourke, G. J. (2000). *Interpretation and uses of medical statistics* (5th ed.). Oxford: Blackwell Science Ltd.

Dunn, H. L. (1959). High-level Wellness for Man and Society. *American Journal of Public Health and the Nation's Health, 49*(6), 7.

Fowler, J., Jarvis, P., & Chevannes, M. (2002). *Practical Statistics for Nursing and Health Care* (1st ed.). Chichester: John Wiley and Sons.

Harris, M., & Taylor, G. (2003). Medical Statistic Made Easy. In A. Bosher (Ed.), Taylor & Francis e-Library.

Health Level 7 (1997). Retrieved January 31, 2008, from http://www.hl7.org/

Health Promotion Glossary Update. Retrieved May 29, 2007, from http://www.who.int/health-promotion/about/HPR%20Glossary_New%20Terms.pdf

Heart Rate Monitor. Retrieved December 20, 2007, from http://www.omronhealthcare.com/enTouchCMS/app/viewCategory?catgId=33

Introduction to Medical Statistics. (2001, November 6, 2001). Retrieved January 23, 2008, from http://www.brettscaife.net/statistics/introstat/index.html

Jantachume, W. (1999). สถิติที่ใช้ในการวิเคราะห์ข้อมูล: การวิจัยทางการพยาบาล (1 ed.). Khon kaen: Faculty of Nursing, Khon kaen University, Thailand. Keogh, E., Lin, J., & Fu, A. *Datasets*. Retrieved January 31, 2008, from http://www.cs.ucr.edu/~eamonn/discords/

Martens, R., Hu, W., Liu, A., Mahovsky, J., Saenchai, K., Schauenberg, T., et al. (2001). *TEEMA TRLabs Execution Environment for Mobile Agents*. Regina: Telecommunication Research and Laboratories (TRLabs) Regina.

Mirkin, B. (2005). *Clustering for Data Mining: A Data Recovery Approach* (1st ed.). London: Chapman & Hall/CRC. *Monitoring asthma symptoms*. Retrieved July 4, 2007, from http://chealth.canoe.ca/channel_section_details.asp?text_id=3405&channel_id=2014&relation_id=18605

Munro, B. H. (2005). *Statistical Methods for Health Care Research* (5th ed.). Philadelphia: Lippincott Williams & Wilkins.

Omron, H. *J-720ITC Pocket Pedometer with Advanced Omron Health Management Software*. Retrieved December 20, 2007, from http://www.amazon.com/Omron-HJ-720ITC-Pedometer-Advanced-Management/dp/B000MN92WM/ref=pd_sbs_sg_title_3

Raymond, S. A., Gordon, G. E., & Singer, D. B. (1998, July 14, 1998). *US Patent 5778882 - Health monitoring system*. Retrieved July 4, 2007, from http://www.patentstorm.us/patents/5778882/fulltext.html

The six dimensional wellness model. Retrieved May 29, 2007, from http://www.nationalwellness.org/index.php?id=391&id_tier=381

Walker, G. A. (2002). *Common Statistical Methods for Clinical Research with SAS® Examples* (2nd ed.). Cary, North Carolina, USA: Institute Inc.

What is wellness. Retrieved June 12, 2007, from http://www.hooah4health.com/overview/wellness.htm

Chapter 9
Using Probabilistic Neural Network to Select a Medical Specialist Agent

Vijay Kumar Mago
DAV College, India

M. Syamala Devi
Panjab University, India

Ajay Bhatia
CTIM&IT, India

Ravinder Mehta
Mehta Childcare Center, India

ABSTRACT

The authors aim to design the Multi-agent system, in which the software agents interact with each other to diagnose a disease and decide the treatment plan(s). In this chapter, the authors present a novel approach of applying Probabilistic Neural Network (PNN) to classify the childhood disease and their respective medical specialist. Normally this classification is performed by the pediatricians. The system that has been presented here, imitates the behavior of a pediatrician while selecting super specialist doctor. This decision making mechanism will be embedded in an agent called Intelligent Pediatric Agent. To design the PNN, a database consisting of 104 records has been gathered. It includes 17 different sign symptoms and based on their values, one of the five super specialists is selected. A Back propagation Neural Network (BPNN) has also been designed to compare the results produced by the PNN and it is found that PNN is more promising.

INTRODUCTION

In medical domain, there are conditions which demand participation of different super specialists

DOI: 10.4018/978-1-60566-772-0.ch009

to handle the situation. A specialist has to decide whom to consult for advice. For instance, if a child is suffering from heart stroke as well as dyspnoea (see Appendix A) then, the pediatrician may decide to consult the cardiac surgeon. Medical specialists face such circumstances quite frequently and they tend to learn this decision making through their experiences and keep updating their medical knowledge.

There are number of researchers around the world, from various streams viz. operation research, computer science, mathematics and statistics, trying to design a system that can emulate the behavior of any specialist for such decision making. In the next section, we shall discuss some of the decision making systems. These systems are primarily based on Neural Networks.

This chapter is a part of the Multi-agent system described by Devi (2005).Let us briefly describe the terms used for healthcare professionals in India. A General Doctor (GD) is one who holds basic medical degree like MBBS and is usually positioned at the rural areas to provide general medical treatments. A specialist doctor/physician holds higher postgraduate degree (like M.S., M.D.) after his/her graduation. These specialists are posted at the district level and serve as referral centers. Super Specialist physician holds further specialization degrees (like DM, MCh) in medical or surgical fields and are usually placed at the research institutes and the laboratories.

For each level of healthcare center, we develop the agents to assist the doctors. The basic definition and attributes of an agent are described by Bradshaw (1997). The agent that supports GD is termed as User Agent (UA), and the agent that behaves as a pediatrician is named as Intelligent Pediatric Agent (IPA). During normal diagnosing procedure, UA and IPA communicate with each other (Mago & Devi, 2007). But in some cases the IPA seeks help from the Super Specialist Agent (SSA) to diagnose the disease and then to decide the treatment plan. The situation involves the decision making on the part of the IPA to select an appropriate SSA. This decision making is very crucial for the effectiveness of healthcare delivery system. Hence, the aim of this chapter is restricted to decide which SSA is to be contacted as per the given sign symptoms provided by the

UA. To solve this complex problem, Probabilistic Neural Network (PNN) and Back Propagation Neural Network (BPNN) based decision making system is developed.

In order to understand the whole system, an abstract view of the system is described in the subsequent sub section.

Abstract View

The Multi Agent System (MAS) is a system in which the agents are connected in an intelligent fashion so as to achieve their pre-defined objectives (Wooldridge, 2002). These agents interact with each other, according to their capabilities, and try to produce the desired result. Moreover, there may or may not be any human interference as the intelligence is supposed to be embedded in them (as a software code).

There are numerous papers describing usage of MAS in healthcare. All these papers are domain specific; for instance, they provide assistance to patients for the appointments or support the doctors in diagnosing some specific diseases. They are also used to give advice to health care personnel dealing with the traumatized patients, and to improve vaccination rates, etc. All these systems are aimed at improving the medical delivery system. Similarly, we also aspire to create an agent based environment to provide medical assistance for childhood diseases.

Figure 1 depicts an abstract view of the system wherein, the UA, IPA and the SSA are shown. The UA supplies the sign-symptoms; the IPA using its knowledge tries to provide the assistance by providing treatment plan(s). In certain cases, the IPA finds it difficult to diagnose a disease, it utilizes the PNN and the BPNN based decision making system to decide the SSA. Mago (2007), describes a system based on Bayesian Network (BN) to handle the same problem, but it lacks future enhancement. The BN based systems are inflexible in nature, i.e. one needs to re-work on the prior probabilities altogether if there is any

Figure 1. Abstract view of the MAS System

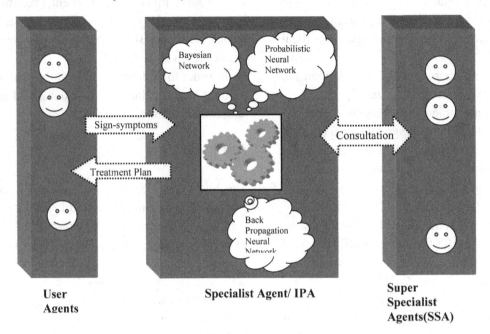

User Agents · **Specialist Agent/ IPA** · **Super Specialist Agents(SSA)**

modification in the network.

The current work presented in this chapter deals with the decision making based on the PNN and the BPNN. It does not suffer from the above mentioned anomaly; instead it provides a mechanism for future enhancements. The IPA here is fully automated and it does not require human intervention at all, whereas the UA does require human interaction with the system.

Capabilities of Agents

In this subsection, we discuss the roles and capabilities of each agent of the system.

- **User Agent:** This agent is designed to interact with the GD on one end and the IPA on the other. It also provides a graphical user interface to the GD. The main tasks performed by it in chronological order are discussed below.
  - Register the general doctor with the IPA.

  - Pose some basic questions related to the condition of the patient to the general doctor,
  - Receive information filled by the GD and pass that to the IPA,
  - Display further queries asked by the IPA,
  - Again receive the inputs and pass the information to the IPA, and
  - Finally display the treatment plan suggested by the IPA.

- **Intelligent Pediatric Agent:** This agent is fully automated, i.e. no human intervention is required. It imitates the behavior of a pediatrician. The pediatrician serves as a referral physician to GD and helps in diagnosing the disease and suggests the treatment plan. All these functionalities have been kept while designing this agent. The capabilities and role that it performs are discussed below:
  - Interact with the UA on one side and the SSA on the other.

- ○ Suggest the treatment plan as per the sign-symptoms provided by the UA.
- ○ During complicated case, either use BN based technique to decide which SSA is to be contacted or use NN based techniques to decide about the SSA.
- ○ Pass the values of sign-symptoms to the SSA for diagnosing the disease and the treatment plan.
- ○ Contact the UA with the treatment plan as suggested by the SSA.
- **Super Specialist Agent:** This agent is designed to accept sign-symptoms from IPA and display them to the super specialist physician. The specialist decides the disease by asking more questions to the IPA and finally it passes the diagnosed disease and its treatment plan to IPA. The capabilities and roles performed by it are listed below:
  - ○ Interact with the IPA on one side and super specialist physician on the other.
  - ○ Display the sign-symptoms provided by the IPA.
  - ○ Using the interface of this agent, the super specialist physician may ask for more values of various sign-symptoms to the IPA.
  - ○ Pass the diagnosed disease and its treatment plan to the IPA.

The main task of this agent is to provide an interface between IPA and super specialist physician.

In the next section, we shall discuss the applications which have been developed by using NN techniques to classify the problem domain in different categories.

BACKGROUND

It is essential to understand that the NN based techniques are producing promising results in the decision making systems in general and particularly in medical domain. And we shall argue that these techniques can be useful in the MASs too.

The use of the PNN has been noticed in medical domain with the aim of classifying the intensity of the disease or monitoring of vital parameters. There is a discussion by Orr (1997) on a system that implements a PNN to estimate mortality risk following cardiac surgery. The aim is to predict the patient survivability after open-heart surgery. Similarly, Huang and Liaq (2004) discuss the classification results for two types of acute leukemias and five categories of embryonal tumors of the central nervous system. They found the computation speed to be satisfactory and 100% recognition accuracy in classifying the type of leukemia.

There is another system in medical sphere (Sakane & Tsuji, 2004), which utilizes the PNN for monitoring vital parameters of patients for diagnosing purpose. This paper proposes a method to discriminate the vascular conditions from biological signals by using the PNN, and develops the diagnosis support system to judge the patient's conditions on-line.

A modified PNN for brain tissue segmentation with magnetic resonance imaging is proposed by Song and Jamshidi (2007). In their research, a new method is proposed which is based on a novel self-organizing map–weighted probabilistic neural network structure, to estimate the probability density function of pixels from brain MR images.

In another research by Sung-Neil and Kaun-To (2008) the methods to integrate independent component analysis (ICA) and neural network for electrocardiogram (ECG) beat classification have been developed. The ICA is used to decompose ECG signals into weighted sum of the basic components which are statistically mutual independent. Two neural networks, the PNN and the BPNN, are employed as classifiers. The ECG samples attributing to eight different beat types are sampled from the MIT-BIH arrhythmia database for experiments. The results show high classification accuracy of over 98% with either of the two classifiers.

Similarly, in some researches expert system is also used along with PNN, like in (Karabatak & Ince, 2008). It utilizes association rule (AR) for reducing dimension of the breast cancer database and NN is used for intelligent classification. This research demonstrated that the AR can be used for reducing the dimension of feature space and proposed AR+NN model can be used to obtain fast automatic diagnostic systems for other diseases.

Other investigators, Li, Chiu and Jian (2000), describe the use of the NNs in decision making for surgery to traumatic brain injury patients. This system aids physician and other medical professional in making uncertain medical decisions. It consists of three mathematical models for generating traumatic brain injury medical decision support system on clinical database. The result suggests that the NN may be a better option for complex, non-linear medical decision support systems than conventional techniques.

In another study conducted by Patel and Hanley (1995), an object oriented Artifical Neural Networks (ANN) is used for dermatological decision making. It demonstrates the clinical decision making process to analyze the skin lipid data from patients having microbial skin diseases.

Vartziotis, Fotiadis, and Lagaris (2003) developed a tool on the decision making for health professionals based on the NN. It supports the GUI for visualizing 2-D and 3-D data for biomedical problems. Apart from medical domain, the NN techniques are used in other fields too for decision making as discussed in (Tian, Azimi-Sadjadi & Haar, 2000), (Mao, Tan & Ser, 2000) and (Xin, Dipti, & Long, 2001).

All these systems are efficient and effective but, are domain specific and independent in nature. There is immense scope of utilizing such systems in the Multi-agent environment. That is why; we present the NN based decision making system for the agent.

In the next section we shall discuss the basics of the NN and the construction of the NN as per our requirements.

METHODOLOGY

Introduction to Neural Networks

Neural Network is the interconnection of the neurons. The connection between two neurons is also called synapses. In computers, the NN is nothing but simulation of Biological Neuron Network (BNN). The BNN is in the brain of human beings and helps to process the information from one neuron to another. And hence it develops reasoning capability and other forms of intelligence. In computer terminology, the NN is also called Artificial Neural Network (ANN). The ANN is an adaptive system that changes itself based on information that flows through it. The ANN is used for applications like pattern recognition, classification and function approximation. The usage of the NNs is not only limited to the branch of computing but also widely used in other fields like physics, chemistry, mathematics, economics, psychology, neurophysiology, medicine, and many others.

In the proceeding sub section, we discuss the working of the BPNN and the PNN.

Back Propagation Neural Network

A back propagation neural network is a fully connected, feed-forward neural network. The flow of data is unidirectional: from input layer to output layer through hidden layer. Every neuron in a layer is connected to each neuron of next layer in forward direction. The BPNN may contain multiple hidden layers. Knowledge of the network is encoded in the weights between neurons. The activation levels of the output layer neurons determine the output of the whole network.

The BPNN commences with a random set of connection weights. The network regulates its weights according to some learning rules each time it observes a pair of input-output vector. Every pair of vectors goes through two phases of activation: a forward pass and a backward pass. The forward pass implicates producing the network a sample input to the network and allowing activation flow until they reach the output layer. During the backward pass, the network's actual output is compared with the target output and errors are compared for the output layer neurons. The weights connected to the output neurons can be adjusted in order to reduce those errors. The error estimates of the output layer neurons are then used to obtain error estimates for the neurons in the hidden layer. After, all errors are back propagated to connections originating from the input layer neurons. After each round of forward–backward passes, the system learns incrementally from the input-output pair and gradually reduces the error between the network's predicted output and the actual output.

Although one can adjust the neural network to lower its errors but can never be sure of lowering of the error. The aim of network training is to find the lowest point in this many-dimensional surface. Since the NN error surfaces are very complex so it is impossible to determine analytically where the global minimum of the error surface is, so the NN training is essentially an exploration of the error surface. Typically, the slope of the error surface is calculated at the current point, and used to make a downhill move. Finally, the algorithm stops in a low point, which may be a local minimum.

The algorithm, shown in Figure 2, progresses iteratively through a number of epochs. On each epoch (an epoch corresponds to a given number of training cycles).

This error, together with the error surface gradient, is used to adjust the weights, and then the process repeats. The initial network configu-

ration is random and training stops when a given number of the epochs pass by, or when the error reaches at an acceptable level, or when the error stops improving. Figure 3 describes the basic the input-output structure of the BPNN.

Probabilistic Neural Network

Probabilistic Neural Network is a type of the NN, which consists of three layers of nodes; the Input Layer, the Hidden Layer and the Output Layer (Specht[1], 1990). More specifically, PNN is a type of the NN which uses probability factor for pattern recognition problems. It uses supervised training to assemble distributed functions contained by a pattern layer. These functions are used to approximate the possibility of an input class vector being a part of the learned group. Now these patterns can be combined with the probability of each category to determine the most likely class for the input vector. A pattern layer is an implementation of Bayes Classifier (Specht[2], 1990); in which probability functions are approximated, using a Parzen estimator (Parezen,1962). This is optimum approach of pattern classification and it minimizes the risk of wrong classification. The basic structure of the PNN is shown in figure 4. The PNN training is much simpler than the BPNN. However, the pattern layer can be fairly huge if the distinction between categories is varied and at the same time quite similar in special areas.

Design of Probabilistic Neural Network and Back Propagation Neural Network

In this sub section, we discuss the various sign-symptoms, their respective causes and the super specialist doctors that can be consulted by the pediatrician. It is necessary to understand the sign-symptoms because the presence of one can affect the occurrence of another and hence may result in causing a disease.

Figure 2. Back Propagation Algorithm

Start : begin epoch
    for inp=1 to m
      for each training vector Xp
        Execute **Forward Pass**
        Execute **Backward Pass**
      end for
    end for
    end epoch

    Calculate the error $\text{Err} = \sum_{p-1}^{p} E_P$

    if Err is acceptably low
      then stop
    else
      goto start
    end if
End

Description of Sign Symptoms

Signs and symptoms can be termed as diagnostic indicators which help the doctor determine the condition of the patient. In simple terms, signs are those things that the doctor can see or observe, and symptoms are those feelings that the patient explains. For instance: Pain would be a symptom (a doctor can't see it, but the patient can tell the doctor that he has pain and the extent of it). Tenderness of that area is a sign that a doctor can observe.

Figure 3. Applying inputs to the neural network

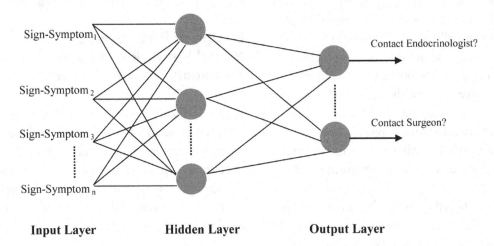

Figure 4. Basic structure of probabilistic neural network

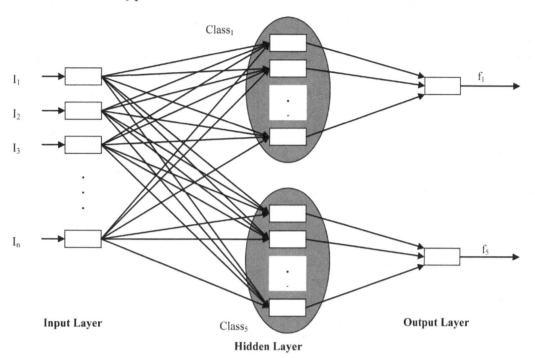

We decide to consider only those sign-symptoms which occur frequently in children. The presence of some sign-symptoms causes uncertainty in the selection of the super specialist doctors. These sign symptoms are listed in Appendix A.

Definition of Consultants

It is necessary to understand the super specialist doctors who can be consulted by child specialist during intense conditions. These doctors work in only one branch. A brief definition of these consultants is given in Appendix B.

Design of Algorithms and Implementation

We took 104 records of 17 different sign-symptoms, for creation of both PNN and BPNN. The values of these sign-symptoms are normalized in the range of 0-1. For instance, if any sign-symptoms have value Yes/No, then it is assigned value 1/0. Similarly for Severe/Moderate/Mild condition, the values assigned are 1, 0.67, and 0.33 respectively. The values of attributes are collected in MS-Excel file. The coding and analysis of the PNN and the BPNN is conducted in the MATLAB (http://www.mathworks.com/). The step wise procedures for creation of the NN and usage of the NN are given below:

Algorithm to create BNN and PNN

Start:

Step 1: Read sign-symptoms and consulted super specialist in vector S_i and P_i respectively

Step 2: Normalize S_i and P_i to map all the values in [0,1]

Step 3: Create PN and BN as PNN and BPNN network respectively

Step 4: Train both PN and PN with S_i and P_i

End

Algorithm to simulate BNN and PNN

Start:

Step 1: Select sign-symptoms from User Interface provided and fetch them into vector I_i

Step 2: Supply I_i to PN and BN (created in above algorithm)

Step 3: Simulate PN and BN

Step 4: Fetch the resultant statistics

End

Application Scenario

The UA and IPA interact with each other to diagnose the disease but during uncertainty, the IPA flashes the screen that is shown in figure 5. The general doctor then using the GUI of the UA selects the sign-symptoms and the reasoning algorithm. For instance, he chooses the sign-symptoms as Chest Pain to Yes, Vomiting to Moderate, Cough to Moderate, Dyspnoea to Severe, and Fever to Severe. The PNN is chosen as the decision making mechanism. These algorithms are part of the IPA which is currently behaving as a server. In this example, the PNN produces the result "Contact Pulmonologist" This result is then passed back to the UA and hence the GD The same output is achieved through the BPNN.

FUTURE TRENDS

The current research aims at the selection of a super specialist, more precisely, a SSA for consultation. The UA supplies the sign-symptoms and the IPA tries to recommend the treatment plan according to its own knowledge. Up to this point, only general doctor using interface of the UA needs to interact with the system but if the IPA, emulating as a child specialist, finds it difficult to respond back, then the pediatrician himself needs to intervene and decide for a super specialist. We aim to automate this decision making. In this direction, we have demonstrated that the PNN and the BPNN provide a sound decision making mechanism. But the system has so far not included the following factors:

- After the selection of the super specialist, the IPA and the SSA interact with each other to decide about the disease and its treatment plan. The UA is not involved in this discussuion or it is not aware of the dialogues. This is a grave problem as the system lacks transparency.
- The system is restricted to the selection of a single specialist only, whereas in real-life problems, a child specialist consults various specialists for diagnosis. The system fails to take into account this complex scenario.

We intend to incorporate these above mentioned features in our future works.

CONCLUSION

We have developed a decision making system; Graphical User Interface for an agent called Intelligent Pediatric Agent. The intelligence behavior of this agent is based on ANNs. The GD uses the system to choose the sign-symptoms and the method for the decision making. One can use either the PNN or the BPNN for getting the results. We use both methods for comparing the results and efficiency of the system developed. During trial period, the system is used by a number of the users and based on their feedbacks; we conclude that PNN is more robust and reliable as compared to the BPNN. The PNN classifies the data and flags the result by using the concept of probability and Bayes' Theorem. But on the other hand the BPNN train itself again and again on the set of data for the result. Overall, the system aims to select the medical super specialists intelligently.

Figure 5. Interface of IPA for selection of sign-symptoms

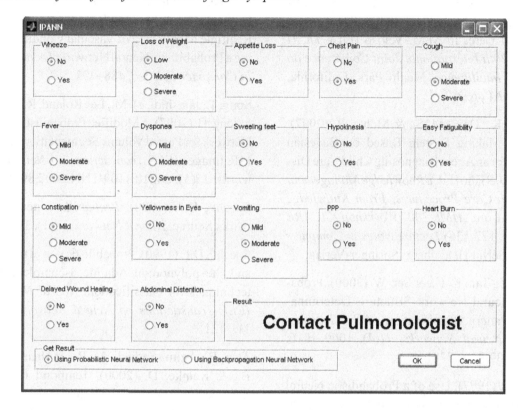

REFERENCES

Bradshaw, J. M. (1997). Software agents. In J. Bradshaw (Ed.), *An introduction to software agents* (pp. 3-46). Cambridge, MA: MIT Press.

Devi, M. S., & Mago, V. (2005). Multi-agent model for Indian rural health care. *Leadership in Health Services*, *18*(4), i–xi. doi:10.1108/13660750510625724

Huang, C. J., & Liao, W. C. (2004). Application of Probabilistic Neural Networks to the Class Prediction of Leukemia and Embryonal Tumor of Central Nervous System. *Neural Processing Letters*, 211–226. doi:10.1023/B:NEPL.0000035613.51734.48

Jin, X., Srinivasan, D., & Cheu, R. L. (2001). Classification of Freeway Traffic Patterns for Incident Detection Using Constructive Probabilistic Neural Networks. *IEEE Transactions on Neural Networks*, *12*(5), 1173–1187. doi:10.1109/72.950145

Karabatak, M., & Ince, M. C. (2008). An expert system for detection of breast caner based on association rules and neural network. *Expert System with Applcations*. Elsevier.

Li, Y. C., Liu, L., Chiu, W. T., & Jian, W. S. (2000). Neural Network modeling for surgical decisions on traumatic brain injury patients. *International Journal of Medical Informatics*, (57): 1–9. doi:10.1016/S1386-5056(99)00054-4

Mago, V. K., & Devi, M. S. (2007). A Multi-Agent Medical System for Indian Rural Infant and Child Care. In M.M. Veloso (Ed.), *IJCAI-07, The 20th International Joint Conference on Artificial Intelligence.* Menlo Park, California, USA: AAAI press

Mago, V. K., Devi, M. S., & Mehta, R. (2007). Decision Making System Based on Bayesian Network for an Agent Diagnosing Child Care Diseases. In D. Riaño (Ed.), *Knowledge Management for Health Care Procedures, From Knowledge to Global Care, AIME 2007 Workshop K4CARE 2007,* (pp. 127-136) *Lecture Notes in Computer Science.* Berlin Heidelberg: Springer-Verlag.

Mao, K. Z., Tan, K. C., & Ser, W. (2000). Probabilistic Neural-Network Structure Determination for Pattern Classification . *IEEE Transactions on Neural Networks, 11*(4), 1009–1016. doi:10.1109/72.857781

Orr, R. K. (1997). Use of a Probabilistic Neural Network to Estimate the Risk of Mortality after Cardiac Surgery. *Medical Decision Making,* (17): 178–185. doi:10.1177/0272989X9701700208

Pan, J., Yung, C., Liang, C., & Lai, L. (2007). An Intelligent Homecare Emergency Service System for Elder Falling. *IFMBE Proceedings,* 424–428. doi:10.1007/978-3-540-36841-0_114

Parzen, E. (1962). On estimation of a probability density function and mode . *Annals of Mathematical Statistics, 33,* 1065–1076. doi:10.1214/aoms/1177704472

Patel, D., Patel, S., & Hanley, D. (1995). Object Oriented Artificial Neural Network in Decision Support Systems for Dermatological Research. *Health Informatics Journal,* (1): 56–68. doi:10.1177/146045829500100206

Sakane, A., Tsuji, T., Yoshiyuki Tanaka, Y., Shiba, K., Saeki, N., & Masashi Kawamoto, M. (2004). Realtime Monitoring of Vascular Conditions Using a Probabilistic Neural Network. *Lecture Notes in Computer Science,* 488–493.

Song, T., Jamshidi, M. M., Lee Roland, R., & Mingxiong, H. (2007). A Modified Probabilistic Neural Network for Partial Volume Segmentation in Brain MR Image. *IEEE Transactions on Neural Networks, 18*(5). doi:10.1109/TNN.2007.891635

Specht[1], D.F. (1990). *Probabilistic* neural networks Source. *Neural Networks, 3*(1), 109-118.

Specht[2], D.F. (1990). Probabilistic neural networks and the polynomial Adaline ascomplementary techniques for classification. *Neural Networks, IEEE Transactions on Neural Networks, 1*(1). 111-121.

Tian, B., Azimi-Sadjadi, M. R., & Haar, T.H.V., B., & Reinke, D. (2000). Temporal Updating Scheme for Probabilistic Neural Network with Application to Satellite Cloud Classification. *IEEE Transactions on Neural Networks, 11*(4), 903–920. doi:10.1109/72.857771

Vartziotis, F., Fotiadis, D. I., Likas, A., & Lagaris, I. E. (2003). A Portable Decision making tool for Health Professionals based on neural networks. *Health Informatics Journal,* (9): 273–282. doi:10.1177/1460458203094005

Wooldridge, M. (2002). *An Introduction to Multiagent Systems.* Chichester, England: John Wiley & Sons

Yu, S. N., & Chou, K. T. (2008). Integration of independent component analysis and neural networks for ECG beat classification. *Expert Systems with Applications,* (34): 2841–2846. doi:10.1016/j.eswa.2007.05.006

APPENDIX A

Abdominal distention: Abdominal distention is often caused by intestinal gas. This may result from eating fibrous foods such as fruits and vegetables. Legumes & beans are common sources of intestinal gas. Abdominal distention may also occasionally result from the accumulation of fluid in the abdomen, which can be a sign of serious medical problems (peritonitis).

Chest Pain: Discomfort/pain in and around the chest. Pain may be caused by physical over-exertion and muscle strains. If pain is associated with shortness of breath, cold sweat, and fatigue, it may be due to heart disorder, lung infection, etc.

Constipation: Constipation is usually subjective. For many people, it simply means infrequent stools. For others, meaning of constipation varies from hard stools, difficulty passing stools (straining), or a sense of incomplete emptying after a bowel movement. The cause of each of these types of constipation is different, and the approach to each should be aimed at specific type of constipation. Medically speaking, constipation usually is defined as fewer than three bowel movements per week. Severe constipation is defined as less than one bowel movement per week.

Cough: Coughing is an important protective reflex of the body & it is a way to keep ones throat and airways clear. However, excessive coughing may point towards some disease & may cause injury also. There are numerous causes, some of them are: Cold, flu, or sinus infection, tuberculosis, Pneumonia, Asthma, Chronic Obstructive Pulmonary Disease or Congestive Heart Failure.

Delayed Wound Healing: It is body's natural defense to restore the integrity of injured tissues by replacement of dead tissues with viable tissues. This starts immediately after an injury, may continue for months or years, and mechanism is essentially the same for all types of wounds. Wound healing may be delayed in conditions where essential mechanisms for the same are denied. Causes include: Infections, Lack of primary wound care, Lack of rest, Weakened General Health, Hypoprotenemia, Insulin Deficiency- diabetes Mellitus, etc.

Dyspnoea: It is difficulty in breathing. A person with this condition usually keeps his head elevated to be able to breathe comfortably. In severe cases, a person wakes up suddenly during the night, feeling shortness of breath- that is called paroxysmal nocturnal dyspnoea. Its main causes are: Chronic obstructive pulmonary disease, Heart failure, Hypertensive heart disease, Obesity (does not directly cause difficulty in breathing while lying down but often aggravates other causes).

Easy Fatigability: In some conditions, body gets easily fatigued & tired in routine work. It is not a symptom of any particular disease. Rather, tiredness can be a symptom of many different diseases and conditions. Reasons of tiredness range from lack of sleep and over exercise to medical cause. The lack of energy can sometimes cause difficulty with normal daily activities, leading to attentive and concentration problems.

Fever: The average normal body temperature is 98.6°F (37°C). Normal body temperature varies by person, age, activity, and time of the day. A rectal temperature of > 100.4°F (38°C) is considered as fever.

Some of the main causes of fever are: Cold or flu-like illnesses, Pneumonia, Appendicitis, Tuberculosis, Meningitis, Sore throats and step throat, Acute bronchitis, AIDS and HIV infection, Cancer, Leukemia, etc.

Heart Burn: Heartburn is a painful burning sensation in the food-pipe, esophagus, which lies just behind the breastbone. The pain often rises in chest and may radiate to neck or throat. Heartburn is more likely to occur if you have a hiatal hernia, which is when the top part of the stomach protrudes upward into the chest cavity. Heartburn can be brought on or worsened by pregnancy and by many different medications.

Hypokinesia: Hypokinesia means slowness in body movements. There is slowed ability to start and continue movements, and impaired ability to adjust the body's position. It can be a symptom of neurological disorders, particularly Parkinson's disease, or a side effect of medications.

Loss of weight: It can be described as decrease in body weight that is not voluntary, i.e. unintentional. There are many causes of unintentional weight loss. Some are: Diarrhea that is chronic (lasts a long time), Eating disorders, including anorexia nervosa and bulimia, Hyperthyroidism, Infections like Tuberculosis, Loss of appetite, etc.

Loss of appetite: A reduced desire to eat, despite the body's basic energy needs. Any illness can affect a previously normal appetite. It can cause weight loss, emotional upset, anxiety, bereavement, and depression.

Polyphagia /Polyuria /Polydipsia: Polyphagia means increased appetite, Polyuria means increased passage of urine, while Polydipsia means increased thirst. Increased appetite is having an excess desire for food. Hyperphagia and polyphagia refer to being focused only on eating excessively. These can be treated as symptoms of different diseases like: Bulimia, Diabetes mellitus, Hyperthyroidism, Hypoglycemia, Premenstrual syndrome, Anxiety, Certain drugs (such as corticosteroids, cyproheptadine, and tricyclic antidepressants), etc.

Swelling Feet: In an ambulatory patient, lower limbs being the dependent part, abnormal buildup of fluid occurs in feet, and legs. It is also called dependent edema. Painless swelling of the feet and ankles is a common problem, particularly in older people. Lower limb swelling is common with the diseases: heart failure, kidney failure, or liver failure.

Vomiting: Vomit is an unintentional discharge of stomach and sometimes intestinal contents from the mouth. The main causes are: Hyperthyroidism, Tumors in the brain, Gastroenteritis, Gastric ulcers and Gallstones

Wheeze: Wheezing is a whistle-like sound during breathing. Wheezing indicates that a person may be having respiratory problems. It is heard when air flows through narrowed-down airways. The main causes are: Asthma, Pneumonia, Bronchitis, Heart failure (cardiac asthma), and Viral infection, especially in infants younger than 2 years.

Yellowness in Eyes: The white part of eyes i.e sclera turns yellow typically in jaundice, which is often related to a liver disorder such as hepatitis. These conditions can be serious and require prompt professional medical diagnosis and treatment. Acute viral hepatitis is the most common cause of jaundice. Hepatotoxic viruses may affect various age groups.

Appendix B

Cardiologist: Cardiology is the super specialist branch in internal medicine dealing with disorders of the heart and its blood vessels. Physicians specializing in this field of medicine are called cardiologists. Cardiac surgeons are those doctors who perform cardiac surgery - operative procedures on the heart and great vessels e.g. Bypass Surgery. The field is commonly divided into different branches according to the type of disease, like congenital heart defects, coronary artery disease, valvular heart disease, and heart failure.

Endocrinologist: Endocrinology is a branch of medicine which deals with disorders of the endocrine system (Glands) and its secretions called hormones. Endocrinology is concerned with the study of the synthesis, storage, and physiological function of hormones and with the cells of the endocrine glands and tissues that secrete them.

Gastroenterologist: Gastroenterology is the branch of medicine which deals with the digestive system and its disorders. Diseases affecting the gastrointestinal tract (i.e. organs from mouth to anus) are included in this specialty. Doctors specializing in the field are called gastroenterologists.

Pulmonologist: Pneumology is the specialty that deals with diseases of the lungs and the respiratory tract. It is also called respiratory medicine and chest medicine. Pulmonology is generally considered a branch of internal medicine, dealing with lungs & pleura. Pulmonology is concerned with the diagnosis and treatment of lung diseases, as well as secondary prevention (tuberculosis). Physicians specializing in this area are called pulmonologists.

Surgeon: A surgeon is a person who performs operations on patients. Surgery deals with surgical treatments that are operative, manual and instrumental techniques on a patient to investigate and/or treat a disease or injury, to help improve body functions or appearance, or sometimes for some different reason.

Chapter 10
A Multi–Agent Simulation of Kidney Function for Medical Education

Kin Lik Wang
University of Hawaii, USA

Nancy E. Reed
University of Hawaii, USA

Dale S. Vincent
University of Hawaii, USA

ABSTRACT

This chapter describes a multi-agent system to simulate kidney function for the purpose of teaching renal physiology to healthcare students. Renal function is modeled with agents. Agents represent molecules and fluids and the environment represents the structures, membranes and volumes of the nephrons in the kidneys. The agents move dynamically through their environment, responding appropriately depending on their surroundings. The authors describe how this multi-agent system is used in research and teaching medical students about the renal system. Results of heuristic and usability testing by medical students show improved visualization of the function of the renal system and self-confidence in learning renal physiology.

INTRODUCTION

Renal physiology is exceptionally difficult to learn. The countercurrent exchange system of the kidney was ranked number one in basic science difficulty and number two in clinical difficulty in a 1990 survey of medical educators (Dawson-Saunders, Feltovich, Coulson, & Steward, 1990). Project TOUCH was a multiyear collaboration between the University of Hawaii and the University of New Mexico in which virtual reality (VR) applications were developed to advance medical education. One application was a 3D VR fly-through model of the kidney (Alverson & Saiki, 2006). Each kidney is composed of millions of nephrons. Our simulation shows the details of one nephron, while adjacent nephrons are shown without detail for context. The simulation prototype has subsequently been enhanced with a new user

DOI: 10.4018/978-1-60566-772-0.ch010

interface and gaming motifs. The new system underwent heuristic and usability tests that are described in this chapter.

The kidney's function is to eliminate water soluble wastes from the body (Banasik, 2000). We chose a multi-agent system implementation because it results in more realistic and detailed model. Agents represent the motion of molecules and fluids within a nephron's tubules. The agents move dynamically and intelligently within their environment to simulate different kidney function, such as water reabsorption and waste secretion.

The rest of this paper is organized as follows. First, multiagent systems and the renal system are described. Second, we describe the implementation and characteristics of our simulation system. Then the visualization of difficult concepts to aid understanding is described. Finally, the usability experiments conducted and the results obtained are described followed by future trends for agents in medical simulations and finally, the conclusion.

BACKGROUND

Multi-Agent Systems Applied in Healthcare

A multi-agent system (MAS) is composed of agents, each of which selects its own course of action based upon its goals (Weiss, 1999; Wooldridge, 2002). Most definitions of agents include the following characteristics: a) An agent perceives its environment, decides on actions, and uses its effectors to perform the selected actions. b) An agent is active over a period of time, taking action based on the world it senses at the moment, c) Agents interact with one another directly through messaging or indirectly through their actions on their common environment, d) An agent has goal(s) as well as some latitude as to how to achieve those goals (Barber et al., 2003). A multi-agent system may be incorporated in a physical (robotic) body, or sense and act upon the world entirely in software simulations, or computer applications, often called softbots.

Multiagent systems have been used in a broad range of applications including soccer games (Robocup, 2008), search and rescue operations (Robocup Rescue, 2008), space (Bernard et al., 1999; NASA, 2008), and military applications (Zafar, Qazi, & Baig, 2006; Sklar, Davies, & Co., 2004) describe SimEd, a simulation of the interactions that occur among students, teachers and administrators. Their aim is to create a toolkit that will allow policy makers to experiment with their decisions.

Agents have also been used in medical applications. The journal *Artificial Intelligence in Medicine* recently published a special issue on software agents in health care (Moreno & Garbay, 2005). *IEEE Intelligent Systems* and *AI Communications* did similar special issues recently.

Examples of agents in medicine include Hudson & Cohen (2006), who use agents to support rural healthcare of the elderly. Poulopoulos, Gortizis, Bakettas, and Nikiforidis (2001) use intelligent agents to track patient information in large databases for use in a telemedicine system. Experience with agent systems in the GruSMA research group is described by Moreno, Valls, Isern, & Sanchez (2006). Vicari et al. (2003) designed a multi-agent system to support the training of diagnostic reasoning and modeling of domains with complex and uncertain knowledge. Prado, Roa, Reina-Tosina, Palma, & Milan (2001) describe a telemedicine system to support patients with end stage renal disease. This system focuses on the monitoring and treatment/therapy for patients with advanced renal disease.

Most agent applications in medicine, including those above, are focused on decision-support for physicians and/or patients. In contrast, the goal of our system is to teach physiological concepts to health care professionals. When health care workers have a better understanding of the physiology of the human body, they can also understand the effects of disease processes in patients, which can improve the quality of care delivered to the patient. Knowing the specific changes that occur in a disease's progression, physicians are able to watch more carefully for signs that the patient is worsening. Hopefully this results in earlier treatment and less severe outcomes. Our program encourages the user to experiment with renal function by changing parameters and viewing the results in a 3D VR environment.

Why use agents for this project? There are many ways to represent moving molecules, which form the basis of our renal simulation. Reeves (1983) introduced a particle system method for modeling fuzzy objects such as fire, clouds, and water. The resulting model is able to represent motion, changes of form, and dynamics, but this approach does not produce the randomness needed in the kidney domain.

Chenney (2004) used flow tiles to represent and design velocity fields. Each flow tile contains small fields, and many tiles can be combined to produce a larger flow. He describes three applications: a crowd on a city street, a river flowing between banks, and swirling fog. We could apply the flow tile concept to the particle, but the problem is that flow tiles use a pre-defined path, so it is hard to use flow tiles to model reabsorption and secretion that are necessary in the kidneys.

One type of multiagent system algorithm is swarm intelligence. Baumgartner, Magele, and Renhart (2004) proposed using particle swarm optimization which imitates the social behavior of birds in a flock flying and sitting down on a pylon. Yoon & Maher (2005) describe a tool to generate path finding aids in a dynamic virtual ant colony. Ants look for food by wandering randomly from their home colony. If they find food, they return to their colony while laying down pheromone (scent) trails that can be followed by other ants. The pheromones are a simple but effective means of communication. Ants are behaviorally unsophisticated and yet, collectively, they perform complex tasks. The ant colony algorithm can run continuously and adapt to changes in real

time. In another example, Schmickl, Thenius, & Crailsheim (2005) modeled honey bees foraging for nectar in a dynamic environment. Without any global decision making, the bees are able to select optimal paths to and from multiple available nectar sources, for example those offering the best ratio of food to cost.

The swarm intelligence models have an advantage over simulated annealing and genetic algorithm approaches in dynamically changing environments (Janson, Merkle, & Middendorf, 2008). Simulated annealing and genetic algorithms are computationally expensive, which may prevent the simulation from running in "real time".

Thomas, Layton, Layton & Moore (2006) provide a summary of the contributions of mathematical models of the kidney. The models are at various levels of detail and their purpose is to obtain a comprehensive understanding of renal function. To that end, the authors are creating new resources (given the name Physiome) to provide general access to current and future models to enhance collaboration between researchers.

The agents in our multi-agent system are similar to the insects described above. Each agent has simple behavior rules that govern their movement. Even though the actions of the agents individually are simple, the resulting behavior is complex. The agent paradigm provides a distributed, robust framework ideal for modeling the renal system. The graphics engine displays the environment and the movement of the agents in 3D.

The Structure and Function of the Kidneys

Humans have two kidneys that each contain more than a million nephrons. A nephron contains eight functional parts as shown in Figure 1: (A) glomerulus, (B) Bowman's capsule, (C) proximal convoluted tubule, (D) descending loop of Henle, (E) ascending loop of Henle, (F) distal convoluted tubule, (G) the collecting tubule, and (H) vasa recta. Thus, fluid flows from A – G in

Figure 1. The eight parts of a nephron in a kidney. (A) glomerulus, (B) Bowman's capsule, (C) proximal convoluted tubule, (D) descending loop of Henle, (E) ascending loop of Henle, (F) distal convoluted tubule, (G) the collecting tubule, and (H) vasa recta (blood vessels).

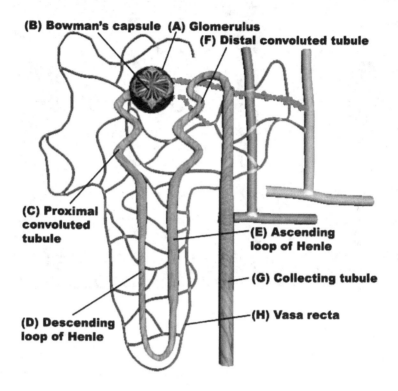

the figure. The parts and functions of the kidneys are described next.

Blood from the body enters nephrons in the kidney from the renal artery. Urea is a waste product of metabolism and is carried by the blood to the kidneys. The kidneys are responsible for removing waste products from the blood, however when removing the wastes, electrolytes and water are also removed, and thus must be recovered. The process occurs in the following five steps.

The concentration of urine permits animals to survive on much less water than they would otherwise need to get rid of metabolic waste. This process is unique to mammals. The movement of urea is responsive to the hormone aldosterone.

First, the glomerulus (A in Figure 1) filters fluid (plasma) from the blood into Bowman's capsule (B) while preventing the passage of blood cells and proteins from the blood. Second, the proximal convoluted tubule (C) reabsorbs two thirds of the filtered water and electrolytes and all of the filtered bicarbonate, glucose, amino acids, and vitamins. Third, the descending loop of Henle (D) reabsorbs more water and delivers a concentrated filtrate to the ascending loop of Henle (E). Fourth, the ascending loop of Henle actively reabsorbs sodium ions to produce a concentrated filtrate. Fifth, the distal convoluted tubule (F) reabsorbs additional sodium ions, chlorine ions, and water. Finally, the collecting tubule (G) reabsorbs water under the influence of antidiuretic hormone, and secretes hydrogen ions and potassium ions.

Figure 2. A screenshot of our simulation, showing the structure of nephrons and molecules in the kidney. The small dots show the location of particles within the kidney.

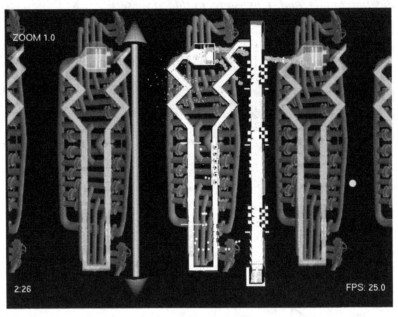

Design and Implementation of the Multi-Agent System

This research was initially funded by Tele-health Outreach for Unified Community Health (TOUCH) (Alverson & Saiki, 2008) and implemented in the software development environment called Flatland (Flatland, 2008). The aim of Project TOUCH was to help develop a virtual reality simulation for medical education (Alverson & Saiki, 2005).

This chapter describes further work on the system including the addition of gaming motifs, as well as heuristic and usability testing. This work was supported under a grant to the University of Hawaii Telehealth Research Institute by the U.S. Army's Telemedicine and Advanced Technology Research Center (TATRC) to develop virtual reality applications.

Figure 2 shows the user's view of our simulation, including three complete nephrons. The agents (details) are visualized for only one nephron. Connections among nephrons are not modeled in the current implementation, as they work in parallel. The agents, plus the environment, form the multi-agent system. Kidney processes are displayed when the agents move within the environment. This uses one of the plugins in Flatland (Flatland, 2008; Alverson & Saiki, 2006). The system is written in the C programming language with OpenGL.

Each particle in the system is an agent. The agent's sensors obtain the particle's current location in its environment. Based on this data, each agent decides the direction and velocity for its next move in the simulation. Particles thus move through the environment modeling the physiological processes.

The Environment: Nodes, Edges and Pools

The environment is analogous to a railroad system where cars and passengers (agents) move along tracks and among stations. A node is analogous to a train station, while an edge is analogous to tracks.

Figure 3. Movement of the agents in their environment modeling renal processes

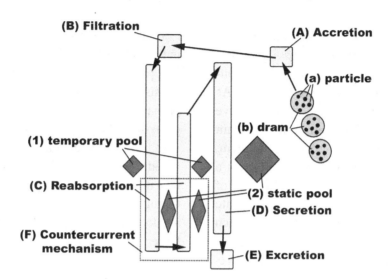

Agents move along the tracks (edges) and from station to station (node to node). The agents can only move along paths where an edge exists.

Each node has a plane perpendicular to the edge attached to its immediate predecessor. The dot product of this plane and the agent's position determines whether the agent passes through the node or not. For example, in a Turn-Right node, all agents moving through the node change their direction vector to the right, following the edge. The agent uses the dot-product to change its direction attribute at the node.

Two pools of agents are used to model the reabsorption and secretion functions in the kidney. The *temporary pool* models reabsorption and the *static pool* models secretion. When an agent moves from inside the tubule (lumen) to outside the tubule (interstitium), it enters a temporary pool, "disappearing" from the tubule.

A static pool uses agents from outside the tubule (interstitium) and moves them into the tubule (lumen). The agent then joins the other agents inside the tubule, thus simulating secretion.

Agents: Particles and Drams

There are two types of agents: particles and drams. We will use *agent* to refer to a particle agent and *dram agent* to refer to dram agents when a distinction is necessary. Agents model either molecules including water, sodium, urea, and potassium, or fluid, including whole blood, plasma, water and filtrates.

Each agent possesses the following attributes: an identifier, type, location, velocity and direction. Agents are grouped into dram agents to simplify the calculations since agents of multiple types move through the system together. Agents can enter or exit a dram agent or other structure during the simulation.

A dram agent contains a group of agents representing molecules and/or fluids in a volume of liquid. Dram agents have attributes including an identifier, location, direction, and speed. Dram agents move through the environment over time, modeling the flow of liquid through the renal system. The ratio of reabsorption and secretion is based on characteristics of the agent and its environment. A group of agents in a dram act together which greatly reduces the number of computations necessary to model processes such as reabsorption and secretion.

Processes: Flow

The flow of agents in the system is accomplished with six actions: *enter, update, separate, reabsorb, secrete,* and *transfer.* One or more agents can enter a dram and form a flow inside the tubule. As agents move through the tubule, they can move in different directions; separate from one dram and enter another dram or create a new dram, reabsorb from a dram to a pool; secrete from a pool into a dram; or transfer to another part of the nephron. The agents and dram agents update their current positions with every move at each step in the simulation.

The *transfer* action implements the movement of urea from the collecting tubule to the ascending loop of Henle, via gradient pools. Physiologically, the process is done through active transport, since the movement goes from an area with lower concentration of urea to one with higher concentration.

Urea in the gradient pools can flow back to the loop of Henle. The gradient pools contain different concentrations of urea. Concentrating urea in the output conserves water while enabling more urea to be excreted.

KIDNEY FUNCTIONS

Accretion

As shown in Figure 1, blood enters the kidney via the afferent arterioles and flows to the glomerular capillaries. From there, fluid enters (accretes to) the (A) glomerulus. Accretion is modeled by agents coming in from vessels outside of the tubule. The agents form a dram and create a flow into the tubule. This is the starting point for renal processing.

Filtration

Filtration occurs in the glomerulus (A) as shown in Figure 1. Two paths leave the glomerulus with one path going to Bowman's capsule (B) and consisting of small, usually uncharged molecules, primarily molecules of water, urea, sodium, and potassium (WUSP). The other path goes to the vasa recta (H) and then exits the kidney. Larger blood components such as red or white blood cells take this path and exit the nephron without going through the tubules. The plasma and molecules that are not recovered in the tubules combine with the larger components of blood in the vasa recta and the resulting filtered blood returns to the body.

In the glomerulus node, agents model the filtration process by sensing information about their environment, and choosing one of the available paths. Then, a dram of whole blood is split into two dram agents with filtered blood in one dram and WUSP in the other dram. Once the WUSP is separated, there is no further movement of agents between the blood dram and the WUSP dram. In this way, the large components in the blood go directly to the vasa recta (H) where it returns to the body and is combined with molecules recovered in the nephrons (WUSP).

Reabsorption

WUSP that has actively or passively left the tubule can be reabsorbed into the nephron at the proximal tubule (C), descending loop of Henle (D), or ascending loop of Henle (E).

In a reabsorption node, a dram senses its current status and is absorbed (disappears). This is accomplished when the agents leave the dram and move into a particle pool, and are thus reabsorbed.

Secretion

In secretion, potassium agents move from plasma into the collecting tubule (G), primarily by active transport. In active transport, energy is expended

Figure 4. The absorption process. Agents move from drams in a node in the tubule to a pool in the nephron.

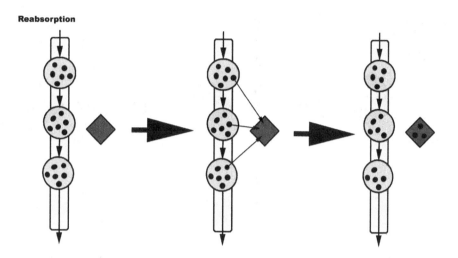

in the cells to force molecules through a barrier. Passive transport (diffusion) also occurs. This maintains homeostasis (pH and other properties of the blood within normal values) and rids the body of metabolic by-products and toxins. In the simulation, pre-defined pools of agents are available. When needed, the agents move into the tubule.

Excretion

The molecules remaining in the distal tubule (F) after passing through the collecting tubule (G) leave the body as urine in the process called excretion. Excretion is modeled by dram agents that move from the collecting tubule to the bladder. Once in the bladder, the dram dissolves in the pool and all agents inside are deleted.

Countercurrent Mechanism

A countercurrent exchange occurs when adjacent currents flow in opposite directions and a property (such as concentration of a substance) is exchanged. There are several countercurrent flows demonstrated in this simulation. The descending

loop of Henle (D) and ascending loop of Henle (E) are adjacent structures, and particles flow in opposite directions and are exchanged between the two sections. Other countercurrent exchanges occur between the ascending loop of Henle (E) and the collecting tubule (G).

Countercurrent flows also exist between the descending loop of Henle (D) and the vasa recta (H), and between the ascending loop of Henle (E) and the vasa recta (H). These flows are depicted in the model. The movement of agents in the simulation gives users a dynamic way to visualize this difficult physiologic concept.

VISUALIZATION SYSTEM TOOLS

Menu

The user's menu is shown in Figure 6. Parameters including which types of molecules are visible are easy to control using a paddle, and changes can be made during the simulation. The paddle interface is a fan with an attached inertia cube (InterSense, 2008). The paddle detects rotation and moves the laser pointer in order to select items shown as

Figure 5. The secretion process. Agents from a pool move into drams in the tubule.

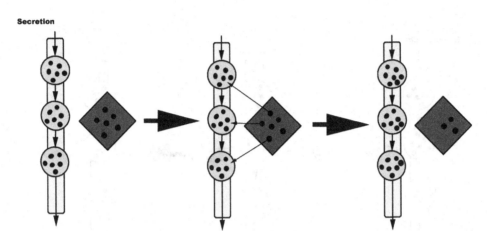

small circular dots in Figures 2 and 6. A student is holding the paddle in front of the projection screen in Figure 7.

The menu presents the user with the choice of which agents will be displayed in the simulation, including water, urea, sodium, potassium, or/and whole blood. The user can focus on one type of agent at a time. The user can also select whether to start or stop the flow. A new "game mode" allows the user to *explore, question, walkthrough,* or *jump* to different sequences in a simulation.

The *explore mode* is used to highlight and display different parts of the nephron. The *question mode* presents the user with a question and allows the user to answer by selecting the correct part of the nephron with the paddle.

Walkthrough mode runs a pre-defined sequence, enabling the user to view the different parts of the nephron from different angles. In *sequence mode,* the user is able to jump to 15 different locations directly, and switch between a mechanical view and an organic view of the nephron. The mechanical

Figure 6. The menu enables the user to choose which particles to display as shown in the upper section of the figure. The user also has control over starting and stopping the flow, viewing a sequence or walk through, or answering a question.

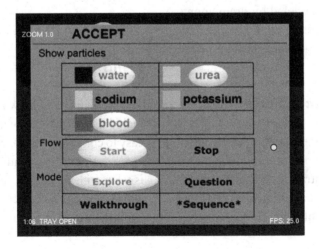

Figure 7. A problem-based learning session using the nephron simulation and a 3D rear-mounted projector. A single medical student controls the simulation using a handheld device. The session was mediated by a faculty member

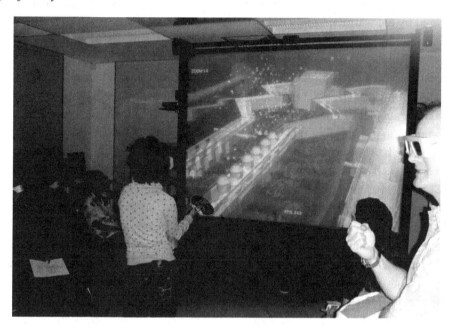

view gives medical students a visual representation of the function of the nephron as in Figure 2. The organic view shows a biological representation of the nephron, similar to Figure 1.

VISUALIZATION OF DIFFICULT CONCEPTS

Filtration in Bowman's Capsule

Small particles are filtered from the blood into a tubule in the kidneys via a semi-permeable membrane in Bowman's capsule (B in Figure 1). This is visualized by showing the particles of Urea, Sodium and Potassium along with water moving out of the blood coming into the kidneys and into a tubule. The rest of the blood, containing all large cells and proteins, continues to flow through the small vessels in the nephron and leaves the kidneys.

Initially the size of the particles was propor-

tional to their actual size (molecular weight). Urea is the largest and sodium(Na+) is the smallest. Users mentioned that they could not see the Na+ particles, so their size was increased.

Reabsorption of Water and Electrolytes

The reabsorption of water and electrolytes is visualized by the agents rejoining the blood after passing through the kidneys. The particles "disappear" into the blood. They are separated from the urea and other wastes that go to the bladder.

Counter-Current Exchange and Multiplication

The structures in the tubules generate a gradient where the concentration of particles increases (increasing osmolality). This occurs in the loop of Henle, in an elegant manner using the opposite direction fluid flows in the adjacent parts of the tubule to concentrate the urine. It functions like a heat exchanger. The intake and outflow tubes are next to each other. In cold climates, the incoming cold air is warmed by the warm air going out. At the same time, the air that was warm in the building is cooled before it exits. The most elegant part is that the coldest incoming air is directly across from the coolest outgoing air. The air at the inside ends of the pipes have about the same temperature. Thus, heat is retained in the building rather than expelled with the air when bringing fresh air into the building.

If the inflow tube was separate from the outflow, room temperature air would be expelled and cold air would come in, with no heat savings.

This is one of the key concepts to understand about the renal system. Our simulation shows the movement of the agents, but does not visually represent the gradients. We plan to add this to future versions of the system. A change in color intensity could represent different levels of particles at the different parts of the gradient.

Usability Study Design

A sample of medical students and one faculty member were recruited via email for the study. Two sessions were planned separated by approximately one month of software development. Open-ended comments by the evaluators were collated and categorized as gaming or content issues.

The studies took place in the medical school simulation center at the University of Hawaii. Data for the group user evaluation were collected anonymously using an audience response polling system. Data for the heuristic evaluation and the individual user evaluations were collected through interviews and written surveys. The research protocols were approved by the University of Hawaii Committee on Human Studies and the United States Army Medical Materiel and Research Command Office of Research Protection.

Usability testing is critical to the development of an effective software application to ensure that the learner is able to focus on the educational objective rather than the process of completing tasks in the virtual environment.

Group User Evaluation

First year medical students viewed the virtual reality nephron simulation during planned laboratory sessions as part of their problem-based learning curriculum. All participants donned active 3D glasses, and a single student used a paddle interface to navigate the scene as it was projected on a rear mounted 3D projector. One or two faculty members mediated each 45-minute session.

Students were surveyed before and after the sessions using an audience response system that collected anonymous paired responses.

Responses were rated using a 5-point Likert scale, from 1 = *strongly disagree* to 5 = *strongly agree* to the following statements:

1) "I feel confident in my understanding of nephron physiology";
2) "I have a good mental image of renal physiology"; and
3) "Renal physiology is hard to visualize."

Observations and comments made during the group sessions were collated and organized into action items for the software developers. During the study, programmers added gaming motifs, on-screen navigation controls, a simple scoring system, as well as enhancements in the visualization of selected particles.

Heuristic Evaluation

The heuristic usability evaluation is a systematic approach to software development that is designed to identify significant usability issues early in the software development life cycle. The heuristic evaluation of this application was modeled on the method proposed by Nielsen & Landauer (1993).

They found that each new evaluator contributes progressively less new information regarding usability issues and problems. By the fifth usability tester, 85% of problems have been identified, and additional testers mostly replicate information that has already been discovered.

Tang, Johnson, Tindall and Zhang (2006) found that a second iteration of the heuristic methodology demonstrated additional improvement in the user interface that was being developed.

Individual User Evaluation

Users were given a group of seven tasks to perform with the simulation before completing a survey. The survey consisted of five domains, each rated on a 7-point Likert scale from 1=unacceptable to 7=exceeds expectations. An acceptable level was defined as a score ≥ 4.

The domains were *learnability, efficiency, memorability, errors,* and *satisfaction.* The task list for users was:

1. Login to the virtual nephron game;
2. Orient to the environment: within the first person view, change the orientation to identify proximal, distal, cortical, and medullary perspectives.
3. Use the paddle interface to find and select the glomerulus, proximal convoluted tubule, and collecting duct.
4. Use the paddle interface to change the view from a hovering view to a head-up view, and from a hovering view to a foot view;
5. Use the paddle interface to change the functional representation of the nephron, and to activate sodium particles and urea particles;
6. Use the paddle interface to navigate to different sites of active transport, depicted in the mechanical view as moving pistons.
7. Exit the virtual environment.

Data Analysis

Before and after survey data were analyzed using a paired, t-tailed Student's t-test. Descriptive statistics are presented next.

RESULTS

Group User Evaluation

Sixty-one students (98% of the class) each interacted with the system six times. Of these, 18% had frequently used videogames and 16% were frequent users of a Nintendo Wii. While 72% had watched a movie using 3D glasses, only 32% had experienced an educational game as part of medical school.

The motion-tracking interface that obtained input from both a head-mounted tracker and a hand-held, paddle-mounted tracker proved to be problematic for those who were also watching the projected images. Observers became disoriented while the device was being used. This problem was resolved by eliminating the head-mounted motion tracker.

Students reported that some of the particles modeled were difficult to see. One suggestion was to increase the size of the white particles (simulating sodium ions) to make them more visible. Particle dynamics in the proximal convoluted tubule was incomplete and subject to misinterpretation. These, as well as other, content and usability issues were recorded and forwarded to software programmers for further development.

Students agreed that the exercise gave them a good mental image of nephron physiology, with a mean rating increasing from 2.90 to 3.75 on a 5-point Likert scale (1=strongly disagree to 5=strongly agree), $p < 0.01$ (Figure 8). After the experience, they disagreed that nephron physiology was hard to visualize, with a mean rating changing from 3.38 to 2.75 on the Likert scale, $p < 0.01$ (Figure 8). Participants agreed that their self-confidence improved as a result of the exercise, with the mean rating increasing from 2.76 to 3.36, p < 0.01 (Figure 8). Overall, students found the game interesting (80%) and thought that it should be made a regular part of the curriculum (70%) (Figure 8).

Heuristic Evaluation

Four medical students and one computer science faculty member completed the evaluation. In the initial session, gaming/interface issues constituted 64% (36/56) of the open-ended comments. This increased to 93% (50/54) of the open-ended com-

ments during the second session, suggesting that important content issues had been addressed in the revised version of the software.

Individual User Evaluation

Five medical students participated in one user evaluation session each. All domains received ratings that "exceed[ed] expectations" on the Likert scale (Figure 8D). This suggests that the iterative approach to software development was successful.

Figure 8. Before/after group results, n=61, 1=strongly disagree to 5=strongly agree. Vertical and horizontal bars are 95% confidence intervals. (A) "I feel confident in my understanding of nephron physiology." (B) "I have a good mental image of renal physiology." (C) "Renal physiology is hard to visualize" (D) Individual usability study, n=5, 1=unacceptable to 7=exceeds expectations.

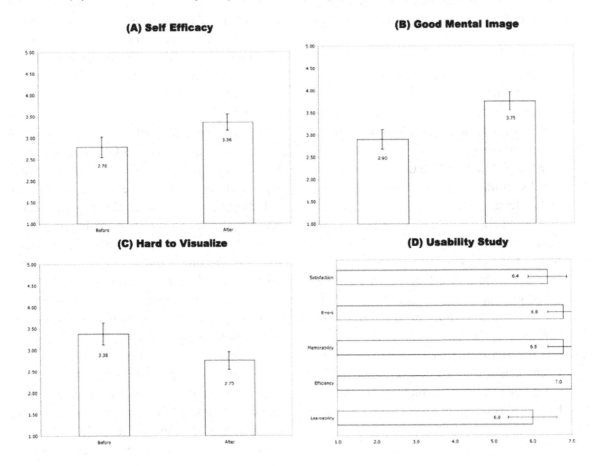

FUTURE TRENDS

Simulations have increasingly provided a realistic and effective method of teaching difficult concepts to medical/healthcare students. Human physiology is very complex, and still not completely understood (Thomas, Layton, Layton & Moore, 2006). By creating models and performing simulations, students gain a more complete understanding of how the body works, and ultimately improve patient care.

Both the modeling of physiologic variables and the stylistic components of the interface in our prototype have room for improvement. Based on feedback from the students, the current version of the nephron game is most suitable for novice learners of renal physiology. Although users felt that the interface was easy to learn, optimal use of the present software may require a knowledgeable technical facilitator. Development of the virtual reality application for use with a large 3D screen makes the system amenable to integration in a problem-based learning curriculum that emphasizes small group interaction and formative assessment facilitated by a faculty member.

Our future plans are to integrate the kidney simulation with a more dynamic game engine. For example, using Monte Carlo processes we could extend the simulation using random variables and statistics to predict how different states of kidney function respond to changing physiologic conditions (Roberts, 1992).

Additional future studies would assess the contribution of gaming elements to student learning and satisfaction, as well as comparing the impact of immersion in this virtual system to traditional non-immersive forms of education.

CONCLUSION

A working prototype that simulates processes in renal physiology was created for use in medical research and education. Using Flatland (2008), agents model molecules and volumes in a virtual 3D simulation of the kidneys. Initial usability study results are encouraging. They show that this multi-agent simulation reduced the learning curve and increased the confidence of medical students learning renal physiology. Future work is planned to add additional features to the simulation.

ACKNOWLEDGMENT

This work has been supported by grant # 06083002 from the United States Army Medical Research and Materiel Command (USAMRMC) Telemedicine and Advanced Technology Research Center (TATRC).

The authors wish to thank the study participants and the following three colleagues at the Telehealth Research Institute: Dr. Andrei Sherstyuk, for programming advice and assistance; Dr. Lawrence Burgess, for mentoring in virtual reality applications; and Kathleen Kihmm Connolly, for grant preparation and administration. In addition we would like to thank the anonymous reviewers and JML for their comments. This paper improved substantially as a result.

REFERENCES

Alverson, D. C., & Saiki, S., Jr. (2008). *Telehealth outreach for unified community health (Project TOUCH)*. University of New Mexico and University of Hawaii. Retrieved August 7, 2008, from http://hsc.unm.edu/som/projects/touch/.

Alverson, D. C., Saiki, S Jr, Caudell, T. P., Goldsmith, T., Stevens, S., Saland, L., Colleran, K., Brandt, J., Danielson, L., Cerilli, L., Harris, A., Gregory, M. C., Stewart, R., Norenberg, J., & Shuster, G., Panaoitis, Holten, J., Vergera, V. M., Sherstyuk, A., Kihmm, K., Lui, J., & Wang, K. L. (2006). Reification of abstract concepts to improve comprehension using interactive virtual environments and a knowledge-based design: a renal physiology model. *Studies in Health Technology and Informatics, 119*, 13–18.

Alverson, D. C., Saiki, S. Jr, Caudell, T. P., & Summers, K., Panaiotis, Sherstyuk, A., Nickles, D., Holten, J., Goldsmith, T. E., Stevens, S. M., Kihmm, K., Mennin, S., Kalishman, S., Mines J., Serna, L., Mitchell, S., Lindberg, M., Jacobs, J., Nakatsu, C., Lozanoff, S., Wax, D. S., Saland L., Norenberg, J., Shuster, G., Keep, M., Baker, R., Buchanan, H. S., Stewart, R., Bowyer, M., Liu, A., Muniz, G., Coulter, R., Maris, C., & Wilks, D. (2005). Distributed immersive virtual reality simulation development for medical education. *Journal of International Association of Medical Science Educators, 15*(1), 19–30.

Banasik, J. L. (2000). Renal Function (2nd ed.). In *Pathophysiology: Biological and Behavioral Perspectives* (pp. 626–648). Philadelphia, PA: W.B. Saunders Company.

Barber, K. S., Goel, A., Han, D. C., Kim, J., Lam, D. N., & Liu, T. H. (2003). Infrastructure for Design, Deployment and Experimentation of Distributed Agent-based Systems: The Requirements, The Technologies, and An Example. *Autonomous Agents and Multi-Agent Systems, 7*(1), 49–69. doi:10.1023/A:1024124804035

Baumgartner, U., Magele, Ch., & Renhart, W. (2004). Pareto optimality and particle swarm optimization. *IEEE Transactions on Magnetics, 40*(2), 1172–1175. doi:10.1109/TMAG.2004.825430

Bernard, D., Dorais, G., Gamble, E., Kanefsky, B., Kurien, J., Man, G. K., et al. (1999). Spacecraft Autonomy Flight Experience: The DS1 Remote Agent Experiment. *Proceedings of the American Institute of Aeronautics and Astronautics Conference* (pp. 28-30). Albuquerque, NM: AIAA Space Technology Conference.

Cavazza, M., & Simo, A. (2003). A virtual patient based on qualitative simulation. *In IUI '03: Proceedings of the 8th international conference on Intelligent user interfaces* (pp. 19–25). New York, NY: ACM Press.

Chenney, S. (2004). Flow tiles. *In SCA '04: Proceedings of the 2004 ACM SIGGRAPH/Eurographics symposium on Computer animation* (pp. 233–242). New York, NY: ACM Press.

Dawson-Saunders, B., Feltovich, P. J., Coulson, R. L., & Steward, D. E. (1990). A survey of medical school teachers to identify basic biomedical concepts medical students should understand. *Academic Medicine, 65*(7), 448–454. doi:10.1097/00001888-199007000-00008

Eberhart, R. C., & Shi, Y. (1998). Comparison between genetic algorithms and particle swarm optimization. *Evolutionary Programming VII: Proceedings 7th annual conference on Evolutionary Programming conference* (pp. 611-616). Berlin: Springer-Verlag.

Flatland (2008). University of New Mexico. Retrieved August 7, 2008, from http://www.hpc.unm.edu/homunculus/.

InterSense. (2008). InterSense Inc. Reterieved August 28, 2008, from http://www.intersense.com/.

Janson, S., Merkle, D., & Middendorf, M. (2008). Molecular docking with multi-objective Particle Swarm Optimization. *Applied Soft Computing, 8*(1), 666–675. doi:10.1016/j.asoc.2007.05.005

Kumar, S., & Berl, T. (1999). Chapter 1: Diseases of Water Metabolism. *Atlas of Diseases of the Kidney, 1*, 1–22. Philadelphia, PA: Current Medicine, Inc.

Moreno, A., & Garbay, C. (2003). Editorial: Software agents in health care. [Amsterdam, The Netherlands: Elsevier.]. *Artificial Intelligence in Medicine, 27*, 229–232. doi:10.1016/S0933-3657(03)00004-6

Moreno, A., Valls, A., Isern, D., & Sanchez, D. (2006). Applying Agent Technology to Healthcare: The GruSMA Experience. [New York, NY: IEEE Press]. *IEEE Intelligent Systems, 26*(6), 63–67. doi:10.1109/MIS.2006.108

NASA. (2008). *The Remote Agent Project*. Retrieved August 28, 2008, from http://ti.arc.nasa.gov/projects/remote-agent/.

Nielsen, J., & Landauer, T. K. (1993). A mathematical model of the finding of usability problems. *Proceedings of the INTERACT '93 and CHI '93 Conference on Human Factors in Computing Systems* (pp. 206-213). New York, NY: ACM Press.

Poulopoulos, V., Gortizis, L., Bakettas, I., & Nikiforidis, G. (2006). *In Proceedings of the International Conference on Information Technology: Research and Education* (pp. 253-257). New York, NY and Piscataway, NJ: IEEE Press.

Prado, M., Roa, L., Reina-Tosina, J., Palma, A., & Milan, J. A. (2001). Virtual Center for Renal Support: Definition of a Novel Knowledge-Based Telemedicine System. *Proceedings of the 23 Annual IEEE Engineering and Medicine in Biology Society Conference* (pp. 3878-3881). New York, NY and Piscataway, NJ: IEEE Press.

Reeves, W. T. (1983). Particle systems - a technique for modeling a class of fuzzy objects. *In SIGGRAPH '83: Proceedings of the 10th annual conference on computer graphics and interactive techniques* (pp. 359–375). New York, NY: ACM Press.

Roberts, M. S. (1992). Markov process-based Monte Carlo simulation: a tool for modeling complex disease and its application to the timing of liver transplantation. *In WSC '92: Proceedings of the 24th conference on winter simulation* (pp. 1034–1040). New York, NY: ACM Press.

Robocup (2008). *Robocup Federation homepage*. Retrieved August 22, 2008, from http://www.robocup.org/

Robocup-rescue. (2008). *Robocup Rescue homepage*. Retrieved August 7, 2008, from http://www.rescuesystem.org/robocuprescue/

Schmickl, T., Thenius, R., & Crailsheim, K. (2005). Simulating swarm intelligence in honey bees: foraging in differently fluctuating environments. *In GECCO '05: Proceedings of the 2005 conference on genetic and evolutionary computation* (pp. 273–274). New York, NY: ACM Press.

Sklar, E., Davies, M., & Co, M. S. T. (2004). SimEd: Simulating Education as a Multi Agent System. *In AAMAS '04: Proceedings of the Third International Joint Conference on Autonomous Agents and Multiagent Systems* (pp. 998-1005). New York, NY: ACM Press.

Tang, Z., Johnson, T., Tindall, D., & J. Zhang (2006). Applying heuristic evaluation to improve the usability of a telemedicine system. *Telemedicine and e-Health, 12*(1), 24-34.

Thomas, S. R., Layton, A. T., Layton, H. E., & Moore, L. C. (2006). Kidney Modeling: Status and Perspectives. *Proceedings of the IEEE, 94*(4), 740–752. doi:10.1109/JPROC.2006.871770

Vicari, R. M., Flores, C. D., Silvestre, A. M., Seixas, L. J., Ladeira, M., & Coelho, H. (2003). A multi-agent intelligent environment for medical knowledge. *Artificial Intelligence in Medicine, 27*(3), 335–366. doi:10.1016/S0933-3657(03)00009-5

Weiss, G. (1999). *Multiagent Systems: A Modern Approach to Distributed Artificial Intelligence.* The MIT Press.

Wooldridge, M. (2002). *An Introduction to Multiagent Systems.* John Wiley & Sons (Chichester, England).

Yoon, J. S., & Maher, M. L. (2005). A swarm algorithm for wayfinding in dynamic virtual worlds. *In VRST '05: Proceedings of the ACM symposium on virtual reality software and technology* (pp. 113–116). New York, NY: ACM Press.

Zafar, K., Qazi, S. B., & Baig, A. R. (2006). Mine detection and route planning in military warfare using multi agent system. *In COMPSAC '06: Proceedings 30th annual international computer software and applications conference* (pp. 327-332). Los Alamitos, CA: IEEE Computer Society Press.

Section 4
Population Modeling Systems

196

Chapter 11
Role of Multi–Agents System in Creation of Collaborative Environments within Mental Health Domain

Maja Hadzic
Curtin University of Technology, Australia

Darshan S. Dillon
Curtin University of Technology, Australia

ABSTRACT

Mental illness is becoming one of the major problems of our society. The World Health Organization predicted that depression would be the world's leading cause of disability by 2020. The exact causes of many mental illnesses are still unknown, mainly due to the complex nature of mental health. In this paper, the authors propose a multi-agent system designed to assist in effective and efficient management, retrieval and analysis of mental health information. They utilize the TICSA approach to define different agent Types, their Intelligence, Collaboration paths, address Security problems and Assemble individual agents. They use UML 2.1 Sequence and Composite diagrams to model social and goal-driven nature of the multi-agent system. The proposed multi-agent system has the potential to provide and expose the knowledge that will increase our understanding and control over mental health and help in development of effective prevention and intervention strategies.

INTRODUCTION

Mental illness is becoming one of the major problems of our society. The World Health Organization predicted that depression would be the world's leading cause of disability by 2020 (Lopez & Murray, 1998). The number of mentally ill people is increasing globally each year. This introduces major costs in economic and human terms, to the individual communities and the nation in general, both in rural and urban areas. The recognition that many mental illnesses may not become chronic if treated early has led to an increase in research in the last 20 years.

DOI: 10.4018/978-1-60566-772-0.ch011

Research into mental health has increased and resulted in a wide range of information and publications covering different aspects of mental health and addressing a variety of problems. A huge body of information is available within the mental health domain. This information is dispersed over various information sources which are heterogeneous in structure and content. As the research continues, new papers or journals are frequently published and added to various databases. Portions of this data may be related, overlap or semi-complementary with one another. No tool exists which helps us identify these kinds of relationships, overlaps, complementarities and redundancies.

Retrieving specific information is very difficult with current search engines as they look for the specific string of letters within the text rather than its meaning. In a search for "genetic causes of bipolar disorder", Google provides 95,500 hits which are a large assortment of well meaning general information sites with few interspersed evidence-based resouces. Medline Plus (http://medlineplus.gov/) retrieves 53 articles including all information about bipolar disorder plus information on other mental illnesses. A large number of articles is outside the domain of interest and is on the topic of heart defects, eye and vision research, multiple sclerosis, Huntington's disease, psoriasis etc. PubMed (http://www.ncbi.nlm.nih.gov/pubmed) gives a list of 1,946 articles. The user needs to select the relevant articles as some of the retrieved articles are on other illnesses such as schizophrenia, autism and obesity. Moreover, the user needs to read each article individually and establish the links between the selected articles manually. We need to take a systematic approach to making use of the available information that cannot reach its full value unless it is systematically analysed and linked with other available information from the same domain.

Wilczynski *et al.* (2006): "General practitioners, mental health practitioners, and researchers wishing to retrieve the best current research evidence in the content area of mental health may have a difficult time when searching large electronic databases such as MEDLINE. When MEDLINE is searched unaided, key articles are often missed while retrieving many articles that are irrelevant to the search." Wilczynski *et al.* (2006) developed search strategies that can help discriminate the literature with mental health content from articles that do not have mental health content. Our research ideas go beyond this. We go a step further and apply data mining algorithms on mental health data. We propose the design of a multi-agents system that will give a consistent format to all mental health information. This will bring the mental health information under one umbrella and enable us to organize this information in a systematic way. This will allow automatic data analysis techniques such as data mining to effectively use mental health data, reveal data patterns hidden within the large body of the mental health data, and expose the knowledge that will help medical practitioners develop better prevention and intervention strategies.

LITERATURE REVIEW

Complexity of the Mental Health

The increase in mental health research has resulted in increase of information but the exact causes of many mental illnesses remain unclear. However, it has been proven that mental illness is a causal factor in many chronic conditions such as diabetes, hypertension, HIV/AIDS resulting in higher cost to the health system (Horvitz-Lennon *et al.* 2006).

As mental illness is still a grey area of medical research, and the exact causes of mental illness are unclear, precise treatment strategies cannot be developed at this stage. Doctors are often forced to prescribe medication which may provide temporal relief but in reality mask the real issue and often result in side effects that will make the patient's situation even worse (Pacher & Kecskemeti, 2004; Check, 2004; Friedman & Leon, 2007; Werneke *et al.* 2006). The drugs used to treat mental illness have negative effects on both physical and mental health. Specifically, the negative effect on cardiovascular health is evident (Pacher & Kecskemeti, 2004). The mental health of patients taking drugs often becomes worse. The drug may mask one mental problem, but another mental problem that has never existed before may appear. Suicidal thoughts (Check, 2004; Friedman & Leon, 2007) are the most common and dangerous side effect of the drugs. Additionally, sexual dysfunction (Werneke *et al.* 2006) is another side effect that may negatively effect marital relationships of the patient and, in turn, create additional problems and pressure.

Researchers believe that mental illness is caused by various factors. For example, genetic analysis has identified candidate loci on human chromosomes 4, 7, 8, 9, 10, 13, 14 and 17 (Liu *et al.*, 2003). There is some evidence that environmental factors such as stress, lifecycle matters, social environment, climate etc. are important (Craddock & Jones, 2001; Smith *et al.* 2005). Some researchers suggest that a bacterial or viral infection may cause mental illness (Wenner, 2008). More research is required to explain why mental illness appears to be transmittable; is it really caused by a microorganism and why the wellness/illness appears to be 'contiguous'? Additionally, interest in the relationship between religion and spirituality and mental health has increased in recent years. Hill and Pargament (Hill & Pargament, 2003) illustrate that dimensions such as closeness to God, religious or spiritual orientation, source of motivation, religious and spiritual support and religious and spiritual struggle, are significantly tied to physical and mental health. Schumaker (1992) reviews the work of various scientists who examined the relationship between religion and spirituality with various aspects of psychological well-being including depression, suicidal thoughts, substance abuse, anxiety, fear

of death, sin and guilt, self-esteem, meaning of life etc. Research into mental health has been made even more complicated through the existence of various types of specific mental illnesses such as chronic, postnatal and psychotic types of depression.

Identification of the precise patterns of causal factors responsible for a specific type of mental illness still remains unsolved and is therefore a very active research focus today. Many research teams focus only on one factor and perhaps one aspect of a mental illness. For example, in the paper "Bipolar disorder susceptibility region on Xq24-q27.1 in Finnish families" (PubMed ID: 12082562), the research team Ekholm *et al.* (2002) examined one genetic factor (Xq24-q27.1) for one type of mental illness (bipolar disorder). As mental illnesses do not follow Mendelian patterns but are caused by a number of genes usually interacting with various environmental factors, ever factor for all aspects of the illness needs to be considered. We believe that data mining techniques have the power to simultaneously analyse the data and expose the data patterns invisible to human eye simply because of the large volume of mental health information.

Multi-Agent Systems

Multi-agent systems (Wooldridge, 2002) are being used more and more in the medical domain. One of the main advantages of agents is their autonomy. They can act independently from the user and from the rest of the system, and make decisions on their own. Even though the agent is able to act autonomously, it has to be sociable and collaborate with other agents of the system in order to address more complex problems. Only through cooperation, coordinating their actions, sharing tasks and results with other agents, can multi-agent systems reach their full potential. The collaborative nature of agents enables the multi-agent system to find solutions to complex problems through carrying out distributed problem solving. Some agents are mobile i.e. they are capable of migrating to different places. This feature can increase dynamics and efficiency of the whole system.

Being goal-driven is a feature of many different agents. The fact that an agent has an overriding goal, regardless of the specifics of its processing, endows it with many other features. Specifically, it is proactive, i.e. it takes actions on its own initiative, and it is intelligent, i.e. it reasons and chooses to perform the most beneficial actions towards achieving its goals.

The multi-agent systems greatly contribute to the design and implementation of complex health information systems. Effective implementation of multi-agent systems within the health domain could result in a revolutionary change that will positively transform the existing health systems. Some of these agent-based systems are designed to use information within specific medical and health organizations, others use information from the Internet.

The information available to organization-based systems is limited to a specific institution and these multi-agent systems help the management of the already available information. They do not have a purpose of gaining new knowledge regarding the disease in question. For example, Agent Cities (Moreno & Isern, 2002) is a multi-agent system composed of agents that provide medical services. The multi-agent system contains agents that allow the user to search for medical centres satisfying a given set of requirements, to access his/her medical record or to make a booking to be visited by a particular kind of doctor. AADCare (Huang *et al.*, 1995) agent architecture is a decision support system for physicians. It connects patient's records with the predefined domain knowledge such as knowledge regarding a specific disease, a knowledge base of clinical management plans, a database of patient records etc. MAMIS (Fonseca *et al.*, 2005) is a Multi-Agent Medical Information System facilities patient information search and provides ubiquitous information access to physicians and health professionals.

Other multi-agent systems retrieve information from the Internet. BioAgent (Merelli *et al.*, 2002) is a mobile agent system where an agent is associated to the given task and it travels among multiple locations and at each location performs its mission. At the end of the trip, an information integration procedure takes place before the answer is deployed to the user. Holonic Medical Diagnostic System (Ulieru, 2003) architecture is a medical diagnostic system that combines the advantages of the holonic paradigm, multi-agent system technology and swarm intelligence in order to realize Internet-based diagnostic system for diseases. All necessary/available medical information about a patient is kept in exactly one comprehensive computer readable patient record called computer readable patient pattern (CRPP) and is processed by the agents of the holarchy. Different web crawling agents (Srinivasan *et al.*, 2002) have been designed to fetch information about diseases when given information about genes that when mutated may cause these diseases.

We have highlighted the importance of multi-agent systems within mental health domain in our previous works (Hadzic & Chang, 2008a; Hadzic & Chang, 2008b). In this paper, we go a step further by (1) describing such system in greater detail and (2) using the UML 2.1 diagrams to expressing the ideas more effectively.

Data Mining

Data mining is a set of processes that is based on automated searching for actionable knowledge buried within a huge body of data (Han & Kamber, 2006). Data mining algorithms have great potential to expose the patterns in data. Data mining help to extract information, to find hidden patterns and knowledge, and to make predictive models for decision making and new discoveries. Data mining draws work from areas including database technology, machine learning, statistics, pattern recognition, information retrieval, neural networks, knowledge based systems, artificial intelligence, high-performance computing and data visualization (Sesito & Dillon, 1994). Some advantages of data mining over the traditional approaches include:

- efficient processing of large and complex data (scalability)
- automatically analysing, detecting errors and inconsistencies, classifying, and summarizing the data with no human intervention (automation)
- extracting novel and useful patterns which leads to new knowledge and discoveries (knowledge extractions)
- combining the advantages of various disciplines (multi-disciplinary nature)
- reducing costs and time associated with the data analysis (cost and time efficiency)

Within the health domain, data mining techniques have been predominantly used for tasks such as text mining, drug design, gene expression analysis, genomics and proteomics. The data analysis necessary for microarrays has necessitated data mining (Piatetsky-Shapiro, & Tamayo, 2003). The data mining algorithms can be applied to derive patterns specific to mental illness, such as exposing a unique combination of causal factors responsible for onset of the illness in question and providing an indication of influence. This can greatly contribute in the identification of precise patterns of genetic and environmental factors and in development of prevention and intervention strategies. The extracted data patterns can provide useful information to help in mental illness prevention, and assist in delivery of effective and efficient mental health services.

Much of the mental health information is not in strictly structured form and the use of traditional data mining techniques developed for relational data is not appropriate in this case. The majority of available mental health information can be meaningfully represented in XML format,

which makes the techniques capable of mining semi-structured or tree structured data more applicable. In our previous works (Hadzic *et al.*, 2008a; Hadzic *et al.*, 2008b; Hadzic *et al.*, 2008c), we have demonstrated the potential of the tree mining algorithms to derive useful knowledge patterns in mental health domain. We have used our previously developed IMB3-Miner algorithm and showed how tree mining techniques can be applied on mental health data represented in XML format. We discussed the implications of using different mining parameters within the current tree mining framework and demonstrated the potential of extracted patterns in providing useful information.

Ontology

Ontology is an enriched conceptual model for representing domain knowledge. Ontology captures and represents specific domain knowledge through specification of meaning of concepts including definition of the concepts and domain-specific relationships between those concepts. Ontologies provide a shared common understanding of a domain and have been suggested as a mechanism to provide applications with domain knowledge and support knowledge integration, use and sharing by different applications, software systems and human resources (Gómez-Pérez, 1998).

An ontology, particularly in medicine, grew out of a perceived need for a controlled vocabulary (Cimino, 2006; Smith, 2006). The importance of ontologies has been recognised within the biomedical domain and work has begun on developing and sharing biomedical ontologies (Ceusters *et al.*, 2001; Burgun, 2006). The Gene Ontology (GO) (http://www.geneontology.org/) project works on establishing consistent descriptions of gene products in different databases by using the GO to annotate major repositories for plant, animal and microbial genomes. The Unified Medical Language System (UMLS) (Kim & Park, 2004) is a collection of many biomedical vocabularies and it consists of Metathesaurus, Semantic Network, SPECIALIST Lexicon and a number of software tools. There are one million biomedical concepts in UMLS, and 135 semantic types and 54 relationships are used to classify these concepts. Human Disease Ontology (Hadzic & Chang, 2005) captures and represents the knowledge about human diseases. It consists of disease types, symptoms, causes and treatments subontologies. Protein Ontology (http://proteinontology.info/) (Sidhu *et al.*, 2006) provides a unified vocabulary for capturing declarative knowledge about protein domain and to classify that knowledge to allow reasoning. It acts as a mediator for accessing not only relational data but also semi-structured data such as XML or metadata annotations and unstructured information. A great variety of biomedical ontologies is available via The Open Biomedical Ontologies (http://obofoundry.org/) covering various domains such as anatomy, biological processes, biochemistry, health and taxonomy.

UML

Multi-Agent Systems (MAS) are increasingly being proposed and used within the biomedical domain. One of the ongoing issues within the modelling of multi-agent systems is the lack of a standardized modelling language. Some research groups have proposed the use of UML to model agent-based systems. Others have extended UML to suit modelling requirements specific to multi-agent systems. We have noticed a number of problems with the existing approaches. The major problems relate to the inconsistent semantics of the existing UML Diagrams, and the unintuitive and complex notation.

Kavi *et al.* (2003) propose to extend UML with a number of modeling constructs. Next to the Agent, the additional modeling constructs include (1) Belief, Goal and Plan - to enable modeling of the reactive and proactive behaviors of agents, and (2) FIPA Performative, KQML

Performative and Blackboard - to model agent's communication. The authors give an impression of using the Sequence Diagram. However, they have changed the semantics of the Sequence Diagram by using smiley faces, thought clouds, and the like. Da Silva *et al.* (2004) propose MAS-ML as a modeling language to support modeling of multi-agents systems. MAS-ML is an extension of UML and uses Organization, Role and Class Diagrams to model static aspects of an application while Sequence Diagrams are used to model the dynamic aspects of an application. We notice changes in the semantics of rectangles without the use of a stereotype. Additionally, the use of <<role_change>> is syntactically correct but the resulting diagram appears complex and is difficult to follow. VisualAgent (De Maria *et al.*, 2005) is a Java-based development environment which uses the MAS-ML and is composed of three tools: a graphical tool, a transformation tool and a code generation tool. The VisualAgent can be used to present some preliminary ideas, but does not allow for detailed presentation as it virtually lacks existing UML diagrams or stereotypes. Da Silva *et al.* (2005) use UML2.0 Activity Diagrams to model agent plans and actions. They consider a plan to be an activity, decompose them into a number of actions and define the action execution sequence. The strength of this approach is that it allows definitions of stereotypes for Activity Diagrams. However, the chosen notation appears to be difficult to understand and to follow.

Odell *et al.* (2001) uses non-standard extensions of UML since they do not use stereotypes and changes the semantics of existing UML constructs. In particular, (1) no use of stereotypes was made to define an agent and (2) the definition of classes and instances are mixed up in sequence diagrams. It was specified that one defines agent as Agent: Role/Class in Figure 6, but names of classes in Figures 8-10 were underlined which implies that they were instances. We will not use underlining throughout this paper in order for it to be clear that we refer to classes, not instances.

As a third point we notice in sequence diagrams a rectangle to be defined as a Agent/Role combination. In particular, this meant that a single Agent was represented by multiple rectangles, each one representing a single role. On contrary, we use a single rectangle to represent a composite class (which corresponded to an Agent) with ports (see UML 2.1) to represent roles. Thus we work within the existing framework of UML 2.1 whilst only making extensions within the framework of UML (i.e. by use of stereotypes).

The latest version of UML, UML 2.1, has greater expressive power over previous UML versions. This allows representing more complex scenarios and introducing greater details into the modeling process enabling effective capture and representation of multi-agent actions and inter-actions. We use UML2.1 to define and describe multi-agent systems by not changing the semantics of the diagrams, which is a critical point that makes our use of UML 2.1 valid. In this paper we illustrate how UML 2.1 can be used to model a multi-agent system specifically designed to intelligently store, use, manage, analyze and retrieve mental health information. We believe that UML 2.1 has not only enabled the introduction of a notation for MAS, but also effective capture and representation of the dynamic processes associated with these MAS.

TICSA APPROACH TO THE MULTI-AGENT SYSTEM DESIGN

In this project we focus on creating a collaborative environment for the mental health research domain. Different mental health researchers working on different aspects of the shared problem would be able to come together, share their information effectively, cooperate with each other and jointly build solutions to common problems. This is of vital importance for the mental health research community as mental illnesses are caused by different factors, and most researchers work on

a single causal factor. Sharing of the information will enable the examining each factor in the context of other factors.

In our previous work (Hadzic & Chang, 2008c), we have described five important aspects (TICSA) that need to be addressed during the design of multi-agents systems. These include:

1. Identify Agent **T**ypes According to Their Responsibilities
2. Define Agent's **I**ntelligence
3. Define Agent's **C**ollaborations
4. Protect the **S**ystem by Implementing Security Requirements
5. **A**ssemble Individual Agents

In this paper, we will use this approach to design a multi-agent system that will help to use mental health information effectively and efficiently.

Identify Agent Types According to Their Responsibilities

A multi-agent system is a community of agents. Each agent type plays an unique function within the multi-agent system. The different agent types have different but complementary capabilities and are cooperatively working towards the shared goal. The agents are required to work in unity and coordinate their actions.

When identifying agent types, it is important to:

- establish intuitive flow of problem solving, task and result sharing
- identify agent types that will match their responsibilities within the system needed to establish this kind of flow

We propose a system that will make use of different types of agents to add and retrieve information from the system. It will be possible to add information in two different ways. Human users as well as computer programs will be able to add

Figure 1. Different ways of adding and retrieving information from the system

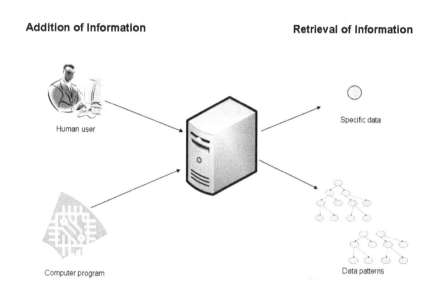

information. Additionally, the information may be retrieved in two different ways. Human users will be able to retrieve specific data as well as to retrieve data patterns specific to problem at hand. This main idea is represented in Figure 1. The resulting system is a combination of human and software agents working together creating a collaborative and mutually beneficial environment. The users of the system are not only information consumers but are also information providers.

We want to design a system where users are able to (i) add information to the system as well as (ii) query the system for the specific information or for data patterns. Additionally, a program will be designed to automatically add data to the system.

A range of actions is required to establish this flow. To add information to the system, these include (1) user login, (2) validation of data, and (3) data storage. To retrieve information from the system, it is required to (1) translate the user's query into a machine-understandable language,

(2) activate appropriate agents to retrieve the target information, (3) select appropriate information, and (4) present the retrieved information to the user. For automatic population of the database, (1) search must be activated, (2) retrieved results validated, and (3) the data added to the database.

Our next task is to identify agent types that will have different responsibilities within the system and help us establish the intuitive flow of problem solving, task and result sharing. *Interface agent* is required to assist the user to add information to the system and to retrieve information. *Database agent* is needed to store, access and retrieve the data when needed. As the system will be queried for data patterns, a *Data Mining* agent is necessary to find the patterns hidden in the data. For the automatic addition of the data, two additional agent types are needed: *Controller agent* to request scout and *Spider agent* to find and retrieve data.

In this first step, we have identified five different types of agents. In the following step, we will discuss their intelligence.

Define Agent's Intelligence

The agents need to be equipped with the knowledge that will enable them to perform their task intelligently e.g. to communicate with each other, to retrieve relevant information, to analyze and manipulate information, present information in a meaningful way, etc. Currently, knowledge bases have been predominantly used to provide agents with intelligence and enable them to perform their action efficiently and effectively. Ontologies are high expressive knowledge models and use of ontologies over knowledge bases is preferred (Maedche, 2003).

We have designed Mental Health Ontology (Hadzic *et al.*, 2008d), and this ontology can be used to increase the overall intelligence of the system. Mental Health Ontology provides a shared common understanding of the mental health domain. It captures and represents mental health knowledge. It is organized according the following three sub-ontologies:

(1) disorder types (such as psychotic disorders, anxiety disorders, personality disorders, mood disorders, substance-related disorders, etc.) which define different types of mental disorders;

(2) causal factors, which are classified under 5 categories (genetic, physical, environmental, personal and microorganisms) and describe various causes of mental disorders

(3) treatments (such as pharmacotherapy, psychotherapy, group and family therapy, electroconvulsive therapy and psychosurgery) and describe various treatments of mental disorders.

Mental Health Ontology can be used for different purposes within our system. Firstly, the ontology can be used to meaningfully organize mental health data within the dedicated database. All information on a specific ontology concept can be put together. For example, all publication

claiming that a mental illness is cased by a virus can be put together. This will greatly facilitate data access and retrieval. Secondly, ontology can significantly help in deriving meaningful data patterns form the data. This approach is described in greater detail in (Hadzic *et al.*, 2008b) where the tree mining algorithms were used to mine ontological data. Thirdly, ontology can be used to present the retrieved information to the user in a meaningful way. The use of ontologies adds an extra dimension to the results and makes it possible to present the user with the map of related answers.

Define Agent's Collaborations

In the first stage of the TICSA approach, we described how to identify different agent types according to their different functions and roles within the multi-agent system. Here, we focus on structural organization and position of agents within the system. The aim of this step is to:

- define system architecture that will enable the most optimal performance of agents
- establish correspondence between different agent types and positions of these agents within the multi-agent system

Here it is important to organize the agents so that the problem solving process can easily flow towards its completion and that the communication between different agents can be easily established. In combination with capabilities of individual agents, these two features are major factors determining efficient and effective system performance.

The agents of the proposed system are sociable. This means that they are able to interact with each other in order to cooperate, collaborate and negotiate with respect to information, knowledge and services. The agents are cooperatively working on different levels within this multi-agent system and are dependent on each other with the respect to the same goal. To reduce the complexity of the overall tasks, it is subdivided among various agents. Individual agents work only on their aspect of the problem.

We will discuss each of the four interaction cases in the rest of this section. We will use UML 2.1 diagrams to represent interactions and sequences of actions within the system. A Sequence Diagram is generally defined across the page by a series of rectangles, each of which represents a class. Each of these rectangles has a dotted line running vertically down the page. These dotted lines are known as lifelines. As you go down the page, time passes as messages flow between objects. UML 2.1 allows for a particular class to have more than one lifeline. Namely, a particular class may have many ports, each one with its own lifeline. The agent may be represented by a rectangle, and have many ports, each with its own lifeline.

We will use a Sequence Diagram where Composite Classes have more than one port and represent different roles of the same agent. This will enable us to model the multi-agent system and represent agents which play more than one role concurrently. Each port has its own lifeline. If there are two ports, this signifies two roles that are played by the agent from which the ports come. We use Composite Class as a rectangle at the head of lifelines in a Sequence Diagram, and each port to represent a role played by the Composite Class, rather than repeating rectangles for each class. In the examples shown in Figures 2-5, a number of agents play multiple roles which is represented by multiple ports. Depending on which role the agent is acting in when it sends/receives messages, the sequence diagram shows arrows to/from a particular lifeline for the agent.

There are three points worth noting in our sequence diagram:

(1) the lifelines of agents are solid throughout since agents tend to be persistent.

(2) each rectangle represents a Composite Class which implements an agent type.

(3) each distinct role played by an agent is represented by a distinct port on the rectangle with its own lifeline.

(1) Human User Adds Data to the System

In the Figure 2, we represent a situation where a human user adds data to the system. The Interface Agent will assist the users (mental health researchers) to input their information in the most effective way. Each user who wants to add data into the database will be registered and given unique ID. This will increase control over the addition of data and prevent malicious actions. The user logs into the system and receives a message from the system letting them know that her/his login is a success. To do this the user interfaces with the Interface Agent. The next step is for the user to enter data that will address the validation criteria for the addition of a publication. This data may include publication details such as the journal, the year of publication, and abstract, table of content of the book/journal/paper where the publication appears. Once the Interface Agent has received this information it will Apply Validation Criteria by sending a message to the Database Agent. The Database Agent will send a message back to the Interface Agent confirming that the Validation Criteria have been applied. The human user will then be in a position to attach the publication, and the data will be sent through the Interface Agent to the Database Agent, which will proceed to add the data to the database. The Database Agent will also manage the database content. Once the publication is added, a Publication Added message will be passed through the Database Agent through the Interface Agent to the human user.

Figure 2. Human user adds data to the system

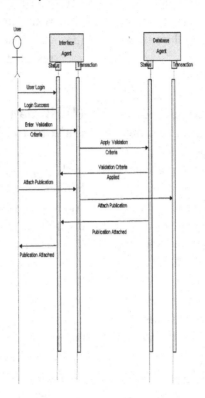

(2) Computer Program Adds Data to the System

Another way of adding the data to the system is using a program. This is shown in Figure 3. The program finds data automatically and adds it to the database without human intervention. A Controller Agent is stationed on the system machine and will make a request to a Spider Agent to scout for papers on the internet. The Spider Agent will be mobile and proceed to act in its role to find papers in many cases. Each time a paper is found it will generate a status message that a paper is found. Once the message has been received the paper will have to be validated before it can be added to the database. This will occur by the Spider Agent sending a message to the Database Agent to validate the paper. The Database Agent will perform the validation (for example, by getting proof that the paper has been refereed and

published) and then send a message back to the Spider Agent that the paper has been validated. The Spider Agent will then send a message through the Database Agent back to the Controller Agent that the paper has been added. This sequence will be repeated for every paper added to the system by the program.

(3) Retrieve Specific Data

In Figure 4, we explain a situation where a human user retrieves simple data from the system. The Interface Agent will assist the user in formulating queries and request the information from the Database Agents. Initially, the person sends a query for data to the Interface Agent. The Interface Agent passes on this query to the Database Agent. The Database Agent interacts directly with the database to execute the query and return the publication(s) requested. The Database Agent then returns the

Figure 3. Computer program adds data to the system

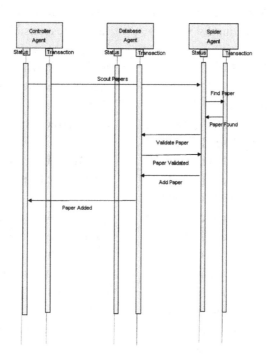

Figure 4. Retrieve specific data

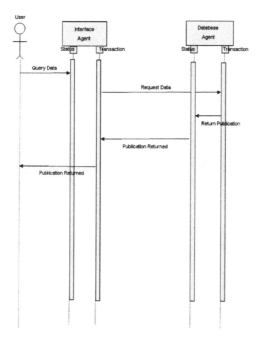

publication through the Interface Agent, to the human user. The Interface Agent will present the information to the user in a meaningful way.

(4) Retrieve Data Patterns

The situation where a human user makes a request for data patterns is represented in Figure 5. Initially the human user will send a pattern query to the Interface Agent, which will send the request to identify a particular pattern to the Data Mining Agent. In order to mine the data, the Data Mining Agent will send a request to the Database Agent to provide data. The Database Agent will interact directly with the database to retrieve the data being mined. A message will then be generated that data has been returned, and data itself will be sent from the Database Agent to the Data Mining Agent in order for it to be mined. The Data Mining Agent will then mine the data by identifying patterns and establishing their rankings. Data Mining Agents will systematically analyse the inputted information and expose the

patterns and knowledge hidden in the data. We are specifically looking for the patterns of causal factors responsible for onset of a specific mental illness. Once the data mining is complete, the Pattern List will be returned back to the Interface Agent from the Data Mining Agent. Finally, the Pattern related information will be displayed by the Interface Agent to the human user.

Protect the System by Implementing Security Requirements

Security plays an important role in the development of multi-agent systems. The risks of jeopardizing the system security must be minimized by providing as much security as possible. The aim of this stage is to:

- identify critical security issues within the multi-agent system
- effectively address the identified issues
- implement the security requirements within the system

Figure 5. Retrieve data patterns

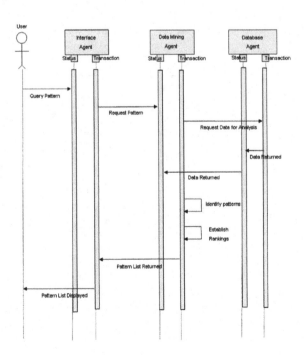

The five security properties defined in (Mouratidis *et al.*, 2003) should be taken into consideration:

1. authentication, proving the identity of an agent

For example, Interface agent forwards validation criteria and publications to the Database agent to be stored in the database. They much provide identification to each other before the exchange of data takes place.

2. availability, guaranteeing the accessibility and usability of information and resources to authorized agents

When a user requests a data pattern, Database agent must provide data to Data Mining agent for the data mining to take place and provide the results to the user.

3. confidentiality, information is accessible only to authorized agents

The data from the database are only accessible to the agents of our system, and inaccessible to external agents.

4. non repudiation, confirming the involvement of an agent in certain action

Spider agent must explain the source of its data.

5. integrity, information remains unmodified from source entity to destination entity

All the information that needs to be added to the database either through the user or through a computer program must not change during the process of data transportation and data exchange.

We have identified some additional characteristics which can greatly contribute to the security of the overall system:

1. compliance, acting in accordance with the given set of regulations and standards
2. service, serving one another for mutually beneficial purposes
3. dedication, complete commitment of the agents to the overall goal and purpose of the multi-agent system

The abovementioned properties are critical inside the multi-agent system as well as outside the multi-agent system, such as during the agent interaction with the environment. After the identification of required security properties, it is necessary to effectively address and implement them within the multi-agent system. As different agents have different functions within the system, some agents will be more critical than others in regard to the security of the system. As a consequence, the critical agents will be assigned more security requirements than the others.

Assemble Individual Agents

In the previous sections, we have discussed functions of agents within a system as well as equipping the agents with intelligence and enabling them to perform these functions optimally, collaborative aspect of agents and security requirements. In this step we focus on bringing these different aspects together and creating a variety of agents. For each agent, it is important to:

- identify required agent components
- assemble the components into an unified system i.e. individual agents

We can use Composite Structure Diagram to define each agent into greater detail. While each Port represents a different role played by the agent, each Part represents a distinct area of processing within the agent. The <<Agent>> stereotype must have a name, at least a Controller part which controls the efforts of the Agent to achieve a goal, and at least one port, which relates to it's playing a role.

The <<Agent>> stereotype based on the Composite Structure Diagram can be used to model each agent within our system. We have chosen to illustrate this on the Interface and Database agents, as shown in Figures 6 and 7.

In Figure 6, we present a Composite Structure Diagram from UML 2.1, which has been stereotyped to represent the Interface Agent that is at the head of a lifeline in the Sequence Diagram discussed earlier. Note that the same two ports (Status and Transaction) that were present in the sequence diagram are also present here. While the Sequence Diagram focuses on the interactions between different Agents in our example, the Composite Structure Diagram illustrates the internal processing within each Agent as well as the different roles played by Agents. In the case of the Interface Agent, there is a Controller part, which would manage state- and goal-related information, a Login part which handles User Login and the

subsequent authentication that would take place, a Communication part that handles the incoming and outgoing messages from the Agent to other Agents, and a Query part which would validate and forward Queries related to data to be extracted and presented to the user. The roles performed by this Agent are shown by the 'Status' and 'Transaction' ports shown on the edge of the Agent.

What applies to the Interface Agent, applies also to the Database Agent. What differs of course is the internal processing. The Controller part is also necessary in this Agent. Additionally, a part to Verify publications to be added to the database is essential. The Database Agent also has to be able to handle requests to store data, and this is performed by a Store part. The opposite side of this is to extract data, and the Retrieve part is present for select queries. The Communicate part is present for the same reason as for the Interface Agent, to handle inter-agent communication. Finally, the roles performed by the Agent are shown by the 'Status' and 'Transaction' ports shown on the edge of the Agent.

Figure 6. Interface agent

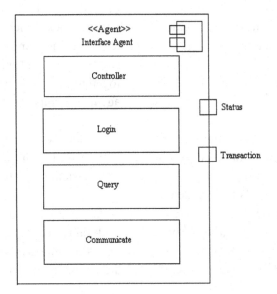

Figure 7. Database agent

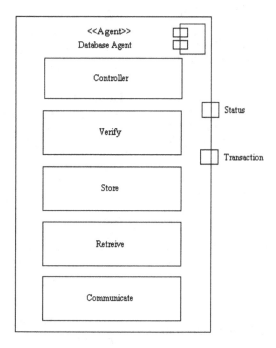

CONCLUSION

In this paper we propose a multi-agent system specifically designed to support the creation of a collaborative research environment and illustrate how UML 2.1 can be used to effectively model this multi-agent system. This chapter has three unique areas of contributions. Firstly, it proposes a solution that will enable mental health researchers to effectively share and use mental health information, and help them jointly derive knowledge and better understand causes of mental illness. This will help mental health professionals to develop effective prevention and intervention strategies, and the general public to gain a better understanding and control over their mental health. Secondly, in this chapter we use the TICSA approach to gives a clear and stepwise insight into the design of multi-agent systems. And thirdly, we illustrate how UML 2.1 can be used to effectively model multi-agent systems in general, contributing to the development of standard notation for modeling multi-agent systems. We have used the UML 2.1

Sequence Diagram to capture and represent the sociable nature of agents and UML 2.1 Composite Diagram to model the individual agents in greater detail. The combination of ports which represent agent's roles, and parts which capture agent's internal processes enable effective representation of the goal-driven nature of agents. Additionally, we have not changed the semantics of the UML 2.1 diagrams which is a critical point that makes our use of UML 2.1 valid.

REFERENCES

Burgun, A. (2006). Desiderata for domain reference ontologies in biomedicine. *Journal of Biomedical Informatics*, *39*, 307–313. doi:10.1016/j.jbi.2005.09.002

Ceusters, W., Martens, P., Dhaen, C., & Terzic, B. (2001). LinkFactory: an advanced formal ontology management System. *Proceedings of Interactive Tools for Knowledge Capture* (KCAP 2001).

Check, E. (2004). Antidepressants:Bitter pills. *Nature, 431*, 122–124. doi:10.1038/431122a

Cimino, J. J. (2006). In defense of the desiderata . *Journal of Biomedical Informatics, 39*, 299–306. doi:10.1016/j.jbi.2005.11.008

Craddock, N., & Jones, I. (2001). Molecular genetics of bipolar disorder. *The British Journal of Psychiatry, 178*(41), 128–133. doi:10.1192/bjp.178.41.s128

Da Silva, V. T., Noya, R. C., & De Lucena, C. J. P. (2004). Using the MAS-ML to model a multi-agent system. *Software engineering for multi-agent systems II: research issues and practical applications . Lecture Notes in Computer Science, 2940*, 129–148.

Da Silva, V. T., Noya, R. C., & De Lucena, C. J. P. (2005), Using the UML 2.0 Activity Diagram to Model Agent Plans and Actions. *Proceedings of the 4ᵗʰ International Conference on Autonomous Agents and Multiagent Systems*. The Netherlands.

De Maria, B. A., Da Silva, V. T., Noya, R. C., & De Lucena, C. J. P. (2005). VisualAgent: A Software Development Environment for Multi-Agent Systems. *Proceedings of the 20th Brazilian Symposium on Databases and 19th Brazilian Symposium on Software Engeneering*, Brazil.

Ekholm, J. M., Pekkarinen, P., Pajukanta, P., Kieseppä, T., Partonen, T., & Paunio, T. (2002). Bipolar disorder susceptibility region on Xq24-q27.1 in Finnish families . *Molecular Psychiatry, 7*(5), 453–459. doi:10.1038/sj.mp.4001104

Fonseca, J. M., Mora, A. D., & Marques, A. C. (2005). MAMIS – A Multi-Agent Medical Information System. *Proceedings of IASTED International Conference on Biomedical Engineering (BioMED 2005)*, Austria.

Friedman, R. A., & Leon, A. C. (2007). Expanding the Black Box-Depression, Antidepressants, and the Risk of Suicide. *The New England Journal of Medicine, 356*, 2343–2346. doi:10.1056/NEJMp078015

Gómez-Pérez, A. (1998). Knowledge sharing and reuse, *The Handbook on Applied Expert Systems* (pp. 1-36). CRC Press.

Hadzic, M., & Chang, E. (2005). Ontology-based Support for Human Disease Study. *Proceedings of the Hawaii International Conference on System Sciences, HICSS38*, 2005.

Hadzic, M., & Chang, E. (2008a). Web Semantics for Intelligent and Dynamic Information Retrieval Illustrated Within the Mental Health Domain. In E. Chang, T.S. Dillon, R. Meersman, & K. Sycara (Eds.), *Advances in Web Semantics: A State-of-the Art*. Springer.

Hadzic, M., & Chang, E. (2008b). An Integrated Approach for Effective and Efficient Retrieval of the Information about Mental Illnesses. In A.S. Sidhu, T.S. Dillon, & E. Chang, (Eds.), *Biomedical Data and Applications*. Springer.

Hadzic, M., & Chang, E. (2008c). TICSA Approach: Five Important Aspects of Multi-agent Systems. *Proceedings of the International IFIP Workshop On Semantic Web & Web Semantics, On The Move Federated Conferences*, Mexico.

Hadzic, M., Chen, M., & Dillon, T. (2008d). Towards the Mental Health Ontology. *Proceedings of the IEEE International Conference on Bioinformatics and Biomedicine, USA*.

Hadzic, M., Hadzic, F., & Dillon, T. (2008a). Tree Mining in Mental Health Domain. *Proceedings of the Hawaii International Conference on System Sciences (HICSS-41)*, USA.

Hadzic, M., Hadzic, F., & Dillon, T. (2008b). Mining of Health Information from Ontologies. *Proceedings of the International Conference on Health Informatics (HEALTHINF2008)*, Portugal.

Hadzic, M., Hadzic, F., & Dillon, T. (2008c). Domain Driven Data Mining for the Mental Health Domain. In P.S. Yu, C. Zhang, & H. Zhang (Ed.), *Domain Driven Data Mining: Domain Problems.* Springer.

Han, J., & Kamber, M. (2006). *Data Mining: Concepts and Techniques* (2nd ed.). San Francisco: Morgan Kaufmann

Hill, P. C., & Pargament, K. I. (2003). Advances in the Conceptualization and Measurement of Religion and Spirituality: Implications for Physical and Mental Health Research . *The American Psychologist*, *58*(1), 64–74. doi:10.1037/0003-066X.58.1.64

Horvitz-Lennon, M., Kilbourne, A. M., & Pincus, H. A. (2006). From Silos To Bridges: Meeting The General Health Care Needs Of Adults With Severe Mental Illnesses. *Health Affairs*, *25*(3), 659–669. doi:10.1377/hlthaff.25.3.659

Huang, J., Jennings, N. R., & Fox, J. (1995). An Agent-based Approach to Health Care management. *International Journal of Applied Artificial Intelligence*, *9*(4), 401–420. doi:10.1080/08839519508945482

Kavi, K., Kung, D. C., Bhambhani, H., & Pancholi, G. & Kanikarla. M. (2003). Extending UML for Modeling and Design of MultiAgent Systems. *Proceedings of the 2nd International Workshop on Software Engineering for Large-Scale Multi-Agent Systems (SELMAS2003), held in conjunction with the International Conference on Software Engineering*, USA.

Kim, J., & Park, J. (2004). BioIE: Retargetable information extraction and ontological annotation of biological interactions from the literature. *Journal of Bioinformatics and Computational Biology*, *2*(3), 551–568. doi:10.1142/S0219720004000739

Liu, J., Juo, S. H., Dewan, A., Grunn, A., Tong, X., & Brito, M. (2003). Evidence for a putative bipolar disorder locus on 2p13-16 and other potential loci on 4q31, 7q34, 8q13, 9q31, 10q21-24, 13q32, 14q21 and 17q11-12. *Molecular Psychiatry*, *8*(3), 333–342. doi:10.1038/sj.mp.4001254

Lopez, A. D., & Murray, C. C. J. L. (1998). The Global Burden of Disease, 1990-2020. *Nature Medicine*, *4*, 1241–1243. doi:10.1038/3218

Maedche, A. D. (2003). *Ontology Learning for the Semantic Web*. Norwell, Massachusetts, Kluwer Academic Publishers.

Merelli, E., Culmone, R., & Mariani, L. (2002). BioAgent-A mobile agent system for bioscientists. *Proceedings of the Network Tools and Applications in Biology Workshop Agents in Bioinformatics*, Italy.

Moreno, A., & Isern, D. (2002). A first step towards providing health-care agent-based services to mobile users. *Proceedings of the First International Joint Conference on Autonomous Agents and Multi-agent Systems* (pp. 589-590).

Mouratidis, H., Giorgini, P., & Manson, G. A. (2003). Modelling secure multi-agent systems, *Proceedings of the Second International Joint Conference on Autonomous Agents and Multiagent Systems* (pp. 859-866).

Odell, J., Van Dyke, H. P., & Bauer, B. (2001). Representing Agent Interaction Protocols in UML. In P. Ciancarini, & M. Wooldridge (Ed.), *Agent-Oriented Software Engineering* (pp. 121-140). Springer-Verlag.

Pacher, P., & Kecskemeti, V. (2004). Cardiovascular Side Effects of New Antidepressants and Antipsychotics: New Drugs, old Concerns? *Current Pharmaceutical Design, 10*(20), 2463–2475. doi:10.2174/1381612043383872

Piatetsky-Shapiro, G., & Tamayo, P. (2003). Microarray data mining: Facing the challenges. *SIGKDD Explorations, 5*(2), 1–6. doi:10.1145/980972.980974

Schumaker, J. F. (1992). *Religion and Mental Health*. Oxford University Press.

Sestito, S., & Dillon, T. S. (1994). *Automated knowledge acquisition*. Sydney: Prentice Hall of Australia.

Sidhu, A. S., Dillon, T. S., & Chang, E. (2006). Integration of Protein Data Sources through PO. *Proceedings of the 17th International Conference on Database and Expert Systems Applications* (DEXA 2006) (pp. 519-527).

Smith, B. (2006). From concepts to clinical reality: An essay on the benchmarking of biomedical terminologies. *Journal of Biomedical Informatics, 39*, 288–298. doi:10.1016/j.jbi.2005.09.005

Smith, D. G., Ebrahim, S., Lewis, S., Hansell, A. L., Palmer, L. J., & Burton, P. R. (2005). Genetic epidemiology and public health: hope, hype, and future prospects. *Lancet, 366*(9495), 1484–1498. doi:10.1016/S0140-6736(05)67601-5

Srinivasan, P., Mitchell, J., Bodenreider, O., Pant, G., & Menczer, F. (2002). Web Crawling Agents for Retrieving Biomedical Information. *Proceedings of International Workshop on Agents in Bioinformatics,* Italy.

Ulieru, M. (2003). Internet-enabled soft computing holarchies for e-Health applications. *New Directions in Enhancing the Power of the Internet* (pp. 131-166).

Wenner, M. (2008). Infected with Insanity: Could Microbes Cause Mental Illness? *Scientific American*. Retrieved from http://www.sciam.com/article.cfm?id=infected-with-insanity.

Werneke, U., Northey, S., & Bhugra, D. (2006). Antidepressants and sexual dysfunction. *Acta Psychiatrica Scandinavica, 114*(6), 384–397. doi:10.1111/j.1600-0447.2006.00890.x

Wilczynski, N. L., Haynes, R. B., & Hedges, T. (2006). Optimal search strategies for identifying mental health content in MEDLINE: an analytic survey. *Annals of General Psychiatry*, 5.

Wooldridge, M. (2002). *An Introduction to Multiagent Systems*. John Wiley and Sons.

Chapter 12
Multi–Agent Systems in Developing Countries

Dean Yergens
University of Manitoba, Canada & University of Calgary, Canada

Julie Hiner
University of Calgary, Canada

Jörg Denzinger
University of Calgary, Canada

ABSTRACT

Developing countries are faced with many problems and issues related to healthcare service delivery. Many factors contribute to this, such as a lack of adequate medical resources, a shortage of skilled medical professionals, increasing clinical demands due to infectious diseases, limited technological systems and an unreliable telecommunications and electrical infrastructure. However, the potential for multi-agent systems and multi-agent simulations to address some of these issues shows great promise. Multi-agent simulations have already been applied to modeling infectious diseases such as HIV and Avian Flu in the developing world. Furthermore, groups of smart agents, by their very design, can function autonomously and act as a distributed service, which greatly enables them to successfully operate in the kind of environments encountered in developing countries.

INTRODUCTION

Developing countries possess an ideal environment for multi-agent systems (MAS). However, most of the published literature around multi-agent systems seems to be focused on projects and systems being developed and implemented in more developed countries; such as in North America, Asia and Europe. This is most likely because most of the multi-agent systems research and activity is conducted and carried out in developed countries.

But recently there has been an increasing amount of literature published about the use of multi-agent simulations in developing countries, most noticeably around simulating the spread of infectious diseases. This is probably a reflection of the increasing awareness that the general public in developed countries has around infectious diseases in developing countries, such as HIV, Tuberculosis and Avian Flu. This awareness is also creating con-

DOI: 10.4018/978-1-60566-772-0.ch012

cerns about the potential spread to the developed world, and due to these concerns more effort and research is occurring in modeling epidemics in order to understand how to react to and contradict these outbreaks.

The application of Multi-agent Simulations to the area of infectious disease management and response is a promising avenue for public health in terms of modeling these potential epidemics. If we were to take a hypothetical SARS epidemic, a multi-agent simulation would be a great method in modeling the spread of the disease and the effects on the general population. Containment strategies could then be applied against the developed model to see what reaction is the most effective and by what time that reaction would need to be executed in order have an impact on counteracting the outbreak. Agents could be created to simulate people in the community and their (relevant) interactions. The infectious disease could then be modeled into the population and various factors examined such as the incubation time of the virus, the period of time that a person is contagious to others, and the mortality rate once infected. Other agents could be designed around transportation activities. Details about transportation mode and transfer locations could then be factored into the model. This would allow public health investigators to answer questions such as: How many people may have been passengers on planes from an infected area? How many other passengers were on those aircraft and might have potentially been infected? What are the destinations of those flights, and should those cities or countries be warned as to the potential threat?

Not only could this hypothetical SARS scenario be implemented as a multi-agent simulation, but it could also be adapted into a multi-agent system acting as a real-time global health warning system. With the creation of agents able to connect to real-time information systems, such as air traffic control and flight scheduling data, comes the possibility of a quicker response to incidents and consequently containment of such incidents

(outbreaks).

In addition to applying MAS to public health issues, there are many other healthcare areas where MAS could be applied in developing countries. Some examples of these include:

- Decision Support applied to direct clinical care.
- Training using agent-based resources.
- Telemedicine, having the ability to access information or other medical personal either nationally or internationally.
- Pharmacy management, including drug interaction alerts and drug treatment compliance monitoring.
- Inventory and logistic management for Medical Supplies.

However, in order to be successful in implementing these systems we also need to understand the environment in which many developing countries exist. Challenges such as not having enough medical personnel or not having the proper equipment or supplies are common problems in many hospitals and clinics. In addition, the working environment and infrastructure may have challenges such as phone lines that are inoperative and electricity systems that are unreliable, especially during certain times of the year such as the rainy season in sub-Saharan Africa.

For many of these challenges, the advantages of using multi-agent systems are rather clear. MAS have the ability to function in a distributed manner and can be designed to act autonomously, making them ideally suited for applications in environments that are lacking a reliable telecommunications or electrical network. Autonomy allows the agents to be opportunistic, waiting for required resources to become available and then acting immediately. Unlike humans, agents are never too tired to realize that there is an opportunity, or too busy to be able to check if the required resources align.

In this chapter, we will further explore the

technological and environmental advantages and disadvantages of developing countries, including a look at what issues are encountered in the implementation of not only MASs but any kind of health-related information technology system. We will then examine the special health care issues that developing countries are encountering. These include such things as limited resources; increasing demand; poverty; a poor overall health status compared to developed countries; and the impact of diseases such as HIV/AIDS, TB, Malaria and increasingly Avian Flu. Based on this, we will explore how MASs have been applied to developing countries from a healthcare perspective.

A key part of this chapter is the presentation of a multi-agent simulation system within a simulation visualization and analysis framework that looks into the pressing issue of the decreasing availability of nurses and other medical professionals in many developing countries, using Sub-Sahara Africa as the case study. We conclude with some areas for future work that we believe will have a great potential in improving healthcare in developing countries, utilizing the advantages of multi-agent systems.

BACKGROUND

The healthcare problems in developing countries are extremely challenging. Issues such as poverty, limited resources, and a shortage of medical professionals all contribute to a challenging environment in which to address the population's healthcare needs.

Many developing countries also have a high incidence of infectious diseases. Vector borne diseases such as malaria and food- and water-borne diseases such as bacterial diarrhea and hepatitis A put a considerable strain on the healthcare systems and the people's health status in such countries. These not only result in sickness that may affect a family's household, but in many cases is a leading cause of death.

HIV/AIDS is another concern in developing countries, especially in Sub-Saharan Africa where its impact has been most felt. In 2003, Malawi had a 14.2% HIV prevalence rate while Zambia had a 16.5% HIV prevalence rate (CIA 2008). Due to these factors, Malawi in 2008 had a life expectancy of just over 43 years compared to life expectancies in Canada of 81 years, 78 years in the United States and 82 years in Japan (CIA 2008).

Developing countries also face extreme shortages of medical professionals such as physicians and nurses for treating the general population. For example, in 2004 it was reported (WHO 2008) that Malawi had only 266 physicians and 7,264 nursing and midwifery personnel. This worked out to 1 physician and 6 nurses/midwifery personnel per 10,000 people. In comparison, Canada in 2006 (WHO 2008) had 62,307 physicians and 327,000 nursing and midwifery personnel, which works out to 19 physicians and 101 nursing/midwifery personal per 10,000 people. In addition, many developing countries are faced with the constant recruitment ("poaching") of their medical professionals by developed countries (Hangoro C., et al. 2004).

Developing countries also face major infrastructure challenges. These infrastructure challenges can have a significant impact on the application of information technology by making the system unreliable, increasing the costs of implementation and complicating on-going support for these systems due to a wide variety of factors including the electrical, telecommunications, and technological environment.

Electrical Infrastructure

Electrical systems in developing countries may be unreliable due to a wide range of factors, including a lack of investment and maintenance in the underlying infrastructure and an over subscription of the capacity of available energy. Severe weather during certain times of the year can also affect the reliability of the electricity grid, such as during the rainy season in Sub-Saharan Africa.

The limited electrical supply and severe weather can often lead to black outs, brown outs and spikes in the electricity grid. There are ways to address these issues, such as with the use of Uninterrupted Power Supplies (UPS) or diesel powered generators. However, often an organization does not have the financial resources to invest in this equipment. Furthermore, this is an additional expense that developing countries need to incur in their operations compared to developed countries. The mentioned events can also permanently damage the computer equipment, making replacement extremely difficult in developing countries reliant on foreign aid and grants for many of their healthcare and technological supplies.

These power outrages also affect the ability of an organization to perform work, as occasional black outs can affect the entire organization's performance. Finally, the electrical grid may also not reach into specific parts of the country due to a lack of investment in the electrical system on a national level.

Telecommunications Infrastructure

The telecommunications infrastructure in developing countries can also be a significant barrier in the implementation of computer systems. The adoption of cellular technology, especially amongst end consumers, is an exciting development as it allows the end user to be in touch with others in a very cost effective manner. Even though the use of cell phones has been widely adopted by most people, there can still be an issue around Internet connectivity in these countries.

Even where Internet connectivity exists, it may be cost prohibitive to many people and projects, or lack capacity (bandwidth) resulting in slow performance accessing the Internet. This may have an impact on the opportunities to perform many tasks relevant to healthcare, such as telemedicine or even downloading journal articles due to band-

width constraints. Even what we might consider basic web page activity may be too bandwidth intensive for developing countries, resulting in the inability to access this content. Options such as satellites (VSAT) allow remote communities' access to the Internet, but cost continues to be a major factor against the wide-spread adoption of satellite technologies.

Technological Environment

Finally, the technological environment is another major challenge for developing countries. Computer equipment is often donated or sourced from a wide variety of countries. The results of this have often been healthcare clinics with computer equipment from multiple countries, with varying levels of capabilities and software consistency across the computers in the facility. Even keyboards from multiple countries with different languages may exist. This can be a challenge for implementing new systems, as the end user computer system may be varied and outdated, therefore incapable of running new application(s). A lack of human resources with the required technical knowledge and skill set is yet another factor that may impact the successful implementation and adoption of new information technology solutions.

Application of MAS in Developing Countries

The application of healthcare-related multi agent systems in developing countries has been rather limited to date. Few clinical systems have been referenced in the literature. One such system that was represented was the use of a multi agent approach for diagnostic expert systems (Shaalana K., et al. 2004). Shaalana (2004) described a system which consisted of several agents, including diagnostic and expert agents that contained autonomous knowledge-based systems and was accessed via the Internet.

The use of agent based systems for creating

simulations has been applied in many applications for studying the impact of infectious diseases in developing countries. Several systems have been created looking at a wide range of diseases, including Trypanosomiasis (Muller G., et al. 2004) otherwise known as sleeping sickness, SARS (Gong J., et al. 2006), Avian Flu (Yergens D., et al. 2006a) and HIV (Teweldemedhin E., et al. 2004).

The role of multi agent systems in humanitarian or disaster response (Scalem M., et al 2004, Yergens D., et al 2006b) has also been discussed. Scalem (2004) describes a decentralized disaster management system utilizing mobile multi agent systems. Yergens (2006b) discussed the collaboration of multi agent simulation for modeling epidemics with a low-bandwidth satellite surveillance system for application in developing countries.

There have also been several applications of multi agent systems applied to other health-related areas such as environmental, international development, and demining activities in developing countries.

Several authors have presented work related to the environmental sector by addressing water management (Adamatti DF., et al. 2004, Berger T., et al. 2002, Ducrot R., et al. 2004). Adamatti (2004) developed an application that integrated both an agent based system and a role playing game approach. This system was called "Jogo-Man", and was used for helping water management decisions with its stake holders. Berger (2002) also looked at water management and land use through a multi agent framework addressing the complex interdependencies that exist between the two. Ducrot (2004) investigated the use of a multi agent system for addressing water management and the issues faced with urbanization.

Due to the close relationship between the reduction of poverty and better health status, we have included international development as a potential area of improving healthcare using multi agent technologies. One application identified was a multi agent simulation used for investigat-

ing development policies in less favored areas in Uganda and Chile (Berger T., et al. 2006).

An additional area of application of multi agent systems has been in a humanitarian capacity of developing robots for clearing minefields (Santana P.F., et al. 2005, Kopacek P., 2002). Kopacek (2002) presented the concept of autonomous intelligent swarms of robots for clearing minefields.

All of these present novel applications of the use of multi agent systems and multi agent simulations in the domain of healthcare in developing countries.

MEDSTAFF: AN EXAMPLE OF THE USE OF MULTI-AGENT SIMULATION IN DECISION MAKING IN DEVELOPING COUNTRIES

The idea behind MedStaff was to create an environment in which health care policy decision makers in developing countries could create and analyze simulations about the impact of healthcare staffing in their region. These simulations are intended to help answer questions such as: How many health care facilities need to be involved? What kind of facilities do they have to be? And how many medical professionals of what types need to be working at each facility?

The staffing component also needed to answer questions such as the effect of aging staff and how retirement would affect a facility and the entire environment. It also needed to address illness amongst staff, especially in countries that have a high prevalence of HIV.

In addition to retirement and disease, we also needed to examine what factors affected staff retention in a healthcare facility. This could include other in-country healthcare facilities recruiting away staff, other in-country organizations such as Non-Government Organizations (NGOs) or Government Agencies recruiting personal. Finally, as indentified in the previous section, we also needed to analyze how external poaching of staff is affecting staffing needs within the country.

The requirements for the simulation model involved many different players, such as the many healthcare facilities and their function and locations, the various kinds of medical staff and issues such as retirement age, illness which might shorten the duration of the healthcare worker's employment, and a multitude of external factors such as recruitment from in-country organizations such as NGOs and the increasing recruitment from the international community. To address this we needed to construct a multi-agent simulation that would allow us to factor in all of these different players and have them act independently and in their own interests, much like in real life.

The MedStaff System Architecture

In the creation of MedStaff, we needed to create several different components that would operate in collaboration to provide the full multi-agent simulation environment. This system not only needed to provide the multi-agent simulation,

but also have the capability to adapt to new data sources, such as data from other countries or other organizations that may have a large number of healthcare facilities and staff that would be facing the same issues. The MAS environment also needed the ability to expand upon itself to factor in new kinds of healthcare facilities, new staffing professionals and also new players that affect those healthcare facilities and staff both in a positive and in a negative way. Finally, the MedStaff system also needed a visualization and reporting environment for analyzing the data created by a multi-agent simulation run.

To accomplish this, the MedStaff multi-agent simulation system architecture was composed of the following components, each of which will be described in detail later in the chapter.

Data Management Component

The data management component provides a repository for all the data that is required in defining a scenario for the MedStaff system, and in

Figure 1. MedStaff multi-agent system architecture

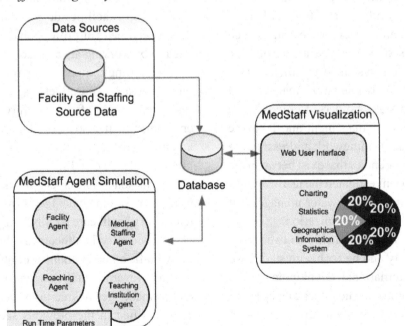

analyzing a simulation within it. This data comes from outside partners such as the Ministry of Health or some other organization that has the relevant information. Relevant data for defining the model includes details about the healthcare facilities, such as type of facility (hospital or healthcare clinic), location (town, province, latitude, longitude) and types of services provided (Emergency Room, Diagnostic Imaging, etc). The second type of data that is required is related to staffing information and includes data elements such as type of position (Nurse, Nurse Assistant, Birth Attendant, etc), age, sex and other factors related to a healthcare worker. The last function that the data management component provides is the collection of the MedStaff multi-agent simulation results. When a simulation scenario is run, all statistics and certain key interactions are logged in the database. This then allows us to analyze the scenario run later.

Multi-Agent Configuration Component

The Multi-agent configuration component is where a user essentially creates all the agents and defines the simulation and its parameters. Agents are created using two methods. The first method is by having the agents automatically generated from the information stored in the database of the data management component. This includes creating all the healthcare facility agents and also creating all the healthcare worker agents. The second method that can be applied is the creation of other kinds of agents. These other kinds of agents include teaching institution agents and poaching agents. The latter two agent types are the ones that will most likely have the greatest effect on the simulation environment.

Multi-Agent Simulation Run-Time Component

This component is the core of the MedStaff environment, as this is where a simulation scenario is

compiled and executed. The run-time environment takes the scenario developed in the multi-agent configuration component in collaboration with the data management component and executes it. Both the results and additional specific logging of the scenario are saved back to the data management component to be used for analysis later.

Visualization and Analysis Component

The last component is the visualization component. This component is a collection of tools that can be used for visualizing and analyzing the data contained in the data management component. This component provides basic charting, a geographical information system and advanced statistical capabilities. In addition, this component is used not only to visualize and analyze the results of a MedStaff simulation but also for understanding the source data before it is used in the generation of the agent simulation scenario.

The Data Management Component in Detail

The first component of the MedStaff system is the data management component. This component provides a repository for storing all of the data required by the MedStaff multi-agent simulation system. The data management component consists of three functions.

The first of these three functions is the management of the data for the creation of the multi-agent system for a scenario. As described later under the Multi-agent Configuration Component section, two types of agents are dynamically created from the database. These two types of agents are healthcare facility agents (FA) and medical staffing agents (MSA). The creation of these types of agents is done dynamically based on the relevant information from external sources. The external sources that were utilized in our MedStaff modeling for Zambia and Malawi were provided by the Malawi Ministry of Health and the Churches Health Association of Zambia (CHAZ), and utilized healthcare survey data produced by the Japanese International Community Agency (JICA).

The source data varied slightly between Malawi and Zambia. However, the core information that we utilized included information about the healthcare facilities, such as type of facility (hospital or healthcare clinic) and geographical information related to location of the healthcare facility (town, province, latitude, longitude). While types of services for the healthcare facilities were available (Emergency Room, Diagnostic Imaging, etc), these were not utilized in the MedStaff MAS we will report on. The second piece of data that was provided by the source databases was related to staffing information, and included information such as type of position (Nurse, Nurse Assistant, Birth Attendant, etc) and some demographic information such as the sex of the medical professional. The staffing information was linked to the appropriate healthcare facility. In several cases we had to generate statistical information for staffing based upon similar facilities to make up for information that was missing from the source databases.

The second function of the data management component is to act in collaboration with the MedStaff MAS. This involved interacting with both the Multi-agent Configuration component and the Multi-agent Runtime component. The Multi-agent configuration component needs to access the information stored in the data management component in the creation and generation of the healthcare facility agents (FA) and the medical staffing agents (MSA). The Multi-agent Runtime component also has to communicate with the data management component which provides the capability of storing the results and logging activities from the multi-agent simulation while it is running.

The final function of the data management component is to act in collaboration with the visualization environment component and to provide the necessary data for the display and analysis of the MedStaff MAS. Not only does the visualization environment component access the results of the MAS, it also has the ability to display and analyze the source data from the data management component to create a graphical interface to the system.

Simulation Environment and Agent Customization

As already stated, there are four main types of agents represented in a MedStaff MAS scenario. The majority of the agents in the MedStaff simulation environment are dynamically created using the information contained in the data management component (i.e. the FAs and the MSAs). The other two types of agents are Teaching Institute Agents (TIA) and Poaching Agents (PA).

The core agent of the MedStaff MAS is the medical staff agent. The MSA is essentially the healthcare worker in the system and basically what we are the most interested in. We are concerned about retaining these medical staff members and we are concerned that we have adequate staffing both short term and long term at our healthcare facilities. Each MSA works at a specific healthcare facility and thus is associated with a Facility Agent. Each FA represents a real hospital or healthcare clinic in the scenario and aggregates information such as location and number of staff (MSA) currently working in that facility.

There also exists Teaching Institute Agents. These are agents that represent universities, colleges and training schools that add supply of medical staff resources into the MedStaff simulation environment. Since teaching institutes vary by what kind of positions they produce, how many students graduate, when these students graduate and which geographical location they are located in, each TIA is unique and created as such. The TIAs feed MSAs into the various FAs.

The last type of agent is the Poaching Agent. We defined a PA for any action that reduces the

Figure 2. Agent interaction

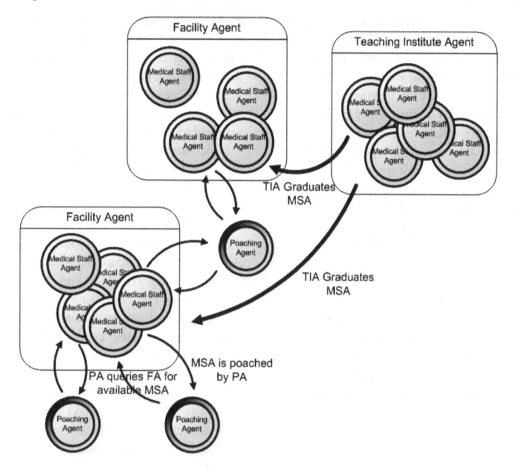

supply of MSA in the MedStaff MAS scenario. A PA may take on various forms such as a Non Government Organization (NGO) that is starting a new project in the country and needs medical professionals to staff the project, or an international agency that recruits medical staff for international assignments, thus removing them from the overall supply of MSAs in the simulation scenario. Another type of PA may be illness or disease related, such as an HIV PA that expires MSAs from the MedStaff MAS scenario.

The following figure shows the general interactions between the different agent types. Notice that for our application (which is one of several for which MedStaff can be used for) the Poaching Agents are the driving force of the interactions between agents (the other agents essentially do

what the PAs want them to do and they provide information for the Visualization Component).

In the following, we will describe the agents and the simulation environment in more detail.

Healthcare Facility Agent Implementation

Every healthcare facility that is to be represented in the MedStaff environment is created as its own agent. The FAs are automatically generated from the data that is stored in the data management component and include information such as name and facility type. In addition, there may be various levels of a healthcare facility such as a Level I or Level II of a hospital which would indicate the severity, acuity or services that a specific level of hospital may have.

The FA is also assigned information about the ownership of the facility. This is used to indicate if the healthcare facility is government-run, such as within the Ministry of Health; whether it is a private hospital and which organization operates it; or if it is part of a larger organization like a faith-based network, which is very common in developing countries. The type of ownership is essential, as often retention or recruitment strategies are organization-specific and need to be modeled with that level of detail. The FA can also be assigned other data such as population catchment. This attribute simply references the population base that that healthcare facility may serve in its community. This also can be used in the model for identifying a baseline of how many medical professionals (per profession) are needed per 1,000 people in the catchment area.

Other information related to the location of the healthcare facility also includes the district/region that the facility is in and, for visualization purposes, the latitude and longitude of the facility. This allows an FA to be displayed within a Geographical Information System.

The following table (Table 1) is a list of the attributes that are assigned to each Facility Agent.

Medical Staff Agent Implementation

As already stated, at the core of a MedStaff MAS scenario is the medical staff agent. The MSA basically functions as the representation of a real-life medical staff professional. At the start of the run of a MedStaff scenario, the MSAs are created dynamically based upon the information in the data management component. This component then populates the MedStaff environment with all the medical staff that the system is aware of assigned to the corresponding FAs.

Once the MSA are created there is only one other way to add more MSA to the simulation scenario, which is through Teaching Institute Agents (TIA) to be discussed later. However, there are multiple ways that MSAs may be removed from the system, which is accomplished via Poaching Agents (PA). Any action or situation that may reduce the supply of MSAs in the scenario is modeled by a PA. For example, there are international and national recruitment PAs, and PAs representing retirement events or disease events that remove MSAs from the model.

A MSA is assigned demographic information such as age and sex (which are used to determine if they can be the target of a PA). In addition, other attributes can be assigned to the MSA such as HIV Status. HIV status, especially in developing countries in sub-Saharan Africa, is a serious issue and has a tremendous impact on the retention of medical professionals in the healthcare facilities. The HIV status attribute also influences how PAs interact with this specific agent.

An example of this could be an International Poaching Agent (Inter-PA) that is responsible for

Table 1. Healthcare facility agent attributes

Attribute	Description
Name	The name of the healthcare facility.
Type	The type of healthcare facility it is. Examples could be a Hospital Level I or a Healthcare Clinic.
Distinct	The district or region that the healthcare facility is located within.
Catchment Population	The number of potential patients that this healthcare facility may serve.
Ownership	The organization or institution that the healthcare facility is associated with.
Latitude	The latitude GPS coordinate of the healthcare facility.
Longitude	The longitude GPS coordinate of the healthcare facility.

recruiting a specific type of medical professional for employment overseas. However, many organizations (and therefore their Inter-PAs) have as a requirement that an MSA to be recruited must have a negative HIV status. Obviously, the Inter-PA for recruiting certain MSAs will not interact with HIV positive MSAs.

An MSA that is removed from the simulation as a result of being poached will naturally inform its FA about this fact. The FA then provides us with the statistics regarding its MASs, and especially with the possibility to identify facilities that do not retain enough MSAs of a certain profession/type.

The following is the list of attributes that are assigned to each Medical Staff Agent (MSA) in our current system. Naturally this list can be extended to allow other simulations. (Table 2)

Training Institute Agent Implementation

Every training institute to be represented in the MedStaff environment is created as its own TIA. Each TIA is created by hand and not created directly from the data management component, as we did with the Facility Agents or the Medical Staff Agents. The reason for this is that each TIA has its own unique characteristics, such whether it is a university or a college, whether it is a public or a private institution, what kind of medical professions it trains, how long the program takes, how many students it can train per class and how many classes graduate per year.

Another factor that we had to build into each unique TIA was the set of details about the internal organization itself. For example, a TIA may have special factors that either make it unique or create some variation in the programs that may vary the number and timing of student graduations. A prime example of this might be a government university that is faced with limited resources and thus incurs strikes from either the students or the faculty and therefore does not produce graduates on a constant basis. Because of this variation, and the limited number of teaching facilities that are often found in a developing country, we took the approach to develop each TIA on its own and again not dynamically from information stored in a database. Being able to handcraft the behavior of a TIA is one of the strengths of a multi-agent simulation approach, although it makes creating scenarios more work intensive. We naturally used a specific TIA in several scenarios, and we also tried to parameterize the behaviors for each TIA as much as possible to allow them to be easily modified.

With regard to interaction with other agents, each TIA performs the task of placing the graduates of its various teaching programs into the various FAs. This is because a specific healthcare facility, represented by the FA, may need a specific type of graduate; or the organizations that run the FA may also run the TIA and therefore recruit from its own TIA. Location may be a factor in the recruitment, as a medical professional trained in one region of the country may prefer to continue working in that same region.

Table 2. Healthcare staff agent attributes

Attribute	Description
Position	The position of the healthcare worker. Examples could be a Registered Nurse or a Nurse Assistant.
Education Level	The educational level of the healthcare worker.
Sex	The Sex of the worker.
Age	The Age of the worker.
Years	How many years the healthcare worker has been at that Healthcare Facility
HIV Status	The HIV Status of the healthcare worker.

Poaching Agent Implementation

We took the approach of defining any kind of action that took a medical professional away from a healthcare facility as a Poaching Agent. Examples of what we consider a PA to be include a Non-Government Organization (NGO) that recruits medical professionals for running various projects within the country. Another example is external organizations or countries that recruit medical professionals away from the country to work internationally. Illness, accident, or disease are also implemented as PAs, as in the case of HIV. HIV has a significant effect on the MSA, just like in real life. The major impact of HIV on the MSA is that the MSA will expire and be terminated from the model. Like in real life, this has a negative impact resulting in less MSAs and a shorter working life.

Again, due to the complexity and variation of the types of actions that could affect employment at the various healthcare facilities we took the approach of creating each PA by hand on its own, like we did for the Training Institute Agents, and not dynamically like we did for the Healthcare facility agents or the Medical Staffing Agents. The advantage of creating individual PAs by hand compared to having the system dynamically create these agents from a database was that we can model more complex behavior of the various PAs. This allows decision makers to do better what-if simulations, which is naturally the goal

of MedStaff.

We developed a generic poaching agent. This generic poaching agent was then used as the foundation for creating specialized poaching agents. The generic agent was extended to address different poaching (i.e. MSA removing) actions that we might see in a developing country. In the following, we will describe several implementations of poaching agents. (Table 3)

The first major type of PA needed in our scenarios was an agent that recruited specific types of medical professionals away from a healthcare facility for international work, which is currently one of the major issues in developing countries. The PA received its own unique name and characteristics and behavior assigned to it. These characteristics include how many and what type of medical professionals were required on a given time basis. In the MedStaff MAS scenarios, we used 1 month as the time slice for the actions to take place. This meant that the agent seeks out specific types of healthcare medical professionals on a monthly time interval; and it can be adjusted for specific healthcare facility criteria such as the type of hospital, the location and also the organization that runs the healthcare facility.

We can also introduce these PAs at various times into the environment simulated by MedStaff. For example, if we know that a specific Non-Government Organization will be starting a new reproductive health and family planning project in the country in two years we can then

Table 3. Types of poaching agents

Poaching Agent	Description
NGO	A Non Government Organization that may recruit medical professionals away from healthcare facilities. There may be many NGO Poaching Agents in the system.
International Recruitment	A country or agency that recruits MSAs for international assignment out of the country. There may be many International Recruitment PAs in the system.
Illness and Disease	Illness and disease, such as HIV would be modeled as a PA. The MSA is then removed from the system if the HIV PA has selected that MSA based upon statistics.
Retirement	Once a medical professional reaches a certain age, he/she is retired and therefore removed from the system.

model that poaching behavior as the project is being implemented. To expand on this scenario, we can then create the PA to become active 1 year prior to the implementation of the project. Second, perhaps from previous experience we know how this NGO operates, we can then factor into the PA that it only poaches specific types of medical professionals from specific kinds of healthcare facilities or from specific kinds of organizations that are represented in the FA. In addition, it might only be targeting FAs in a specific geographical location as that is where the project will be concerned. Each new instance of a PA receives its own unique name..

Another type of PA that can have a major impact on the MedStaff simulations is related to illness and disease. As noted before, HIV has had a major impact on not only the general population in certain developing countries, especially sub-Saharan Africa, but also on the medical professional workforce working in those regions. We implemented an HIV PA that, based upon pre-defined statistics, targets specific types of medical staff agents and renders them inoperative (expired) thus removing them from the MedStaff simulation.

Of course, this HIV PA can become more sophisticated with additional statistics from external sources (that would be added to the data management component). When the Multi-agent Configuration component is initialized, then the HIV statistics could be applied towards the MSA in the system. However, we have not implemented this to date.

Other diseases, illness or even traffic accidents (which are extremely common in developing countries due to less reliable vehicles and poor road infrastructure), could also be factored into the system by the implementation of a new PA.

Multi-Agent Simulation
Run Time Component

The MedStaff Run Time component is where the actual MAS for the simulation runs and sce-

narios are initialized and executed. The Run Time component utilizes the multi-agent configuration component and starts to create the environment that MedStaff will operate in. The first part of the execution is the creation of all the agents that can be created utilizing information from the data management component. This includes the healthcare Facility Agents and the Medical Staffing Agents.

Once those agents are created, the custom agents such as the Teaching Institute Agents and the Poaching Agents are created and activated. These agents then interact with both the FAs and MSAs for the duration of the simulation scenario.

The MedStaff Run Time environment works on a one month time slice and we initialize the MAS to run for a 10 year period as the default. As the scenario is running, various statistics and events are recorded to the data management component. This then allows us after the MAS simulation is performed to display and analyze the results of that specific scenario using the Visualization Environment Component.

Visualization Environment
Component

A visualization environment was included to aid in the display and analysis of the MedStaff MAS simulations. This visualization environment includes basic charting and trending, statistics and a geographical information system component.

The visualization component was implemented as a web-based display that runs separately from the actual MedStaff MAS simulations. This allows multiple decision makers to look at the data and explore the various scenarios that the MedStaff MAS simulation was applied to.

The visualization component utilizes data that is stored in the data management component. This allows the source data that was used to generate MedStaff MAS to be studied and analyzed. In any simulation project, having a good understanding of the source data and (in this case) the current system is essential. The results data generated from the MedStaff MAS simulations can also be viewed and analyzed within the visualization environment.

As mentioned before, several components make up the visualization environment. These are described below.

Basic Charting and Trending

Several charting components were implemented in the web-based framework. These include the ability to graph any piece of data in the data management component in a variety of ways including Line, Bar, Pie, Scatter, Radar and Gantt charts. The customized interface also allows multiple charts to be displayed in the same report or webpage and provides the user with the ability to filter the results. This provides the ability to display various aspects of data, such as reporting on only the healthcare facilities and associated medical staff that are in hospitals belonging to the ministry of heath in a certain region of the country. In addition, the ability to view data as a network chart was also added.

Advanced Statistics

For advanced statistics, the use of R (www.r-project.org) was included to provide statistical analysis for both the simulation data and also for the data that is currently in the system. R was embedded in the web-based framework and also included the provision to filter the data through the interface for the ability to analyze that specific information.

Geographical Information System

The last component of the visualization environment is the inclusion of a Geographical Information System style interface. Two approaches were taken here to display geographical data. The first was through an interface with Google Maps. The

second method was through using R (www.r-project.org) and the mapproj R package (www.r-project.org) for displaying geographical data.

Experimental Evaluation

For our experimental evaluation of the MedStaff MAS simulations we used Malawi as the test country. We chose Malawi because we had a good understanding of the geographical layout of the country and could indentify with the location of the various healthcare facilities and the organizations they belonged to. We also had a pretty good understanding of potential poaching agents. We utilized facility and staffing data provided by the Malawi Ministry of Health. We used this information to create the healthcare Facility Agents and the Medical Staffing Agents. We then created several Teaching Institutes Agents and Poaching Agents to evaluate how poaching agents and teaching institute agents are interacting with the rest of the simulation model.

MULTI-AGENT SIMULATION INITIALIZATION AND RUN

A MedStaff MAS scenario for Malawi was initialized and executed. We limited the scenario to only focus on "Nurse/Midwifes" MSAs. All other medical staffing professions were also created in the model, but were not targeted by any poaching agents or additionally produced by teaching institutions.

574 FAs were created during the initialization of the MedStaff MAS scenario. There were an additional 8336 Medical Staff Agents generated and assigned to the various FA. To include the HIV status attribute in the MSA we used a HIV prevalence rate of 14.2% from Malawi based upon 2003 data (CIA 2008). The details of the FA and MSA can be seen in the following two tables. In addition, region, geographical location, organization membership and population catchment area

Figure 3. Screenshot of the visualization environment

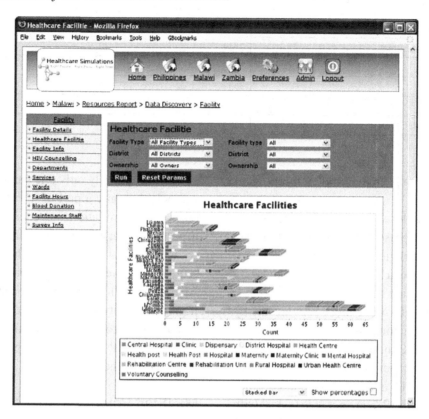

were also included in the FA.

Five Teaching Institute Agents were also introduced in the environment. For demonstration purposes the TIA were initially set at producing 30 "Nurse/Midwives" in two classes every year.

Four Poaching Agents were created and all of them were modeled as Non Government Organizations (PA-NGO) that recruited "Nurse/Midwives" on a system wide (national) scale. In addition, a fifth Poaching Agent (PA) was created to func-

tion as an International Donor that had different poaching behavior than the PA-NGOs described previously.

An important element of the MedStaff MAS simulation is the ability to add new Teaching Institute Agents (TIA) and Poaching Agents (PA) and adjust the parameters and alter the behavior of the agent. As seen in the simulation example, the ability to adjust and focus the scenario on only "Nurse/Midwifes" allows great flexibil-

Table 4. Top 5 healthcare facility types

Healthcare Facility Type	Count
Health Centre	384
Dispensary	64
Rural Hospital	37
Hospital	25
District Hospital	22

Table 5. Top 5 medical staff positions

Medical Staff Position	Males	Females	Total
Health Surveillance Assistants	2849	1417	4266
Nurse/Midwives	50	2404	2454
Clinical Officers	363	15	378
Medical Assistants	342	33	342
Environmental Health Officers	210	22	232

ity in implementing more complex multi-agent simulations.

To look more closely at some of the results, the following figure presents the simulation results for 23 FAs in one regional district in the southern part of Malawi over a 3 year horizon. Of those 23 FAs, 14 facilities are health clinics.

As these results show, most FAs are hit by the simulated poaching; some of them, like the Thondwe Health Centre or the Ngwelelo Health Centre, lose all of their nurses. The standard actions of the one TIA in this region, that becomes visible after month 17.5, are not able to deal with this constant lose of nurses due to the PAs. Decision makers need to come up with different strategies for this TIA, if they want the mentioned FAs to be adequately staffed. Another FA, namely the Makwapaia Health Centre, seems to attract new MSAs, but is not able to keep them.

This is naturally only one simulation run and we looked at only a part of it, but it shows how multi-agent simulations in general and MedStaff in particular can be used to provide decision makers with at least some idea of the potential consequences of their decisions concerning staffing. An obvious follow-up simulation should explore if giving priority to the troubled Health Centers when it comes to recruiting can fix their problems or just provide PAs with more opportunity to move MSAs out of the system.

MedStaff Potential Enhancements

Possible next steps in the evolution of the MedStaff system would be to strengthen the user interaction in terms of defining the simulation scenario. As we detailed previously in this chapter, the Training Institution Agents and the Poaching Agents are

Figure 4. 36 month simulation results for health clinics

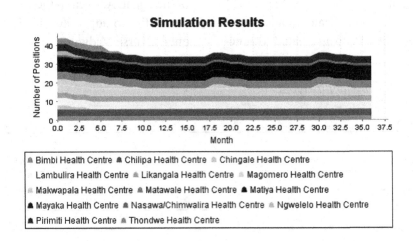

created by hand and not automatically from the database like with the healthcare facility Agents and Medical Staffing Agents. Having the ability for the end user to directly configure TIAs and various PAs would be an added benefit and would help in the deployment of the system to multiple partners or agencies that might not have the required computer skills to directly alter the agents. Another major enhancement that we would like to see would be to have real-time medical staffing information from the various healthcare facilities so that the MSA could be updated remotely. At present, we are relying on medical staffing surveys that often have a long lag time, often years, before they are completed and shared.

In terms of the multi-agent simulation itself, we would like to focus next on retention strategies in the FAs. This would allow the model to investigate what incentives would potentially keep medical staff from accepting other positions (especially international placements).

FUTURE TRENDS

One area that presents a real opportunity for vastly improving healthcare by utilizing multi agent systems is mobile devices, especially the use of cell phones. As cell phones continue to be widely adopted throughout the developing world, most notably in Africa and Asia, the ability to harness them towards medical services and clinical care is very promising (and often not hindered by competing financial demands with other healthcare priorities). As the technology continues to advance in developing countries and the cost of these mobile devices decreases, the possibility of running agent based systems on cheap cellular devices is becoming more of a reality.

There exist many medical applications that could benefit from the distributed and autonomous nature of cellular technology. One example is to use the distributed ability of cellular technology for establishing Public Health surveillance net-

works for monitoring water borne diseases that may appear in the community's drinking supply. Another example might be for monitoring drug treatment and patient compliance for tuberculosis (TB) and Malaria, in an effort to reduce the virus from gaining resistance by treatment plans that are not always fully followed by the patient.

We also envision a greater role in the application of multi-agent systems and simulations in the area of humanitarian response and disaster management. Like the previous example about cellular phones, the ability to have distributed agents that can act autonomously when required presents itself very well to humanitarian relief and disaster management. The intelligent agents could be used for keeping end users in a constant loop and communicating relevant information to other agents within the system. Furthermore, with the increasing use of RFID for tracking materials, these agents could keep track of logistical items such as food and medical supplies and communicate that information back to a central command station when the opportunity presented itself.

The area of privacy and security will also be an increasingly important area of research and implementation, especially in the healthcare domain. This will be just as important in developing countries as it currently is in the developed world.

One final point that should be indentified in the area of healthcare, technology and developing countries is around the ability to implement new systems. As already mentioned healthcare organizations in developed countries have many legacy systems and because of this are often very resistant to new information technology approaches. This is often because they have already invested in a previous technology solution and do not have the resources to implement a new technology solution.

Developing countries often do not have this issue around having to support legacy systems, and are therefore more nimble to adopt the latest technology. A prime example of this is in the area of cell phone adoption in developing countries. Developing countries have essentially jumped over traditional land lines for telecommunications and have moved forward with cellular based telecommunications. This ability to adopt new technology solutions creates an opportunity for technologies like multi-agent systems to be applied that might have faced difficulty moving forward in a traditional developed healthcare facility.

CONCLUSION

Healthcare in developing countries offers both challenges and opportunities for the application of multi-agent systems and general agent technology. The fact that these countries are still developing their healthcare systems allows for the introduction of new technologies without the various obstacles that are presented by legacy systems (and legacy decisions).

But in order to focus, health policy decision makers need to get a good grip on the consequences of the decisions that they have to make. This produces even more of a need for good simulation systems than we have in developed countries. Key requirements for such simulation systems are simplicity that allows easy adaptation of the model, the use of "standard" components, and finally the ability to get results quickly without the need for unnecessary committees and large development groups. Multi-agent based simulations fulfill these requirements nearly by default.

Our MedStaff simulation system is an example of how multi-agent based simulation allows decision makers in developing countries to explore new possibilities. It also helps them by aiding their decision- making process to minimize the impact of outside influences on their jurisdiction. In addition to responding to the health policy makers questions, MedStaff provides the necessary simulation infrastructure, analysis infrastructure and basic agent implementations for answering their questions, but also gives users the flexibility

to enhance existing agents with new behaviors customized for tomorrow's questions.

Finally, due to the absence of healthcare legacy systems in developing countries, systems that solve the unique challenges faced in developing countries will most likely find rapid adoption. This presents a new and untapped environment in which multi agent systems can be applied, and show their true potential.

ACKNOWLEDGMENT

We would like to thank the University of Calgary International Grants committee, the University of Calgary Centre for Health and Policy Studies and the following significant contributors: Dr. Tom Noseworthy, Dr. Simon Mphuka, Mr. Thouse O'Dala, Dr. W.O.O. Sangala, John Ray and Kevin Mackie.

We would also like to thank the Malawi Ministry of Health and Churches Association of Zambia (CHAZ) for helping shape the MedStaff project and also for providing the source databases of all the healthcare facilities and staffing information.

We would also like to acknowledge the Simkit Simulation Kernel developed by the TeleSim Group, Department of Computer Science at the University of Calgary, Canada.

REFERENCES

Adamatti, D. F., Simão Sichman, J., & Ducrot, R. (2004). Using multi-agent systems and role-playing games to simulate water management in peri-urban catchments. *Proc. Sixth International Conference on Social Science Methodology*. Amsterdam, The Netherlands.

Berger, T., & Ringler, C. (2002). Trade-offs, efficiency gains and technical change – Modeling water management and land use within a multiple-agent framework. *Quarterly Journal of International Agriculture, 41*(1-2), 119–144.

Berger, T., Schreinemachers, P., & Woelcke, J. (2006). Multi-agent simulation for development of less-favored areas. *Agricultural Systems, 88,* 28–43. doi:10.1016/j.agsy.2005.06.002

CIA. (2008). CIA World Factbook Washington, D.C.: *Central Intelligence Agency, 2008*. Retrieved September 8, 2008, from https://www.cia.gov/library/publications/the-world-factbook/

Ducrot, R., Le Page, C., Bommel, P., & Kuper, M. (2004). Articulating land and water dynamics with urbanization: an attempt to model natural resources management at the urban edge. *Computers, Environment and Urban Systems, 28,* 85–106. doi:10.1016/S0198-9715(02)00066-2

Gong, J., Zhou, J., Li, W., & Lin, H. (2006). Design and implementation of an intelligent virtual geographic environment for the simulation of SARS transmission. *Proceedings of the 2006 ACM international conference on Virtual reality continuum and its applications* (pp. 383-386). SESSION: Session S2: VR applications

Hongoro, C., & McPake, B. (2004). How to bridge the gap in human resources for health. *Lancet, 364*(9443), 1451–1456C. doi:10.1016/S0140-6736(04)17229-2

Kopacek, P. (2002). Demining robots: A tool for international stability. *15th Triennial World Congress IFAC, 2002.* (pp. 1–5). Barcelona, Spain.

Muller, G., Grébaut, P., & Gouteux, J. P. (2004, January). An agent-based model of sleeping sickness: simulation trials of a forest focus in southern Cameroon. *Comptes Rendus Biologies, 327*(1), 1–11. doi:10.1016/j.crvi.2003.12.002

Santana, P., Barata, J., Cruz, H., Mestre, A., Lisboa, J., & Flores, L. (2005, September). A Multi-Robot System for Landmine Detection. *Emerging Technologies and Factory Automation, 2005. ETFA 2005. 10th IEEE Conference on, 1,* 721-728.

Scalem, M., Bandyopadhyay, S., & Sircar, A. (2004, October). An approach towards a decentralised Disaster Management Information Network. *Lecture Notes on Computer Science, Springer Publications, 3285, AACC2004.*

Shaalana, K., ElBadryb, M., & Rafea, A. (2004). A multiagent approach for diagnostic expert systems via the internet. *Expert Systems with Applications, 27,* 1–10. doi:10.1016/j.eswa.2003.12.018

Teweldemedhin, E., Marwala, T., & Mueller, C. (2004). Agent based modelling: A case study in HIV epidemic. *Proceedings of the 4th International Conference on Hybrid Intelligent Systems (HIS'04)* (pp. 154–159). Washington, DC, USA: IEEE Computer Society.

WHO. (2008). Core Health Indicators the latest data from multiple WHO sources. *WHO Statistical Information System (WHOSIS)*. Retrieved September 8, 2008, from http://www.who.int/whosis/database/core/core_select_process.cfm?country=cai&indicators=healthpersonnel

Yergens, D., Hiner, J., Denzinger, J., & Noseworthy, T. (2006a). IDESS - A Multi Agent Based Simulation System for Rapid Development of Infectious Disease Models. [ITSSA]. *International Transactions on Systems Science and Applications, 1*(1), 51–58.

Yergens, D., Noseworthy, T., Hamilton, D., & Denzinger, J. (2006b, May). Agent Based Simulation combined with Real-Time Remote Surveillance for Disaster Response Management. *5th International Joint Conference on Autonomous Agents and Multi-Agent Systems, (Workshop on Agent Technology for Disaster Management)*, Hakodate, Japan.

Chapter 13

Projecting Health Care Factors into Future Outcomes with Agent–Based Modeling

Georgiy Bobashev
RTI International, Russia

Andrei Borshchev
XJ Technologies, Russia

ABSTRACT

Human behavior is dynamic; it changes and adapts. In this chapter, we describe modeling approaches that consider human behavior as it relates to health care. We present examples the demonstrate how accounting for the social network structure changes the dynamics of infectious disease, how social hierarchy affects the chances of getting HIV, how the use of low dead-space syringe reduces the risk of HIV transmission, and how emergency departments could function more efficiently when real-time activities are simulated. The examples we use build from simple to more complex models and illustrate how agent-based modeling opens new horizons for providing descriptions of complex phenomena that were not possible with traditional statistical or even system dynamics methods. Agent-based modeling can use behavioral data from a cross-sectional representative study and project the behavior into the future so that the risks can be studied in a dynamical/temporal sense, thus combining the advantages of representative cross-sectional and longitudinal studies for the price of increased uncertainty. The authors also discuss data needs and potential future applications for this method.

INTRODUCTION

Risk Factors and Predicted Dynamic Risks

Predicting the future of health outcomes is always a challenge. Almost all specific health outcomes can depend on hard-to-predict factors. For example, the number of new influenza cases in a town depends on the random contacts among its residents. At the same time, some stable causal dependencies can provide robust background for ballpark estimates, qualitative analysis, and often quantitative assessment of relative risks. In the same example, children at school have a much higher chance of getting the flu than a single adult working on a construction

DOI: 10.4018/978-1-60566-772-0.ch013

site. The challenge of modeling is to differentiate between the actual critical factors that shape the outcome and the uncertainty surrounding the prediction. In a few instances it is possible to combine the two approaches (Bobashev et al., 2000) so that a mathematical model part captures the robust dynamics and a statistical part accounts for the unexplained variation.

Naturally, modeling strategy depends on the objectives. Beyond that, a clear understanding of the scales on which the outcome resides drives the modeling approach such as system dynamics, agent-based, process (Colizza, 2007 Riley, 2007).

Often global patterns and relationships are the results of the interactions of many local behaviors and decisions (Epstein, 2007). Thus, the description of these local factors becomes critical for understanding how interventions should be structured and which sub-population is the most responsive to an intervention.

Stable and reliable global patterns of the spread of communicable disease could arise dynamically from local and seemingly unpredictable behavior; for example, random network contacts could lead to exponential growth of HIV prevalence. Thus, the studies of local behavior and contact structure could be critical for the description of global outcomes.

In order to project the outcome into the future, one usually needs the following:

- A clear definition of the initial outcome values and risk factors (i.e., the values of the outcomes at the starting (initial) time point. For example, an individual at the baseline could be either HIV positive or negative;
- A description of the actions that individuals may take in the future (e.g., attending a ball game during a flu epidemic season);
- The collection of factors determining the actions, which could relate to a number of independent variables as well as the past

actions or past states simultaneously (e.g., mixing matrices, which probabilistically describe a choice of a sexual partner, reflect that individuals are more likely to seek partners with some similar and dissimilar qualities to themselves so that, as some studies have shown, individuals who have many sexual partners are likely to have sex with those who themselves have many sexual partners [Turner et al., 2006]); and

- The translator of the behaviors into the outcomes (e.g., HIV is transmitted per direct syringe-sharing with a certain probability, which is lower if the syringe is rinsed in bleach).

Simulation models put the ingredients together and, by iterating behavior over time, provide updated outcome values as the events occur (see Figure 1).

Agent-Based Models as Tools for Projecting Behavior into the Future

Agent-based modeling is a method of developing simulation models that suggests that the modeler focuses on describing the behavior of individual entities (e.g., patients, staff, households, companies). Such entities—agents—are put into a certain environment where they interact, change their state, move, or are created or destroyed. The system level (aggregate) behavior emerges as a result of simulation of multiple individual behaviors (Borshchev & Filippov, 2004). Agents in agent-based models (ABMs) are typically acting under control of a simulation engine on a computer and in virtual (model) time. The agent-based approach is particularly helpful when a researcher considers interaction between the individuals and emerging behavioral patterns.

In many health care applications, ABMs can capture reality in a more natural way and often are easier to develop than models based on differential or difference equations, which require aggregated

Figure 1. A process diagram of the iterative behavior projecting into the future

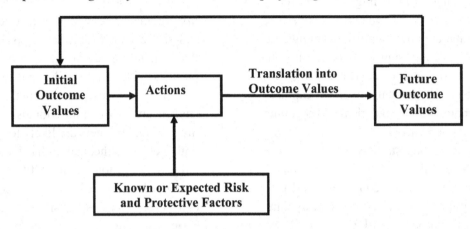

parameter estimates. Because of recent developments in computational hardware and software, realistic agent-based modeling has become quite feasible and thus its popularity has grown in many areas of application.

In this chapter, we consider applications of agent-based modeling in two different health care areas: containment strategies in the spread of infectious diseases and interaction of staff and patients in a hospital.

Examples of Problems that Agent-Based Models can Solve

We start with the system dynamics (differential equations) description of a simple Susceptible-Infectious-Recovered (SIR) model of disease diffusion and show the limitations of such an approach in realistic populations. We then re-conceptualize the model using the agent-based method and demonstrate the basic patterns for specifying behavior of individuals (agents). We then compare the simulation results of system dynamics and agent-based models.

Next we extend an ABM to capture the social network contact structure and illustrate how different network types and parameters affect the results. The further enhancements of the model can include households, working environments, travel, and health interventions such as self-isolation and quarantine.

Another application of network-related behavior is a model of HIV diffusion in a network of drug users with a hierarchy of syringe-sharing and the use of different syringe types. We show which groups of individuals have the highest chance of being infected in the future and thus need the most attention of the public health interventions. We show that even a small percentage of high dead-space syringes could be enough to sustain a high level of HIV in the population.

The last model in this chapter is a model of an emergency department (ED) where patients and staff interact with one another. We use a process modeling method for this model, which can be considered as intermediate between system dynamics and agent ABM. We show that such a model allows ED administrators to optimize the use of the staff and the utilization of other ED resources, and outline how ABMs can help to further enhance the model.

The Modeling Language

Throughout the chapter we use the modeling language of AnyLogic (a software tool for agent-based and mixed-method simulation modeling), which includes several commonly adopted visual notations: stock and flow diagrams, statecharts, and process flow diagrams. All models described in this chapter are available as runnable applets at the AnyLogic Web site (AnyLogic 2008).

How Do Social Networks Affect the Disease Dynamics?

When one gets the flu during a winter epidemic, does one always know who has given them the disease? Probably not. Most people would say that they picked it up "randomly" from "someone" at work, in school, etc. Of course, most people don't want to get sick and do not specifically target a hazardous contact, so there might be an impression that infectious disease are spreading "randomly." However, when it comes to a sexual encounter, could it be considered "random"? Do people randomly pick a sexual partner, or drug-injecting partner, or even a person with whom to socialize at work? A recent study has shown that sexual partnerships are quite different among teenagers than among mature adults, and these structures can dramatically affect the spread of sexually transmitted diseases among these sub-populations. Similarly, among drug injectors, some networks have almost no HIV, while in others the prevalence can reach 80%.

One of the answers is hidden in the network structure of social, sexual, and drug-injecting contacts. In the next section, we show how to explore the impact of such a structure on the disease dynamics using ABMs. Because different diseases have different infectivity, course of disease, mortality, etc., we illustrate the impact of the networks on a generic disease where individuals can be susceptible to, infected with, or recovered from the disease.

A System Dynamics Model

In a "classic" system dynamics model of a disease diffusion (Anderson and May, 1991; Sterman, 2000) we divide the total population into three compartments (categories) with respect to their disease status: Susceptible to the disease, Infectious, and Recovered, hence the three compartments that could be modeled as stocks in the stock and flow diagram used in system dynamics science (see Figure 2). As people are infected they move from the Susceptible category to the Infectious category, and then, as they recover, to the Recovered category. The disease spreads as those who are infectious contact and pass the disease to those who are Susceptible (the positive feedback loop) while at the same time depleting the pool of susceptible (the negative loop). The recovery from the disease creates another negative feedback loop.

Mathematically, the system dynamics model is a system of differential and algebraic equations, in the case of SIR they are:

Initially a fraction of the total population (PercentInitiallyInfected) are Infectious and the rest are Susceptible.

The simulation of the system dynamics SIR model produces a bell-shaped curve of the Infectious population (see Figure 3). However, this model makes a number of simplifying assumptions. One of the strongest assumptions is the homogeneity and perfect mixing of individuals in each compartment (stock): for example, all infectious people are assumed to behave in exactly the same way regardless of their individual history, properties, etc. This assumption implies that any person in the population can contact anyone else with the same probability. This simplification could sometimes be justified when the disease of interest is spread through airborne particles like influenza and the population of interest resides in a large well-connected metropolitan area such as New York or London. However, for structured populations and diseases where the transmission

Figure 2. The stock and flow diagram of the SIR model

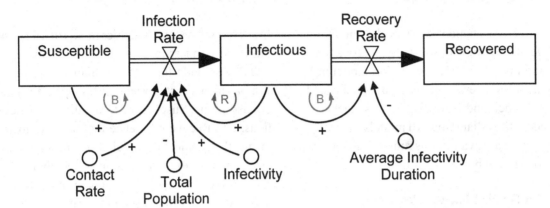

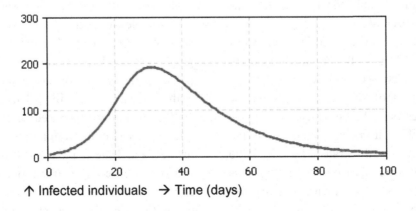

---

depends on the type of contact, such simplification could be misleading. In the ABM of the same problem, such an assumption can be dropped completely.

An Agent-Based Model

In a completely disaggregated ABM, each person is modeled as a separate object with his own parameters, state variables, and behavior rules. The agent's behavior may be continuous over time, discrete (based on events), or hybrid. In this particular model, we distinguish between three different states of a person (Susceptible, Infectious, and Recovered) and assume that state transitions are instantaneous and there are no continuous changes.

A statechart with a sequence of three states naturally describes this behavior. Note that the states of an agent mirror the three stocks in the system dynamics model; however, here the states are mutually exclusive: the agent can be in only one state at a time (see Figure 4). To reflect the fact that some people are already infected at the beginning of the simulation, the statechart entry point has a branch InitiallyInfected. The choice of the initial state can be probabilistic (e.g., based on a global model parameter PercentInitiallyInfected)

Figure 3. The dynamics of infectious population (disease prevalence) in the system dynamics SIR model

Figure 4. The statechart of a person in the agent-based SIR model

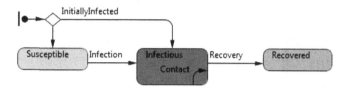

or deterministic (e.g., with infected people placed in particular locations).

The transition to the Infectious state models the event of a disease being passed to the agent from a sick person. In the model terms, the trigger of that transition is the message "Infection." Once in the Infectious state, the agent is able to pass the disease to others; thus, we are interested in his contacts. We assume that ContactRate (a global parameter) is constant while in the Infectious state, and we can use internal transition Contact that will be repeatedly taken until the agent recovers. In the action of that transition, the agent will choose another agent from the people that he knows (this is defined by the social network, which we consider below) and send him the message "Infection." However, we know that not every contact results in infection being passed, so the message should be sent with the probability InfectionProbability, which is yet another global parameter. If the message reaches an agent who is already Infectious or Recovered, it is ignored because there is no transition from those states triggered by such a message. Finally, the transition Recovery is a timeout that defines the illness duration. In the system dynamics model, the timeout is often modeled as exponentially distributed with the mean AverageIllnessDuration. Here we can use the same assumption for the sake of comparison; however, the more realistic approach would be to use a real distribution of the length of the infectious period as was done in Rvachev and Longini (1985) to compare the simulation results with the output of the system dynamics model. However, the ABM gives you absolute freedom in modeling durations of agent states: for example, you can easily use a uniform

distribution between 5 and 15 days.

At the top level of the model, we define the population, the social network type, and the global parameters, which are the same as in the system dynamics model. In this particular model, the agents are homogeneous, i.e., they share the same parameter values and have identical behavior. Again, one is free to add any degree of heterogeneity to agent-based models: from individual parameters with different values to different behavior patterns (e.g., different ContactRate of different people).

We also need to define simulation outcome variables on which to collect the statistics of interest such as the maximum size of the infectious population and the time from initial exposure to the maximum size of the infectious population.

The Network Types

The experiment design for this model follows the pattern suggested in Rahmandad and Sterman (2008). We explore the dynamics of disease diffusion in the following types of networks:

- Fully Connected: Anybody can contact anybody else. This network type fully corresponds to the perfect mixing assumption of the system dynamics model.
- Random: An agent is linked to a random subset of the agent population.
- Scale Free (Barabasi & Albert, 1999): Some people are "hubs" with lots of connections and some are "hermits" with few connections. This type of network is built using a preferential attachment algorithm

Figure 5. Schematic diagrams of different network structures

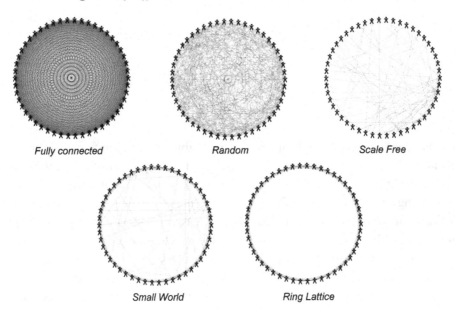

where the probability of a new person linking to the existing people is proportional to the number of links those people already have.

- Small World (Watts, 1999): Most agents are linked to their close neighbors, but there is a certain percentage of long-range links, i.e., links to distant agents. One of the ways to describe such arrangement is to arrange the agents in a circle (ring structure) and define neighbors as agents closest to the left and to the right.
- Ring Lattice: Each person is linked to a fixed number of his closest neighbors on a ring. This type of network is most distant from the fully connected network.

The network structures are illustrated in Figure 5 for a population of 50 agents.

The Simulation Results

Unlike the system dynamics model, which is deterministic and generates a single trajectory,

the ABM is stochastic (in this case due to the contact occurrences, the probability of infection being passed during a contact, the illness duration, and the network structure). Therefore, each simulation run will give different results. We will perform a number of runs for each network structure and assemble the distribution of results in a two-dimensional histogram with highlighted envelopes to indicate the mean realization and variation around it. The solid curve is the number of infected individuals calculated from the base case system dynamics model. The results are qualitatively the same as in Rahmandad and Sterman (2008).

As one can see from the plots in Figure 6, the less a network resembles a well mixed structure, the stronger the discrepancy in the disease dynamics on the networks. This effect is best explained by looking at the extreme setting. When all people are completely connected (Figure 6a), the ABM performs the same as the homogeneously mixed system dynamics model by construction. The epidemic quickly rises and then tails out. Not all people get infected. A percentage of individuals

Figure 6. (a) Disease diffusion in a fully connected network. (b) Disease diffusion in a random network with 10 links per node. (c) Disease diffusion in a scale free network with parameter = 2. (d) Disease diffusion in a small world network with 10 links per node and 5% of long distant links. (e) Disease diffusion in a ring lattice with 10 links per node.

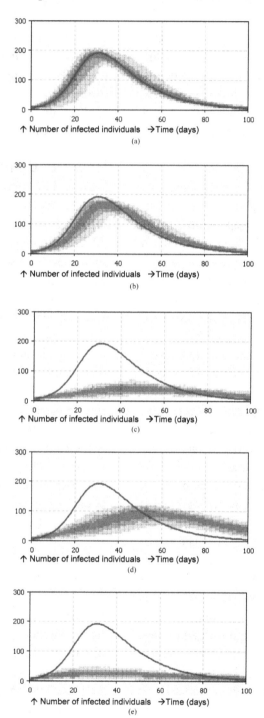

remain susceptible. When the subjects are connected randomly, the epidemic is smaller and spreads more slowly than the completely connected case, because each individual has only a limited number of connections. When all subjects are arranged in a circle, the disease is spread only to the nearest neighbors, and thus the speed of the transmission is much slower, and the epidemic could last for a much longer time and eventually produce an even greater number of infected individuals than under the random mixing case. Small world epidemic shapes could be viewed as a combination of the random mixing and the ring lattice cases, because the small world populations are structured as nearest neighbors with random connections to the rest of the population. One of the main features of the scale free populations is that they have potential "superspreaders" who, if they become infectious, can quickly infect large numbers of people. Although these networks may appear somewhat artificial, they have a direct application to disease prevention programs. Not long ago, Bearman et al. (2004) showed that sexual networks in adolescents and young adults are very different from those among older adults. Most older adults have stable monogamous partnerships, with a small fraction of very active individuals who have a large number of partners concurrently (i.e., network structure with superspreaders). If a sexually transmitted disease enters the population, it could cause a large outbreak (or outbreaks) when people connected to the superspreaders get infected in a short period of time. The rest of the population remains protected because of their monogamous relationships. While the structure of adolescent sexual network is mostly monogamous with no concurrency, the rate of partner change is relatively high. If a sexually transmitted disease enters such a population, it would not cause a quick outburst but would travel slowly from one partnership to another similar to a ring lattice or a small world network with sparse links across the population.

In these examples, we have illustrated the advantage of the ABMs in capturing the network structure. The further enhancements of the agent-based SIR model may include introduction of households, working environments, travel, and self-quarantine.

However, in the SIR example the agents are homogeneous, that is, they do not differ from each other by any specific features. In our next example, we increase the complexity of the agents to illustrate how individual features make a difference in disease dynamics.

How can Being on the Top of Social Hierarchy among Drug Injectors Protect One from HIV?

At the beginning of the HIV epidemic in the United States, heroin users who had been injecting for a longer period of time had a lower prevalence of HIV than drug users with a shorter history of injecting. The answer was unexpectedly simple. Those who had used heroin longer were likely to be higher on the social hierarchy of users and were more likely to procure heroin. Thus they were more likely to inject before others, and an infected syringe would be less likely to reach them (Bourgois, 1998, 2004). Such an effect is difficult to model using conventional methods, but agent-based modeling allows us to incorporate such a modification easily. Below we describe how this could be done in a model of injecting drug users in a single U.S. county.

A Model of HIV Transmission among Injecting Drug Users

An ABM consists of two major structural components: the agents who are performing all the action and the top-level "container" object that defines the structure of the networks, describes the distribution of buddies, prior experiences, etc. In other words, the top-level defines the initial conditions and the global structure for the model.

We first consider a model of a drug user (an

agent). To distinguish between the Susceptible and Infected states of the drug user, we use a statechart with two states (note that, in contrast with the previous SIR model, there is no Recovered state for HIV). A certain percentage of drug users are initially HIV infected; they start in the Infected state. Otherwise, the drug user begins in the Susceptible state and transitions to Infected in the event of using an infected syringe during an InjectingActivity with a certain probability. The corresponding transition Infection is triggered by the message "Infection" coming from the InjectingActivity organizer (the injection behavior is described below). If we plan to run the model for a longer period of time, we can also model the reduced life duration of an infected user. This can be done by adding a transition from Infected to a final state: Dead, triggered by a timeout. The timeout is a draw from the (known) distribution of life duration of an HIV-infected person, and the action of the transition is deleting this user from the model.

The central part of the drug user model is the injection behavior. Each user has a number of "buddies" who periodically get together to use drugs. The number of buddies is defined by the network. Occasionally, an injector would use with a "stranger" who is a random person from the entire population of injectors (Blower et al., 1991). We use a statechart with two states—Idle and InjectingActivity—to model the drug usage behavior. There are two ways to get to the InjectingActivity state: organize an activity or be invited. We assume that anybody can organize an InjectingActivity and invite others. The transition

Organize from the Idle state to the InjectingActivity state occurs after a period of inactivity (in the Idle state) that can be between 1 and 3 days. When this transition is taken, the organizer of the InjectingActivity invites his buddies with a certain probability (FractionInvited) by sending them the message "Invitation." If the user being invited is in the Idle state, he will take the transition Invitation, confirm participation (by sending back the "Confirm" message) and proceed to the InjectingActivity state. The other possibility is that the invited drug user is already at another InjectingActivity, in which case the invitation will be ignored.

The duration of the InjectingActivity itself is not relevant here (we only need to know the participants), but we can set it to 1 hour deterministically for animation purposes. Therefore, the transition InjectingActivityIsOver that brings the drug user back to the Idle state has a constant timeout of 1 hour. The actual injection sequence is modeled in the exit action of the state InjectingActivity of the organizer. The organizer iterates through the list of participants (sorted by the experience, most experienced users at the beginning), starting with the clean syringe. If a user is already infected, the syringe is marked as infected and the subsequent users will get infected with the probability InfectionProbability (in the model terms, the message "Infection" is sent to the user).

An agent can receive three types of messages: "Invitation," "Confirm," and "Infection." The "Invitation" message is forwarded to the DrugUsageBehavior statechart, the "Infection" message is forwarded to the HealthState statechart, and

Figure 7. The HealthState statechart for an injecting agent

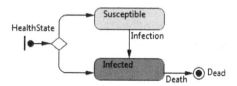

Figure 8. The DrugUsageBehavior statechart and the related drug InjectingActivity data for an injecting agent

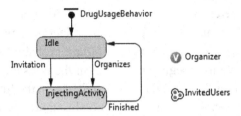

the "Confirm" message causes its sender to be added to the collection InvitedUsers according to his experience. Experience is a parameter that indicates how long the user has been injecting and defines his rank in the social hierarchy of users. The initial value of Experience for a particular user can be set up as a draw from the distribution of experience throughout the drug user population (which, in this case, is the required input data for the model) or deterministically. Note that Experience is the only source of agent heterogeneity in this model.

The Top Level of the Model

At the top level of the model, we need to define the population of injecting drug users, their network of contacts, and some global parameters, namely the following:

- InitialNumberOfUsers: the initial number of agents in the model;
- PercentInitiallyInfected: the percentage of users who are initially HIV positive (for simplicity, we can assume this is not correlated with Experience);
- FractionInvited: the probability that a drug user who is known to the InjectingActivity organizer will be invited;
- InfectionProbability: the probability of getting infected after injection with an infected syringe; and
- ExperiencePDF: the distribution of

experience among the drug user population used to initialize the Experience parameter of individual drug users.

For illustration purposes, here we use a small world network; however, in practical models of HIV transmission, the network structure should be estimated from the data or at least by using a mixing matrix (who injects with whom) as described in the data section below.

Note that if we wish to model the new drug users that join the network during the model runtime, we need to dynamically connect them to the existing users while preserving the network parameters.

The other important model elements that are defined at the top level are various statistics, output visualization, and animation. The following outputs are important in our case:

- the dynamics of the drug user population (if we do not add new users during the simulation),
- the dynamics of the fraction of HIV-infected drug users, and
- the distribution of experience among the users who are infected and not infected at the end of the simulation.

After the model is set up, one can use it to answer important policy and research questions.

Figure 9. Distribution of Experience among Susceptible and Infected users at the end of simulation.

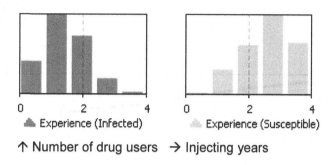

↑ Number of drug users → Injecting years

The Simulation Results

One of the first illustrations of model application results is estimation of the effects that the drug-using experience has on the chances of HIV infection. Because we can track each individual agent in the model, we can make comparisons based on their behavior. After using the simulations to project the behavior over the 3 years ahead, we can compare the distribution of experience among users who are HIV positive and HIV negative (see Figure 9). By running the model many times (e.g., 100) we can collect the necessary statistics and estimate the difference in survival from HIV between those who had more than 2 years of drug-using experience and those who had less (see Figure 10). As both figures show, the survival is indeed better among those who had used drug for a longer period of time. One could use a variety of statistical methods to estimate odds ratios, relative risk, hazard, etc., by applying appropriate statistical methods to the simulated data in the same manner as it would be applied to the real data. However, the main difference is in the interpretation of the variation. In simulation modes, the variation is composed of two sources: uncertainty in the parameters and variation due to the stochasticity of the simulation. We discuss these sources in the discussion section.

This model could be expanded to represent a number of comparisons when agents are supplied with individual characteristics such as demog-raphy, disease status, behavior, etc. The next example illustrates how such models can help evaluate the impact of high dead-space syringes on HIV transmission.

Do All Syringes Pose Equal Risk for HIV Transmission?

William Zule and his coauthors have pointed out the fact that different syringes have different amounts of so-called "dead space," which is a small space in a syringe barrel between the fully depressed piston and the needle (Zule & Bobashev, 2008). This dead space in syringes with detachable needles can retain 50 times more blood after the injection than insulin syringes with built-in needles. While injecting the drug, a user often draws back some blood to fill up the barrel and then injects the drug back into the vein. The syringe could then be passed to the next user, with some blood retained in the barrel. After a couple of rinses, which the injector usually does to prevent the needle from clogging and to reduce the risk of HIV, the relative amount of the virus in the dead space becomes more than 1,000 times higher in the detachable needle syringes compared to insulin syringes. If the concentration of the virus has an impact on the probability of HIV infection, then switching to insulin syringes could reduce the incidence and consequently the prevalence of HIV. But what percentage of injectors would need to switch to more expensive insulin syringes in order

Figure 10. Survival curves among the highly experienced (solid line) and low experienced (dashed line) injectors

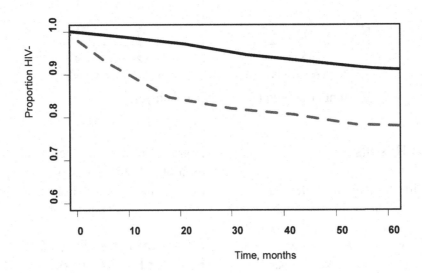

Changes to the Injection Drug Users Model

We assume each drug user always uses a particular type of syringe (safe or unsafe), so we add a Boolean parameter UsesSafeSyringe to the model of the drug user. At the top level of the model we add SafeSyringeUsersFraction—a probability needed to initialize UsesSafeSyringe for each user. We also need another top-level parameter InfectionProbabilitySafe—the probability of getting infected after injection with an infected safe syringe, which is obviously lower than Infection-Probability for a regular (unsafe) syringe.

Another assumption we make is about injection behavior. We assume that if at least one user at the InjectingActivity uses a safe syringe, then that syringe will be used by everyone. Therefore, in the model of the injection sequence in the exit action of the state InjectingActivity of the orga-

nizer, we should first check if anyone has a safe syringe and, if so, use InfectionProbabilitySafe instead of InfectionProbability.

The Simulation Results

Once again, when the model is run a number of times (e.g., 100) we can accumulate the data about the outcomes and summarize it in a form of a statistical analysis or a graph.

Figure 11 shows that even a small percentage of high dead-space syringes can lead to a high prevalence of HIV, which implies that in order for the intervention to be successful, it is necessary to replace the vast majority (>90%) of high dead–space syringes.

By giving the researcher the possibility to track an individual agent, ABMs have the advantage of adding an explicit spatial component. Knowing the location of the individual, it is possible to place them on a Geographical Information System (GIS) map; conduct spatial statistics; and assign various environmental information such as poverty, crime, and education indexes

Figure 11. Dynamics of HIV prevalence in a population of injecting drug users. Solid line corresponds to 100% of high dead-space syringes, dashed line to 50%, dotted line to 10%, and long dashed line to 0%.

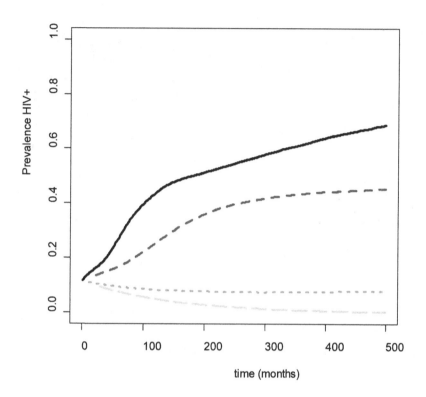

(see Figure 12). This option could have the risk of producing potentially identifiable personal information. However, there are a number of safeguards to protect individual privacy. Some common methods include perturbing the actual location by random spatial noise, aggregating spatial locations up to large spatial areas (from individual addresses to a block group), and using synthetic populations, which are populations of virtual agents that have comparable demographic characteristics to the census at some aggregate level such as county or census tract (Wheaton et al., 2006). The use of virtual populations is thus advantageous because the agents' characteristics are not the characteristics of real people, but at the statistically aggregated level the results of the analysis are similar to what they would be for the real population.

Can ABMs Help to Efficiently Manage the Emergency Department?

The workload in emergency departments is notorious for being extremely high at times. "Physician patient load patterns and ED demand patterns should be taken into consideration when physician shift times are scheduled so that patient load may be balanced among a team. Real-time monitoring of physician patient load may reduce stress and prevent physicians from exceeding their safe capacity for workload" (Levin et al., 2007). The same is true for a number of health care departments that are not EDs.

Because the functioning of an ED is quite complex and the patient cases range widely in the type of care they need, it is often difficult for the management to process the bulk of the

Figure 12. Example of using GIS to map the poverty index and the locations of the injecting drug users in Durham County, North Carolina. The actual locations of the responders have been stochastically scrambled.

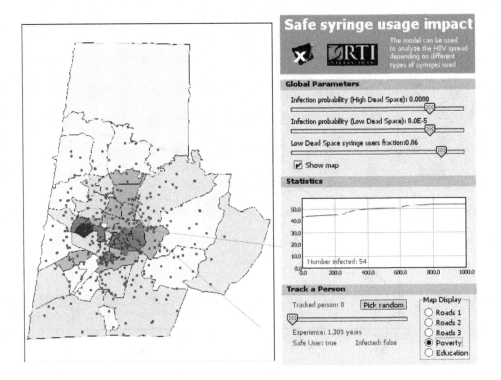

information needed for optimization. A strategy to ease workload in one place can create a bottleneck elsewhere in the process (Miró et al., 2004). Below we demonstrate how ABMs allow one to summarize the processes in the ED and evaluate different strategies to ease the workload.

The Model

Compared to other parts of a hospital, the ED has more clearly defined sequences of operations. Therefore, we can start with a modeling technique that can be considered to be intermediate between system dynamics and agent-based modeling: process modeling, also known as "discrete event" modeling. This modeling method has been known for decades; is well developed; and is widely used in manufacturing, business processes, the service sector, etc. Process modeling suggests that the modeler view the system as a process—a sequence of operations, perhaps with branches and loops—where entities (in this case patients) interact with (and compete for) resources (staff, rooms, equipment). The entities and resource units are modeled as individual objects and may have individual parameter values. Therefore, process models are disaggregated like agent-based ones. However, these objects are passive. They have no independent behavior and thus are completely controlled by the process; and here the process models are fundamentally different from ABMs. We begin by modeling the operations of the ED as a process and then we outline how the model can be extended by adding the agents.

Process models can be designed both bottom up and top down. For this example, we chose the top-down method. The top level of the ED operation model is a sequence of patient admittance, care

Figure 13. The process model of an emergency department

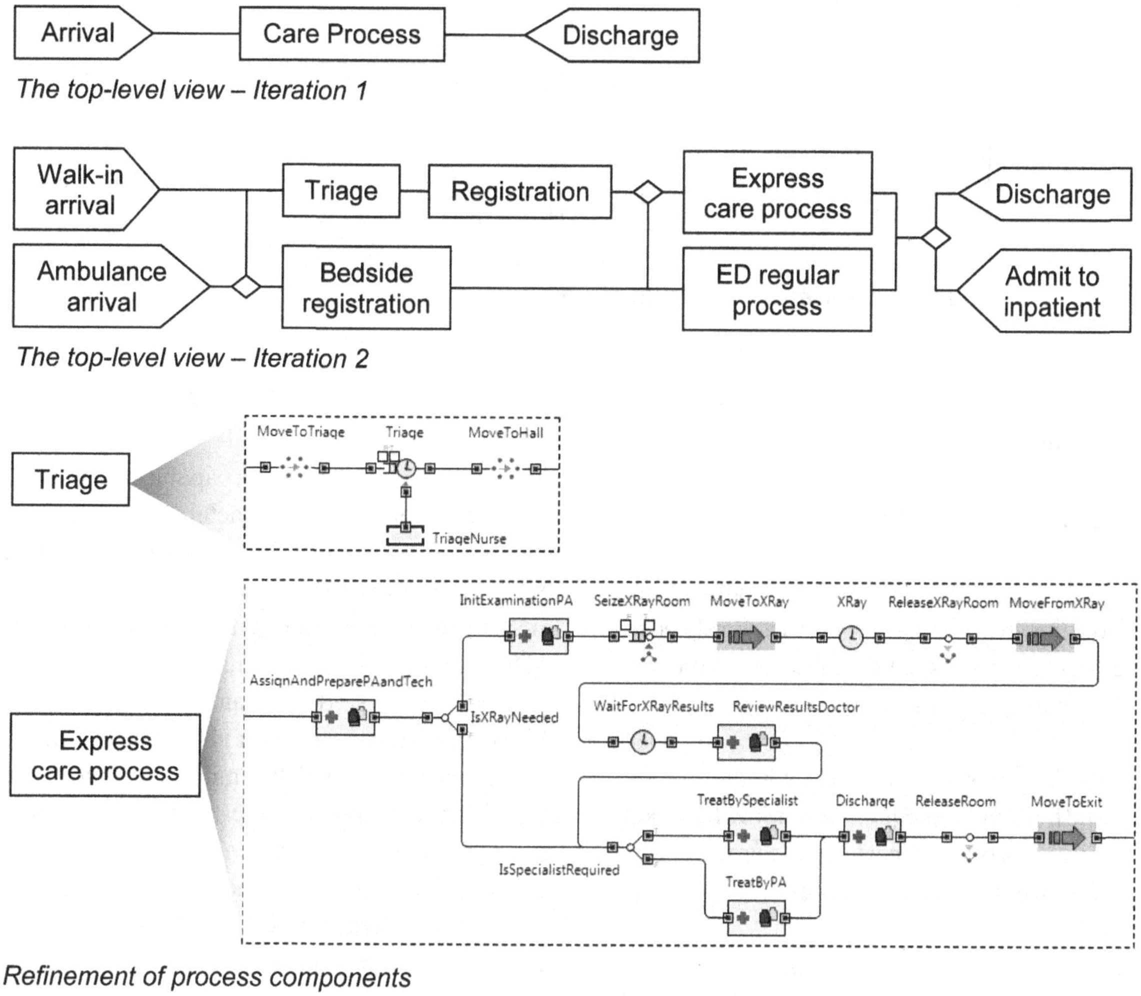

The top-level view – Iteration 1

The top-level view – Iteration 2

Refinement of process components

process, and discharge (see Figure 13). In the next design iteration, we distinguish between walk-in patients and patients brought by ambulance. The walk-in patients go through triage and registration and are then placed into an emergency care room. The ambulance patients are put into a room first and are then registered. There are two types of care process in our ED model: Express Care (open 11AM–11PM) and Regular Care (open 24 hours). These two types have different steps and require different resources. The internals of the Express Care process are shown at the bottom of Figure 13. First, a personal assistant and techni-

cian examine and prepare the patient. Then, if X-rays are needed, they are taken and the results are reviewed by a doctor. After that (or directly after initial examination if X-rays are not needed), a specialist may be needed to treat the patient. After treatment, the express care room is released and the patient is discharged, or, alternatively, admitted to inpatient.

At the bottom level, the process components are built of primitive library objects such as Seize, Delay, Release, MoveTo, ResourcePool, Decision, etc. The properties of patients that flow through the process may affect the branches taken, the

Figure 14. Distribution of patients' length of stay in the emergency room for two different working hours options of Express Care process

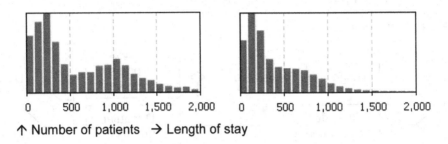

↑ Number of patients   → Length of stay

duration of operations, the type of resources needed, etc.

The Simulation Results

During the simulation of the process model, we are able to collect various kinds of statistics related to patients, staff, rooms, and equipment. Typically, we are interested in the following:

- the length of stay of patients in the ED;
- staff, room, and equipment utilization; and
- locations of bottlenecks in the process, particularly the sizes of queues.

These outputs are used to compare different process improvement strategies, to choose optimal staff levels, and to set working hours. Figure 14 shows the distribution of patients' length of stay in the ED for two different working hours options of the Express Care process.

Another kind of output is animation of the ED operation. Animation can be used to verify the model behavior and to perform rapid what-if experiments. For example, the animation of the ED model could be viewed on a floor plan of the actual ED (applet is available for viewing at the Web site: http://www.xjtek.com/anylogic/demo_models/healthcare/).

Extending the Model with Agents

Although process models are capable of capturing diversity in individual parameters of both entities and resources, the inability to define individual behavior puts a natural restriction on how far the model can go in reflecting reality. In particular, ABMs can help in modeling the longer-term behavior of ED staff. We can associate an agent with each staff resource unit in the process model (a specialist, a technician, a nurse, etc.) and make it persistent throughout the model run, so that the agent exists even when the corresponding resource is not present in the process model. We can then efficiently model the staff knowledge development, trainings, vacations, and even interaction of individual staff members at work, which can affect the ED process. For example, the staff performance and error rates when treating patients may depend on the individual states and properties of the corresponding agents.

FUTURE TRENDS IN DATA COLLECTION

One of the main challenges in the construction of ABMs is obtaining the right data to calibrate and validate the model. It is often *the* main challenge. When conducting health surveys, the focus of the sampling is usually to collect a representative sample of the studied population. The cornerstone

Figure 15. Animation of the emergency department model

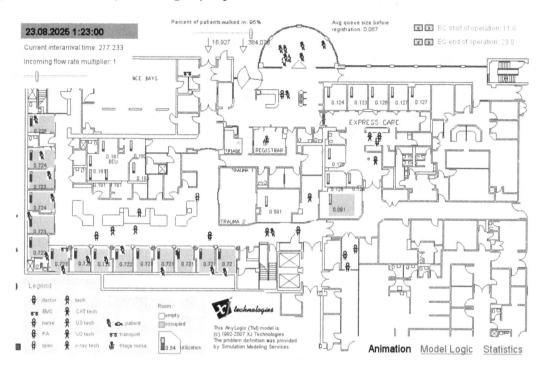

of sampling methods and the resulting models is an assumption of independent and identically distributed subjects where one subject could well be a representative of many other similar subjects. Is this assumption true in the case of sexually transmitted diseases? If sexual partners are seldom picked at random, does the selected partner represent hundreds or thousands of other potential partners? Could a number of partners be averaged for the sake of simplified assumptions? If, over the past month, one person had one sexual partner and another had 9, does that mean that between them they had on average five sexual partners? Similar questions could be asked about a number of other types of contacts, such as injecting drug use contacts and contacts within hospitals and workplaces.

Most often, survey data focused on static and individual estimates is not suitable for the estimations of transition probabilities and network interactions, which are at the center of ABMs. Instead, the surveys for ABMs should focus on collecting data for dynamic and network estimates. Of course, such data pose very serious challenges.

Obtaining network information carries with it the issue of privacy. For example, in order to collect accurate data on sexual networks, one has to ask for identifiable information about sexual partners, which many respondents are reluctant to provide and sometimes do not even have. One compromise between the ease of data collection under the representativeness assumption and the need to obtain partnership information is to collect information about the *types* of partners. For example, sexual partners could be classified into long-term and short-term; their demographics could include age, race, gender, education, and socioeconomic status; and their behavior could include drug use and number of sexual partners as assessed by the respondent. Such information could be then be used to construct a mixing matrix, indicating the probabilities of having a sexual partnership between the representatives of particular categories (Morris, 2004).

Another challenge in obtaining network information is the adequate type of sampling design. Probability surveys are not helpful in identifying target populations, especially if part of the population of interest can be "hidden," such as in the case of injecting drug users. There is no practical way to enumerate all the users to develop a sampling frame. On the other hand, respondent-driven sampling (Heckathorn, 2002) allow one to obtain a representative sample of connected individuals. In this sense, respondent-driven sampling sample links rather than individuals, and following the links combined with the information on the mixing matrices could potentially allow one to reconstruct the network structure.

One critical component that distinguishes ABMs from other types of models is a dynamic scheduling of the events. After the respondents are enrolled, they are usually asked questions regarding their behavior. Some of the typical survey questions deal with the initiation of the behavior ("When was the first time you…?"), recency ("When was the last time you …?"), and frequency ("How often do you…?"). Although these questions somewhat help to schedule the events by estimating the periodicity of particular behavior, they do not help to establish transitions between the types of behavior and its consistency. ABMs often require questions of the type "For how long have you been… ?" or "In what other activities were you involved while…?" Concurrency and the rate of partner change are critical for the transmission of many sexually transmitted diseases. However, such questions are seldom asked in the surveys. For example, knowing how many sexual partners a person had over the last 6 month does not help a researcher to establish how many are stable partners and how many are short-term or occasional.

Nevertheless, a number of tools have been used to collect important behavior data suitable for ABMs. One is a "timeline fall back" where a subject is asked retrospectively about particular events. Prospective ethnographic tools have also been developed to follow-up with respondents and collect information on the scheduling of events (Vahabzadeh et al., 2007). However, these tools were not developed specifically for use in ABMs, and some adaptation might be needed. The use of blogs became very useful in collecting scheduling information. For example, a very sophisticated model of influenza spread in a city, EpiSims (Eubank et al., 2004), used blogs to validate individual movements and contact information.

Additional information that impacts transitions and interactions requires even more detailed ethnographic description. That is why development of ABMs highlights the need for close collaboration with ethnographers and for adapting the old ways of data collection to the new levels of formalizing and using them to project dynamic risk factors into the future.

DISCUSSION

We have presented several simple examples of the uses of ABMs and showed how they could be useful for understanding and projecting risk factors into the future. These models, although quite simplistic, uncover some of the relationships that should be considered when developing health services policy. Because the actual behavior and health-related outcomes could be very complex (detailed, nonlinear, evolutionary, and multiscale), the modes focusing on any specific areas of research are likely to be of a much higher complexity level. In the discussion, we reexamine the utility of agent-based modeling, and modeling in general, to provide some means of safeguarding against misuse and misinterpretation of the models.

Agent-based modeling is a fast-developing area of research, and while numerous models have been developed and utilized, there is not much theory for evaluating ABMs as rigorously as can be done for most system dynamics models. ABMs have a larger number of parameters, each of which has to be evaluated; the stochastic nature of micro-simulation often leads to a broad variety of solutions. Reality, in turn, could be viewed within a similar paradigm: the observed events and behavior are only a single realization of what could have happened out of millions of potential outcomes. The function of ABMs is thus not to reproduce actual observations but rather to capture more general features of the phenomenon. Thus, we would like to warn about a temptation to treat the outcome of an ABM as an imitation of an observed real-life situation. Another application of ABMs is identification of the results that could be rare or unusual. These applications are especially important in risk management, when the objective is to estimate the risks of rare but potentially damaging outcomes. Before the conclusions can be made about ABMs, the outcomes from a large number of realizations should first be processed to reveal the trends and relationships that are general enough to guide future decisions. The same argument applies to modeling in general; however, system dynamics models are often already operating in terms of the aggregated measures such as rates, odds ratios, and risk factors, while ABMs evaluate individual trajectories and thus require an additional aggregation step.

What makes ABMs advantageous in specific cases is the ability to describe local non-linearity and self-organization resulting from a sequence of local events. There is one more important utility of ABMs that makes them attractive to modern modeling: the natural manner in which events are described. ABMs allow the description of events without using sophisticated mathematical apparatus. While system dynamics models require that the aggregated dynamic equations are developed first and then the solution of these equations projects the outcome into the future, in ABMs the behavior is project into the future first and then the results are aggregated. This process is often easier and more natural to formalize and thus more appealing to a researcher. For example, when describing health-related processes in a complex world, one might start with a simple equation-based model

and then increase the description of disease transmission by adding more and more compartments corresponding to various population subgroups. For a simple system of four differential equations described here it is possible to derive important analytical solutions that have a strong impact on health policy (Bailey, 1975; Anderson & May, 1991). When the number of equations becomes too high, the model loses its analytic appeal but becomes more useful as a numeric simulator. An ABM is designed as an efficient numeric simulator from the very beginning. By design, ABMs are naturally expandable to accommodate increasing levels of complexity such as heterogeneity in contacts, variations between individuals, and combinations of processes across physical scales such as molecular, cellular, organ, individual, group, and population.

ABMs also have a number of specific challenges, including the following:

- *Challenge to populate the model with parameter values.* Populating an ABM often requires knowledge of detailed individual decision-making and/or scheduling patterns. For example, in a model of different types of syringes, we did not consider the fact that many drug users change their behavior after they learn about their seroconversion. It takes different lengths of time for different categories of people to admit to the testing clinic and then change the behavior (often depending on the local intervention programs and insurance status). Also, knowledge of the actual network structure would change the actual numerical values of the results. However, the qualitative assessment might remain very similar. Depending on the purpose of the models and the results of sensitivity analysis, one should make decisions about spending large amounts of money to improve the model's numerical values, as opposed to conducting inexpensive qualitative assessment of a simple model.

- *Challenge to validate the model.* Validating ABMs is a topic of numerous discussions. With the large amounts of data that would be available in the industrial setting with repeated processes, validation is not as big a challenge as in the health care environment. The lack of validation data that was discussed in the data collection section prohibits the models from being fully validated. In the presented models we used simplified parameterization when the values of parameters were obtained from published literature and educated guesses. This was done to illustrate that even simple models can provide additional insight into important health-related problems. There is a large body of models and peer-reviewed literature that describes more detailed models that have been calibrated and validated to different degrees (Law, 2007), but the assessment of these much more complex models is not the purpose of this chapter.

- *Challenge to obtain an analytical solution.* Although for equation-based models it is possible in many cases to obtain an analytical solution or an approximation, little has been done yet to obtain an analytical solution for an ABM that could be used instead of numerical simulations. Few exceptions occur when agents are simple, i.e., when they are not involved in complex interactions and do not evolve during the course of the simulation. In such simplified case, the model is reduced to the analysis of the networks that have a more advanced theory behind them (Snijders et al., 2007, Newman, 2002).

- *Computational challenge.* The advantage of system dynamics models is that they deal with aggregated populations and thus do not depend as dramatically on the population size they describe. Conversely, ABMs increase computational demands as the population size increases. The more complex are the agents the stronger becomes the limitation. For example, when agents are organized in a large network, each agent contains information about the individuals that they are likely to meet in the households, workplace, common areas, etc. Advanced computational methods are needed to program such arrangements in an efficient way. The options for conducting large simulation experiments are to use large computational facilities such as supercomputers, distributed computational clusters, and computational networks such as TeraGrid. However, for the purposes of evaluating the impact of policies in smaller locations such as hospitals and health care facilities, user-friendly software packages, such as AnyLogic, which create manageable models, are often sufficient.

Finally, we would like to bring clarity into the "explanatory" and "predictive" sides of modeling. In different subject areas, these terms would have different meanings. For example, in economics, a "predictive" model would produce a predicted value for disease prevalence with a confidence interval, and the same would apply for the estimated forecast of monetary burden. In behavioral and neuroscience, predictive would often indicate a more qualitative way of uncovering a mechanism that governs behavior. Regardless of definitions, we argue that explanatory and predictive are not necessarily conflicting objectives, but rather parts of a larger logical process. For example, the prediction of the national level of HIV prevalence for the next year might be based on a statistical regression trend model. It would probably be the same as this year with small variation that could be explained by the amount of funding spent on prevention and treatment. The linkage between cost and effectiveness could be done with some empirical algebraic equation. What such a model would not be able to tell is why some regions, communities, and individuals are at a higher risk and what would be a better way to change people's behavior. In this sense, a dynamical model powered by ethnographic knowledge may describe the phenomenon qualitatively and thus could be considered "explanatory" or "educational." However, the result of such models would be a qualitative "prediction" aimed at making a suggestion to public health as to which intervention direction is more promising for societal well-being. Thus, explanatory models become useful when their intent and focus is future practical prediction and application. Otherwise, purely explanatory models would have little practical value beyond the casual appeal of computer games.

ACKNOWLEDGMENT

The authors would like to thank Dr. Joshua Epstein for his valuable discussions.

REFERENCES

Anderson, R. M., & May, R. M. (1991). *Infectious disease of humans: Dynamics and control*. Oxford: Oxford Sciences Publications.

AnyLogic. (2008). XJ Technologies and AnyLogic Web site: www.anylogic.com

Bailey, N. J. T. (1975). *The mathematical theory of infectious diseases and its applications*. London: Oxford University Press.

Barabasi, A. L., & Albert, R. (1999). Emergence of scaling in random networks. *Science, 286*(5439), 509–512. doi:10.1126/science.286.5439.509

Bearman, P. S., Moody, J., & Stovel, K. (2004). Chains of affection: The structure of adolescent romantic and sexual networks. *American Journal of Sociology, 110*(1), 44–91. doi:10.1086/386272

Blower, S. M., Hartel, D., Dowlatabadi, H., Andersen, R. M., & May, R. M. (1991). Drugs, sex & HIV: A mathematical model for New York City. *Philosophical Transactions of the Royal Society of London. Series B, Biological Sciences, 331*, 171–187. doi:10.1098/rstb.1991.0006

Bobashev, G. V., Ellner, S., Nychka, D. W., & Grenfell, B. (2000). Reconstruction of susceptible and recruitment dynamics from measles epidemic data. *Mathematical Population Studies, 8*(1), 1–29.

Borshchev, A., & Filippov, A. (2004, July 25–29). From system dynamics and discrete event to practical agent based modeling: Reasons, techniques, tools. *Proceedings of the 22nd International Conference of the System Dynamics Society*, Oxford, England.

Bourgois, P. (1998). The moral economies of homeless heroin addicts: confronting ethnography, HIV risk and everyday violence in San Francisco shooting encampments. *Substance Use & Misuse, 33*(11), 2323–2351. doi:10.3109/10826089809056260

Bourgois, P., Price, B., & Moss, A. (2004). Everyday violence and the gender of Hepatitis C among homeless drug-injecting youth in San Francisco. *Human Organization, 63*(3), 253–264.

Colizza, V., Barthelemy, M., Barrat, A., & Vespignani, A. (2007). Epidemic modeling in complex realities *CR Biologies, 330*, 364-374

Epstein, J. M. (2007). *Generative social science: Studies in agent-based computational modeling*. Princeton, NJ: Princeton University Press.

Eubank, S., Guclu, H., Kumar, V. S. A., Marathe, M. V., Srinivasan, A., Toroczkai, Z., & Wang, N. (2004). Modelling disease outbreaks in realistic urban social networks. *Nature, 429*, 180–184. doi:10.1038/nature02541

Heckathorn, D. D. (2002). Respondent-driven sampling ii: Deriving valid population estimates from chain-referral samples of hidden populations . *Social Problems, 49*(1), 11–34. doi:10.1525/sp.2002.49.1.11

Law, A. M. (2007). *Simulation modeling and analysis* (4th Edition) McGraw-Hill.

Levin, S., Aronsky, D., Hemphill, R., Han, J., Slagle, J., & France, D. (2007). Shifting toward balance: Measuring the distribution of workload among emergency physician teams. *Annals of Emergency Medicine, 50*(4), 419–423. doi:10.1016/j.annemergmed.2007.04.007

Miró, O., Sánchez, M., & Millá, J. (2004). Hospital mortality and staff workload. *Lancet, 356*(9238), 1356–1357. doi:10.1016/S0140-6736(05)74269-0

Morris, M. (2004). Overview of network survey designs. In M. Morris (Ed.), *Network epidemiology: A handbook for survey design and data collection* (pp. 8-24). London: Oxford University Press.

Newman, M. E. J. (2002). The spread of epidemic disease on networks . *Physical Review E: Statistical, Nonlinear, and Soft Matter Physics, 66*, 016128. doi:10.1103/PhysRevE.66.016128

Rahmandad, H., & Sterman, J. (2008). Heterogeneity and network structure in the dynamics of diffusion: Comparing agent-based and system dynamics models. *Management Science, 54*(5), 998–1014. doi:10.1287/mnsc.1070.0787

Riley, S. (2007). Large-scale spatial-transmission models of infectious diseases . *Science, 316*, 1298–1301. doi:10.1126/science.1134695

Rvachev, L. A., & Longini, I. M. (1985). A mathematical model for the global spread of influenza. *Mathematical Biosciences, 75*, 3–22. doi:10.1016/0025-5564(85)90064-1

Snijders, T. A. B., Steglich, C. E. G., & Schweinberger, M. (2007). Modeling the co-evolution of networks and behavior. In K. van Montfort, H. Oud, & A. Satorra (Eds.), *Longitudinal models in the behavioral and related sciences* (pp. 41-71). Mahwah, NJ: Lawrence Erlbaum.

Sterman, J. (2000). Business Dynamics. Systems Thinking and Modeling for a Complex World. Irwin/McGraw-Hill, New York.

Turner, K. M. E., Adams, E. J., Gay, N., Ghani, A. C., Mercer, C., & Edmunds, W. J. (2006). Developing a realistic sexual network model of chlamydia transmission in Britain. *Theoretical Biology & Medical Modelling, 3*(3), 1–11.

Vahabzadeh, M., Jia-Ling, L., Epstein, D. H., Mezghanni, M., Schmittner, J., & Preston, K. L. (2007). Computerized contingency management for motivating behavior change: automated tracking and dynamic reward reinforcement management computer-based medical systems. CBMS '07. Twentieth IEEE International Symposium on June 20–22. Pages: 85-90. Digital Object Identifier 10.1109/CBMS.2007.35

Watts, D. (1999). *Small worlds*. Princeton, NJ: Princeton University Press.

Wheaton, W. D., Allpress, J. L., Chasteen, B. M., Cajka, J. C., Wagener, D. K., Cooley, P. C., & Roberts, D. J. (2006). *Nationwide geographically-explicit synthetic populations using public use microdata.* Presented at Congress of Epidemiology, Seattle, WA, June 21–24, 2006.

Zule, W. A., & Bobashev, G. V. (in press, 2008). High dead-space syringes and the risk of HIV and HCV infection among injecting drug users. *Drug and Alcohol Dependence.*

Compilation of References

Abellán, J. J., Armero, C., Conesa, D., Pérez-Panadés, J., Martínez-Beneito, M. A., Zurriaga, O., et al. (2004). Predicting the Behavior of the Renal Transplant Waiting List in the Pais Valencia (Spain) Using Simulation Modeling. *Proceedings of Winter Simulation Conference* (pp. 1969-1974).

AbsoluteAstronomy. (2009). Retrieved February 25, 2009, from http://www.absoluteastronomy.com/topics/Telemedicine

Ackerman, E., Rosevear, J., & McGuckin, W. (1964). A Mathematical Model of the Glucose-tolerance test. *Physics in Medicine and Biology, 9*, 203–213. doi:10.1088/0031-9155/9/2/307

Adamatti, D. F., Simão Sichman, J., & Ducrot, R. (2004). Using multi-agent systems and role-playing games to simulate water management in peri-urban catchments. *Proc. Sixth International Conference on Social Science Methodology*. Amsterdam, The Netherlands.

Aglets (2002). Retrieved July 27, 2006, from http://www.trl.ibm.com/aglets/

AGREE, C. (2003). Development and validation of an international appraisal instrument for assessing the quality of clinical practice guidelines: the AGREE project. *Quality & Safety in Health Care, 12*(1), 18–23. doi:10.1136/qhc.12.1.18

Alonso, A., Marcos, M., Alonso, J. R., Gelabert, G., Martínez-Salvador, B., & Riaño, D. (2008). (in press). A Knowledge-Acquisition Framework to Facilitate the Development and Reengineering of Care Plans in Electronic Format. *Journal of Telemedicine and Telecare*.

Alverson, D. C., & Saiki, S., Jr. (2008). *Telehealth outreach for unified community health (Project TOUCH)*. University of New Mexico and University of Hawaii.

Retrieved August 7, 2008, from http://hsc.unm.edu/som/projects/touch/.

Alverson, D. C., Saiki, S Jr, Caudell, T. P., Goldsmith, T., Stevens, S., Saland, L., Colleran, K., Brandt, J., Danielson, L., Cerilli, L., Harris, A., Gregory, M. C., Stewart, R., Norenberg, J., & Shuster, G., Panaoitis, Holten, J., Vergera, V. M., Sherstyuk, A., Kihmm, K., Lui, J., & Wang, K. L. (2006). Reification of abstract concepts to improve comprehension using interactive virtual environments and a knowledge-based design: a renal physiology model. *Studies in Health Technology and Informatics, 119*, 13–18.

Alverson, D. C., Saiki, S. Jr, Caudell, T. P., & Summers, K., Panaiotis, Sherstyuk, A., Nickles, D., Holten, J., Goldsmith, T. E., Stevens, S. M., Kihmm, K., Mennin, S., Kalishman, S., Mines J., Serna, L., Mitchell, S., Lindberg, M., Jacobs, J., Nakatsu, C., Lozanoff, S., Wax, D. S., Saland L., Norenberg, J., Shuster, G., Keep, M., Baker, R., Buchanan, H. S., Stewart, R., Bowyer, M., Liu, A., Muniz, G., Coulter, R., Maris, C., & Wilks, D. (2005). Distributed immersive virtual reality simulation development for medical education. *Journal of International Association of Medical Science Educators, 15*(1), 19–30.

Alzheimer's Association. (2009). Retrieved February 7, 2009, from http://www.alz.org/alzheimers_disease_what_is_alzheimers.asp

American Diabetes Association. (2006). Retrieved December 12, 2006 from http://www.diabetes.org

Amoros, P., Corchon, L., & Moreno, B. (2002). The Scholarship Assignment Problem. *Games and Economic Behavior, 38*, 1–18. doi:10.1006/game.2001.0852

Anderson, M., & Sandholm, T. (1999). Leveled Commitment Contracting among Myopic Individually Rational

Agents. [Special Issue on Agent-Based Computational Economics.]. *Journal of Economic Dynamics & Control, 25*, 615–640. doi:10.1016/S0165-1889(00)00039-7

Anderson, R. M., & May, R. M. (1991). *Infectious disease of humans: Dynamics and control.* Oxford: Oxford Sciences Publications.

Anselma, L., Terenziani, P., Montani, S., & Bottrighi, A. (2007). Automatic Checking of the Correctness of Clinical Guidelines in GLARE. In K. A. Kuhn, J. R. Warren & T.-Y. Leong (Eds.), *Proc. of the 12th World Congress on Health (Medical) Informatics, MEDINFO 2007* (pp. 807-811). Brisbane, AUS.

AnyLogic. (2008). XJ Technologies and AnyLogic Web site: www.anylogic.com

Asadachatreekul, S. (2004). *An Agent-based Distributed Inference Engine for Expert System Construction.* University of Regina, Regina.

Baesler, F. F., Jahnsen, H. E., & DaCosta, M. (2003). The Use of Simulation and Design of Experiments for Estimating Maximum Capacity in an Emergency Room. *Proceedings of Winter Simulation Conference* (pp. 1903-1906).

Bailey, N. J. T. (1975). *The mathematical theory of infectious diseases and its applications.* London: Oxford University Press.

Bajo, J., Tapia, D., Rodríguez, S., Luis, A., & Corchado, J. (2007). Nature-Inspired Planner Agent for Health Care. *Computational and Ambient Intelligence, 4507,* 1090-1097. Berlin/Heidelberg: Springer

Banasik, J. L. (2000). Renal Function (2nd ed.). In *Pathophysiology: Biological and Behavioral Perspectives* (pp. 626–648). Philadelphia, PA: W.B. Saunders Company.

Bansal, V., & Garg, R. (2001). Efficiency and Price Discovery in Multi-item Auctions. *ACM SIGecom Exchanges, 2*(1), 26–32. doi:10.1145/844309.844314

Barabasi, A. L., & Albert, R. (1999). Emergence of scaling in random networks. *Science, 286*(5439), 509–512. doi:10.1126/science.286.5439.509

Barber, K. S., Goel, A., Han, D. C., Kim, J., Lam, D. N., & Liu, T. H. (2003). Infrastructure for Design, Deployment and Experimentation of Distributed Agent-based Systems: The Requirements, The Technologies, and An

Example. *Autonomous Agents and Multi-Agent Systems, 7*(1), 49–69. doi:10.1023/A:1024124804035

Barnes, C. D., Quiason, J. L., Benson, C., & McGuiness, D. (1997). Success Stories in Simulation in Health Care. *Proceedings of the 1997 Winter Simulation Conference* (pp. 1280-1285).

Baumgartner, U., Magele, Ch., & Renhart, W. (2004). Pareto optimality and particle swarm optimization. *IEEE Transactions on Magnetics, 40*(2), 1172–1175. doi:10.1109/TMAG.2004.825430

Bearman, P. S., Moody, J., & Stovel, K. (2004). Chains of affection: The structure of adolescent romantic and sexual networks. *American Journal of Sociology, 110*(1), 44–91. doi:10.1086/386272

Becht, M., Gurzki, T., Klarmann, J., & Muscholl, M. (1999). ROPE: Role-Oriented Programming Environment for Multi-Agent Systems. *Conference on Cooperative Information Systems* (pp. 325–333).

Bellifemine, F., Caire, G., & Greenwood, D. (2007). *Developing multi-agent systems with JADE.* Chichester, England: John Wiley and Sons.

Bellifemine, F., Caire, G., Poggi, A., & Rimassa, G. (2003). JADE A White Paper. *EXP in search of innovation - Special Issue on JADE, TILAB Journal, 3,* 6-19.

Bellin, H. T., Fellner, D., & Tchorbajian, N. (1985). *Portable EKG monitoring device for ST deviation.* Retrieved July 4, 2007, from http://www.freepatentsonline.com/4546776.html

Berg, D., Ram, P., & Glasgow, J. (2004). SAGEDesktop: An Environment for Testing Clinical Practice Guidelines. In Z.-P. Liang (Ed.), *Proc. of the 26th Annual Conference of the IEEE Engineering in Medicine and Biology Society, IEEE-IEBMS 2004* (pp. 3217-3220). San Francisco, US.

Berger, T., & Ringler, C. (2002). Trade-offs, efficiency gains and technical change – Modeling water management and land use within a multiple-agent framework. *Quarterly Journal of International Agriculture, 41*(1-2), 119–144.

Berger, T., Schreinemachers, P., & Woelcke, J. (2006). Multi-agent simulation for development of less-favored areas. *Agricultural Systems, 88,* 28–43. doi:10.1016/j.agsy.2005.06.002

Bernard, D., Dorais, G., Gamble, E., Kanefsky, B., Kurien, J., Man, G. K., et al. (1999). Spacecraft Autonomy Flight Experience: The DS1 Remote Agent Experiment. *Proceedings of the American Institute of Aeronautics and Astronautics Conference* (pp. 28-30). Albuquerque, NM: AIAA Space Technology Conference.

Bernon, C., Cossentino, M., & Pavón, J. (2005). Agent-oriented software engineering. *The Knowledge Engineering Review, 20*(2), 99–116. doi:10.1017/S0269888905000421

Bikhchandani, S., & Haile, P. (2002). Symmetric Separating Equilibria in English Auctions. *Games and Economic Behavior, 38*, 19–27. doi:10.1006/game.2001.0879

Bikhchandani, S., & Ostroy, J. (2002). The Package Assignment Model. *Journal of Economic Theory, 107*, 377–406. doi:10.1006/jeth.2001.2957

Blood Pressure Monitor. Retrieved December 20, 2007, from http://www.omronhealthcare.com/enTouchCMS/app/viewCategory?catgId=23

Blower, S. M., Hartel, D., Dowlatabadi, H., Andersen, R. M., & May, R. M. (1991). Drugs, sex & HIV: A mathematical model for New York City. *Philosophical Transactions of the Royal Society of London. Series B, Biological Sciences, 331*, 171–187. doi:10.1098/rstb.1991.0006

Bobashev, G. V., Ellner, S., Nychka, D. W., & Grenfell, B. (2000). Reconstruction of susceptible and recruitment dynamics from measles epidemic data. *Mathematical Population Studies, 8*(1), 1–29.

Borshchev, A., & Filippov, A. (2004, July 25–29). From system dynamics and discrete event to practical agent based modeling: Reasons, techniques, tools. *Proceedings of the 22nd International Conference of the System Dynamics Society,* Oxford, England.

Bourgois, P. (1998). The moral economies of homeless heroin addicts: confronting ethnography, HIV risk and everyday violence in San Francisco shooting encampments. *Substance Use & Misuse, 33*(11), 2323–2351. doi:10.3109/10826089809056260

Bourgois, P., Price, B., & Moss, A. (2004). Everyday violence and the gender of Hepatitis C among homeless drug-injecting youth in San Francisco. *Human Organization, 63*(3), 253–264.

Boutayeb, A., & Chetouani, A. (2006). *A Critical Review of Mathematical Models and Data used in Diabetology.* Retrieved December 6, 2006 from http://www.biomedical-engineering-online.com/

Bradshaw, J. M. (1997). Software agents. In J. Bradshaw (Ed.), *An introduction to software agents* (pp. 3-46). Cambridge, MA: MIT Press.

Brailsford, S. C. (2007). Tutorial: Advances and Challenges in Healthcare Simulation Modeling. *Proceedings of Winter Simulation Conference* (pp. 1436-1448).

Bresciani, P., Giorgini, P., Giunchiglia, F., Mylopoulos, J., & Perini, A. (2004). TROPOS: An Agent-Oriented Software Development Methodology. *Autonomous Agents and Multi-Agent Systems, 8*(3), 203–236. doi:10.1023/B:AGNT.0000018806.20944.ef

Brown, M. (2007). *U of A contributes to all-in-one health device.* Retrieved December 20, 2007, from http://www.expressnews.ualberta.ca/article.cfm?id=8955

Broyles, R. W. (2006). *Fundamentals of statistics in health administration* (1st ed.). Sudbury, Massachusetts: Jones & Bartlett Publishers.

Bui, T. (2000). Agent Based Corporate Information Systems: An Application to Medicine. [Elsevier.]. *European Journal of Operational Research, 122*, 243–257. doi:10.1016/S0377-2217(99)00231-3

Burgun, A. (2006). Desiderata for domain reference ontologies in biomedicine. *Journal of Biomedical Informatics, 39*, 307–313. doi:10.1016/j.jbi.2005.09.002

Campana, F., Moreno, A., Riaño, D., & Varga, L. (2008). K4Care: Knowledge-Based Homecare e-Services for an Ageing Europe. In R. Annicchiarico, U. Cortés, & C. Urdiales (Eds.), *Agent Technology and e-Health* (pp. 95-115). Basel, Switzerland: Birkhäuser Basel.

Canadian Diabetes Association. (2006). Retrieved December 12, 2006 from http://www.diabetes.ca/

Cancer, W. E. B. (2008). *CancerWEB Project.* Retrieved July 29, 2008, from http://cancerweb.ncl.ac.uk/.

Cavazza, M., & Simo, A. (2003). A virtual patient based on qualitative simulation. *In IUI '03: Proceedings of the 8th international conference on Intelligent user interfaces* (pp. 19–25). New York, NY: ACM Press.

CBC News (2006, December 1). *Public vs. private health care.*

CCHBPC. (2006). *Canadian Coalition for High Blood Pressure Prevention and Control.* Retrieved December 12, 2006 from http://hypertension.ca/bpc/

CDC. Centers for Disease Control and Prevention (2006). Retrieved December 11, 2006 from http://www.cdc.gov/diabetes/statistics/prev/national

Centeno, M. A., Giachetti, R., Linn, R., & Ismail, A. M. (2003). A Simulation-ILP based Tools for Scheduling ER Staff. *Proceedings of the 2003 Winter Simulation Conference* (pp. 1930-1938).

Cernuzzi, L., Juan, T., Sterling, L., & Zambonelli, F. (2004). The Gaia Methodology: Basic Concepts and Extensions. In F. Bergenti, M. P. Gleizes, & F. Zambonelli (Eds.), *Methodologies and Software Engineering for Agent Systems* (pp. 69-88). Springer US.

Ceusters, W., Martens, P., Dhaen, C., & Terzic, B. (2001). LinkFactory: an advanced formal ontology management System. *Proceedings of Interactive Tools for Knowledge Capture* (KCAP 2001).

Chaoulli v. Quebec (Attorney General) (2005). 2005 SCC 35. 1 S.C.R. 791, Para 123, Docket 29272, Supreme Court of Canada.

Check, E. (2004). Antidepressants:Bitter pills. *Nature, 431,* 122–124. doi:10.1038/431122a

Chen, Y., & Wang, S. (2007). Framework of agent-based intelligence system with two-stage decision-making process for distributed dynamic scheduling. *Applied Soft Computing, 7,* 229–245. doi:10.1016/j.asoc.2005.04.003

Chenney, S. (2004). Flow tiles. *In SCA '04: Proceedings of the 2004 ACM SIGGRAPH/Eurographics symposium on Computer animation* (pp. 233–242). New York, NY: ACM Press.

Chesani, F., de Matteis, P., Mello, P., Montal, M., & Storari, S. (2006). A Framework for Defining and Verifying Clinical Guidelines: A Case Study on Cancer Screening. In F. Esposito, Z. W. Ras, D. Malerba, & G. Semeraro (Eds.), *Proc. of the Proceedings of 16th International Symposium on Methodologies for Intelligent Systems, ISMIS 2006* (pp. 338-343). Bari, Italy.

Christiansen, J., & Campbell, P. (2003). *HealthSim: An Agent-Based Model for Simulating Health Care Delivery.* Chicago, Illinois: Argonne National Laboratory.

Chun, A., Wai, H., & Wong, R. (2003). Optimizing agent-based meeting scheduling through preference estimation. *Engineering Applications of Artificial Intelligence, 16,* 727–743. doi:10.1016/j.engappai.2003.09.009

CIA. (2008). CIA World Factbook Washington, D.C.: *Central Intelligence Agency, 2008.* Retrieved September 8, 2008, from https://www.cia.gov/library/publications/the-world-factbook/

Ciccarese, P., Caffi, E., Boiocchi, L., Quaglini, S., & Stefanelli, M. (2004). A Guideline Management System. In M. Fieschi, E. Coiera, & J. X. Li (Eds.), *Proc. of the 11th World Congress on Medical Informatics, MEDINFO 2004* (pp. 28-32). San Francisco, USA.

Ciccarese, P., Caffi, E., Quaglini, S., & Stefanelli, M. (2005). Architectures and Tools for innovative Health Information Systems: the Guide Project. *International Journal of Medical Informatics, 74*(7-8), 553–562. doi:10.1016/j.ijmedinf.2005.02.001

Cimino, J. J. (2006). In defense of the desiderata. *Journal of Biomedical Informatics, 39,* 299–306. doi:10.1016/j.jbi.2005.11.008

Clarke, E. H. (1971). Multipart Pricing of Public Goods. *Public Choice, 11,* 17–33. doi:10.1007/BF01726210

Clercq, P. A. d., Blom, J. A., Korsten, H. H. M., & Hasman, A. (2004). Approaches for creating computer-interpretable guidelines that facilitate decision support. *Artificial Intelligence in Medicine, 31*(1), 1–27. doi:10.1016/j.artmed.2004.02.003

Colizza, V., Barthelemy, M., Barrat, A., & Vespignani, A. (2007). Epidemic modeling in complex realities *CR Biologies, 330,* 364-374

Concordia (2004). Retrieved July 27, 2006, from http://www.merl.com/projects/concordia/

Conner-Spady, B. L., & Sanmugasunderam, S. (2005). Patient and physician perspectives of maximum acceptable waiting times for cataract surgery. *Canadian Journal of Ophthalmology, 40,* 439–447.

Core Health Indicators. (2007). Retrieved December 24, 2007, from http://www.who.int/whosis/database/core/core_select_process.cfm

Cossentino, M. (2005). From Requirements to Code with the PASSI Methodology. In B. Henderson-Sellers & P.

Giorgini (Eds.), *Agent-Oriented Methodologies* (pp. 79-106). Idea Group.

Craddock, N., & Jones, I. (2001). Molecular genetics of bipolar disorder. *The British Journal of Psychiatry, 178*(41), 128–133. doi:10.1192/bjp.178.41.s128

Cuesta, P., Gómez Expósito, A., Rodríguez, F. J., & González, J. (2005). Developing a Multiagent System for Mobile Devices. *Revista Iberoamericana de Inteligencia Artificial, 25*, 49–57.

Da Silva, V. T., Noya, R. C., & De Lucena, C. J. P. (2004). Using the MAS-ML to model a multi-agent system. *Software engineering for multi-agent systems II: research issues and practical applications . Lecture Notes in Computer Science, 2940*, 129–148.

Da Silva, V. T., Noya, R. C., & De Lucena, C. J. P. (2005), Using the UML 2.0 Activity Diagram to Model Agent Plans and Actions. *Proceedings of the 4th International Conference on Autonomous Agents and Multiagent Systems*. The Netherlands.

Daly, L. E., & Bourke, G. J. (2000). *Interpretation and uses of medical statistics* (5th ed.). Oxford: Blackwell Science Ltd.

Davis, D., Goldman, J., & Palda, V. A. (2007). *Handbook on Clinical Practice Guidelines*. Ottawa, CA: Canadian Medical Association.

Dawson-Saunders, B., Feltovich, P. J., Coulson, R. L., & Steward, D. E. (1990). A survey of medical school teachers to identify basic biomedical concepts medical students should understand. *Academic Medicine, 65*(7), 448–454. doi:10.1097/00001888-199007000-00008

De Maria, B. A., Da Silva, V. T., Noya, R. C., & De Lucena, C. J. P. (2005). VisualAgent: A Software Development Environment for Multi-Agent Systems. *Proceedings of the 20th Brazilian Symposium on Databases and 19th Brazilian Symposium on Software Engeneering*, Brazil.

Decker, K. (1996). TAEMS: A Framework for Environment Centered Analysis and Design of Coordination Mechanisms. In G. O'Hare & N. Jennings (Eds.), *Foundations of Distributed Artificial Intelligence* (pp. 429-448). Wiley Inter-Science.

DeLoach, S. A. (2004). The MaSE Methodology. In F. Bergenti, M. P. Gleizes, & F. Zambonelli (Eds.), *Methodologies and Software Engineering for Agent Systems:*

The Agent-Oriented Software Engineering Handbook (pp. 107-125). Kluwer Academic Publishers.

DeLoach, S., Wood, M., & Sparkman, C. H. (2001). Multiagent Systems Engineering. *International Journal of Software Engineering and Knowledge Engineering, 11*, 231–258. doi:10.1142/S0218194001000542

Demange, G., Gale, D., & Sotomayor, M. (1984). Multi-Item Auctions. *The Journal of Political Economy, 94*(4), 863–872. doi:10.1086/261411

DeNavas-Walt, C.B.P., & Smith, J. (2007, August). *Income, poverty, and health insurance coverage in the United States: 2006*. U.S. Census Bureau.

Devi, M. S., & Mago, V. (2005). Multi-agent model for Indian rural health care. *Leadership in Health Services, 18*(4), i–xi. doi:10.1108/13660750510625724

Ducrot, R., Le Page, C., Bommel, P., & Kuper, M. (2004). Articulating land and water dynamics with urbanization: an attempt to model natural resources management at the urban edge. *Computers, Environment and Urban Systems, 28*, 85–106. doi:10.1016/S0198-9715(02)00066-2

Dunn, H. L. (1959). High-level Wellness for Man and Society. *American Journal of Public Health and the Nation's Health, 49*(6), 7.

Eberhart, R. C., & Shi, Y. (1998). Comparison between genetic algorithms and particle swarm optimization. *Evolutionary Programming VII: Proceedings 7th annual conference on Evolutionary Programming conference* (pp. 611-616). Berlin: Springer-Verlag.

Ekholm, J. M., Pekkarinen, P., Pajukanta, P., Kieseppä, T., Partonen, T., & Paunio, T. (2002). Bipolar disorder susceptibility region on Xq24-q27.1 in Finnish families . *Molecular Psychiatry, 7*(5), 453–459. doi:10.1038/sj.mp.4001104

Epstein, J. M. (2007). *Generative social science: Studies in agent-based computational modeling*. Princeton, NJ: Princeton University Press.

Esmail, N., Hazel, M., & Walker, M. A. (2008). *Waiting your turn: Hospital waiting lists in Canada* (18th ed.). Fraser Institute.

Eubank, S., Guclu, H., Kumar, V. S. A., Marathe, M. V., Srinivasan, A., Toroczkai, Z., & Wang, N. (2004). Modelling disease outbreaks in realistic urban social networks. *Nature, 429*, 180–184. doi:10.1038/nature02541

Ferrin, D. M., Miller, M. J., Wininger, S., & Neuendorf, M. S. (2004). Analyzing Incentives and Scheduling in a Major Metropolitan Hospital Operating Room Through Simulation. *Proceedings of Winter Simulation Conference* (pp. 1975-1981).

Field, M. J., & Lohr, K. N. (Eds.). (1990). *Clinical Practice Guidelines: Directions for a New Program*. Washington, DC: National Academy Press.

Flatland (2008). University of New Mexico. Retrieved August 7, 2008, from http://www.hpc.unm.edu/homunculus/.

Flexsim Software Products, Inc. (2008). Retrieved Nov. 20, 2008, From http://www.flexsim.com/

Fonseca, J. M., Mora, A. D., & Marques, A. C. (2005). MAMIS – A Multi-Agent Medical Information System. *Proceedings of IASTED International Conference on Biomedical Engineering (BioMED 2005)*, Austria.

Fowler, J., Jarvis, P., & Chevannes, M. (2002). *Practical Statistics for Nursing and Health Care* (1st ed.). Chichester: John Wiley and Sons.

Fox, J., Alabassi, A., Patkar, V., Rose, T., & Black, E. (2006). An ontological approach to modelling tasks and goals. *Computers in Biology and Medicine, 36*(7-8), 837–856. doi:10.1016/j.compbiomed.2005.04.011

Fox, J., Beveridge, M., & Glasspool, D. (2003). Understanding intelligent agents: analysis and synthesis. *AI Communications, 16*(3), 139–152.

Fox, J., Patkar, V., & Thomson, R. (2006). Decision Support for Healthcare: the PROforma evidence base. *Informatics in Primary Care, 14*, 49–54.

Friedman, R. A., & Leon, A. C. (2007). Expanding the Black Box-Depression, Antidepressants, and the Risk of Suicide. *The New England Journal of Medicine, 356*, 2343–2346. doi:10.1056/NEJMp078015

Fuchs, B.C., & Sokolovsky, J. (1990, February). *The Canadian health care system, CRS Report for Congress.* Congressional Research Service: Library of Congress.

Ganendran, G., Tran, Q., Ganguly, P., Ray, P., & Low, G. (2002). An Ontology-driven Multi-agent approach for Healthcare. *Proceedings of the Health Informatics Conference (HIC2002)*, Melbourne.

Garcia, M. E., Valero, S., Argente, E., Giret, A., & Julian, V. (2008). A FAST Method to Achieve Flexible Production Programming Systems. *IEEE Transactions on Systems, Man and Cybernetics. Part C, Applications and Reviews, 38*(2), 242–252. doi:10.1109/TSMCC.2007.913921

Gérard, P., Massin, M. M., Maeyns, K., Withofs, N., & Ravet, F. (2000). Circadian Rhythm of Heart Rate and Heart Rate Variability. *Archives of Disease in Childhood, 83*, 179–182. doi:10.1136/adc.83.2.179

Ghoreishi-Nejad, S., Martens, R., & Paranjape, R. (2008). An Agent-Based Diabetic Patient Simulation, KES-AMSTA. In N.T. Nguyen (Ed.), *Lecture Notes in Artificial Intelligence, 4953*, 832–841.

Gibbs, C. (2000). *TEEMA Reference Guide, Version 1.0*. Saskatchewan: TRLabs Regina.

Gilpin, A., & Sandholm, T. (2007). Information-theoretic Approaches to Branching in Search. *Proceedings of the International Joint Conference on Artificial Intelligence (IJCAI)*.

Gómez-Alonso, C., Isern, D., & Moreno, A. (2007). *Software Engineering Methodologies to Develop Multi-Agent Systems: State-of-the-art* (Research Report No. DEIM-RR-07-003). Tarragona, Catalonia: University Rovira i Virgili.

Gómez-Pérez, A. (1998). Knowledge sharing and reuse, *The Handbook on Applied Expert Systems* (pp. 1-36). CRC Press.

Gómez-Sanz, J., Gervais, M. P., & Weiss, G. (2004). A Survey on Agent-Oriented Software Engineering Research. In F. Bergenti, M. P. Gleizes, & F. Zambonelli (Eds.), *Methodologies and Software Engineering for Agent Systems* (Vol. 11, pp. 33-64): Springer US.

Gong, J., Zhou, J., Li, W., & Lin, H. (2006). Design and implementation of an intelligent virtual geographic environment for the simulation of SARS transmission. *Proceedings of the 2006 ACM international conference on Virtual reality continuum and its applications* (pp. 383-386). SESSION: Session S2: VR applications

Gracanin, D., Bohner, S. A., & Hinchey, M. (2004). Towards a Model-Driven Architecture for Autonomic Systems. *Proceeding of 11th IEEE International Conference and Workshop on the Engineering of Computer-Based Systems (ECBS'04)* (pp. 500-505).

Graham, J. R., Decker, K. S., & Mersic, M. (2003). DECAF – A Flexible Multi Agent System Architecture. *Autonomous Agents and Multi-Agent Systems, 7*(1-2), 7–27. doi:10.1023/A:1024120703127

Group, D. S. (2008). Retrieved Nov. 20, 2008, http://www.3ds.com/products/delmia/welcome/

Groves, T. (1973). Incentives in Teams. *Econometrica, 41*, 617–631. doi:10.2307/1914085

Groves, T., & Ledyard, J. (1977). Optimal Allocation of Public Goods: A Solution to the 'Free Rider' Problem. *Econometrica, 45*, 783–809. doi:10.2307/1912672

Guo, M., Wagner, M., & West, C. (2004). Outpatient Clinic Scheduling – A Simulation Approach, *Proceedings of Winter Simulation Conference* (pp. 1981-1987).

Hadzic, M., & Chang, E. (2005). Ontology-based Support for Human Disease Study. *Proceedings of the Hawaii International Conference on System Sciences, HICSS38*, 2005.

Hadzic, M., & Chang, E. (2008a). Web Semantics for Intelligent and Dynamic Information Retrieval Illustrated Within the Mental Health Domain. In E. Chang, T.S. Dillon, R. Meersman, & K. Sycara (Eds.), *Advances in Web Semantics: A State-of-the Art*. Springer.

Hadzic, M., & Chang, E. (2008b). An Integrated Approach for Effective and Efficient Retrieval of the Information about Mental Illnesses. In A.S. Sidhu, T.S. Dillon, & E. Chang, (Eds.), *Biomedical Data and Applications*. Springer.

Hadzic, M., & Chang, E. (2008c). TICSA Approach: Five Important Aspects of Multi-agent Systems. *Proceedings of the International IFIP Workshop On Semantic Web & Web Semantics, On The Move Federated Conferences*, Mexico.

Hadzic, M., Chen, M., & Dillon, T. (2008d). Towards the Mental Health Ontology. *Proceedings of the IEEE International Conference on Bioinformatics and Biomedicine, USA.*

Hadzic, M., Hadzic, F., & Dillon, T. (2008a). Tree Mining in Mental Health Domain. *Proceedings of the Hawaii International Conference on System Sciences (HICSS-41)*, USA.

Hadzic, M., Hadzic, F., & Dillon, T. (2008b). Mining of Health Information from Ontologies. *Proceedings of the International Conference on Health Informatics (HEALTHINF2008)*, Portugal.

Hadzic, M., Hadzic, F., & Dillon, T. (2008c). Domain Driven Data Mining for the Mental Health Domain. In P.S. Yu, C. Zhang, & H. Zhang (Ed.), *Domain Driven Data Mining: Domain Problems*. Springer.

Han, J., & Kamber, M. (2006). *Data Mining: Concepts and Techniques* (2nd ed.). San Francisco: Morgan Kaufmann

Harper, P. R. (2002). A Framework for Operational Modelling of Hospital Resources. [Kluwer Academic Publishers.]. *Health Care Management Science, 5*, 165–173. doi:10.1023/A:1019767900627

Harris, M., & Taylor, G. (2003). Medical Statistic Made Easy. In A. Bosher (Ed.), Taylor & Francis e-Library.

Hassine, A. B., & Ho, T. B. (2007). An agent-based approach to solve dynamic meeting scheduling problems with preferences. *Engineering Applications of Artificial Intelligence, 20*, 857–873. doi:10.1016/j.engappai.2006.10.004

Health Canada. (2002). *Diabetes in Canada* (2nd ed.). Center for Chronic Disease Prevention and Control, Population and Public Health Branch, Health Canada

Health Level 7 (1997). Retrieved January 31, 2008, from http://www.hl7.org/

Health Promotion Glossary Update. Retrieved May 29, 2007, from http://www.who.int/healthpromotion/about/HPR%20Glossary_New%20Terms.pdf

Heart Rate Monitor. Retrieved December 20, 2007, from http://www.omronhealthcare.com/enTouchCMS/app/viewCategory?catgId=33

Heckathorn, D. D. (2002). Respondent-driven sampling ii: Deriving valid population estimates from chain-referral samples of hidden populations . *Social Problems, 49*(1), 11–34. doi:10.1525/sp.2002.49.1.11

Henderson-Sellers, B., & Giorgini, P. (2005). Agent-Oriented Methodologies: An Introduction. In B. Henderson-Sellers & P. Giorgini (Eds.), *Agent-Oriented Methodologies* (pp. 1-19). Idea Group.

Hertz, A., & Robert, V. (1998). Constructing a course schedule by solving a series of assignment type problems. *European Journal of Operational Research, 108*, 585–603. doi:10.1016/S0377-2217(97)00097-0

Hill, P. C., & Pargament, K. I. (2003). Advances in the Conceptualization and Measurement of Religion and Spirituality: Implications for Physical and Mental Health Research . *The American Psychologist*, *58*(1), 64–74. doi:10.1037/0003-066X.58.1.64

Hommersom, A., Groot, P., Lucas, P. J., Balser, M., & Schmitt, J. (2007). Verification of the Medical Guidelines using background knowledge in Task Networks. *IEEE Transactions on Knowledge and Data Engineering*, *19*(4), 281–316.

Hongoro, C., & McPake, B. (2004). How to bridge the gap in human resources for health. *Lancet*, *364*(9443), 1451–1456C. doi:10.1016/S0140-6736(04)17229-2

Horvitz-Lennon, M., Kilbourne, A. M., & Pincus, H. A. (2006). From Silos To Bridges: Meeting The General Health Care Needs Of Adults With Severe Mental Illnesses. *Health Affairs*, *25*(3), 659–669. doi:10.1377/hlthaff.25.3.659

Hrabak, K. M., Campbell, J. R., Tu, S. W., McClure, R., & Weida, R. (2007). Creating Interoperable Guidelines: Requirements of Vocabulary Standards in Immunization Decision Support. In K. A. Kuhn, J. R. Warren, & T.-Y. Leong (Eds.), *Proc. of the Proceedings of the 12th World Congress on Health (Medical) Informatics, MEDINFO 2007* (pp. 930-934). Brisbaine, AU.

Huang, C. J., & Liao, W. C. (2004). Application of Probabilistic Neural Networks to the Class Prediction of Leukemia and Embryonal Tumor of Central Nervous System. *Neural Processing Letters*, 211–226. doi:10.1023/B:NEPL.0000035613.51734.48

Huang, J., Jennings, N. R., & Fox, J. (1995). An Agent-based Approach to Health Care management. *International Journal of Applied Artificial Intelligence*, *9*(4), 401–420. doi:10.1080/08839519508945482

Humphreys, B. L., Lindberg, D. A. B., Schoolman, H. M., & Barnett, G. O. (1998). The Unified Medical Language System: An Informatics Research Collaboration. *Journal of the American Medical Informatics Association*, *5*(1), 1–11.

Hurst, J., & Siciliani, L. (2003). *Tackling Excessive Waiting Times for Elective Surgery: A Comparison of Policies in Twelve OECD Countries.*

InterSense. (2008). InterSense Inc. Reterieved August 28, 2008, from http://www.intersense.com/.

Introduction to Medical Statistics. (2001, November 6, 2001). Retrieved January 23, 2008, from http://www.brettscaife.net/statistics/introstat/index.html

Isern, D., & Moreno, A. (2008). Computer-Based Execution of Clinical Guidelines: A Review. *International Journal of Medical Informatics*, *77*(12), 787–808. doi:10.1016/j.ijmedinf.2008.05.010

Isern, D., Sánchez, D., & Moreno, A. (2007). An ontology-driven agent-based clinical guideline execution engine. In R. Bellazzi, A. Abu-Hanna, & J. Hunter (Eds.), *Proc. of the 11th Conference on Artificial Intelligence in Medicine, AIME 2007* (pp. 49-53). Amsterdam, The Netherlands.

Janson, S., Merkle, D., & Middendorf, M. (2008). Molecular docking with multi-objective Particle Swarm Optimization. *Applied Soft Computing*, *8*(1), 666–675. doi:10.1016/j.asoc.2007.05.005

Jantachume, W. (1999). (1 ed.). Khon kaen: Faculty of Nursing, Khon kaen University, Thailand. Keogh, E., Lin, J., & Fu, A. *Datasets*. Retrieved January 31, 2008, from http://www.cs.ucr.edu/~eamonn/discords/

Jin, X., Srinivasan, D., & Cheu, R. L. (2001). Classification of Freeway Traffic Patterns for Incident Detection Using Constructive Probabilistic Neural Networks. *IEEE Transactions on Neural Networks*, *12*(5), 1173–1187. doi:10.1109/72.950145

Karabatak, M., & Ince, M. C. (2008). An expert system for detection of breast caner based on association rules and neural network. *Expert System with Applcations*. Elsevier.

Kavi, K., Kung, D. C., Bhambhani, H., & Pancholi, G. & Kanikarla. M. (2003). Extending UML for Modeling and Design of MultiAgent Systems. *Proceedings of the 2nd International Workshop on Software Engineering for Large-Scale Multi-Agent Systems (SELMAS2003), held in conjunction with the International Conference on Software Engineering*, USA.

Kim, J., & Park, J. (2004). BioIE: Retargetable information extraction and ontological annotation of biological interactions from the literature. *Journal of Bioinformatics and Computational Biology*, *2*(3), 551–568. doi:10.1142/S0219720004000739

Kopacek, P. (2002). Demining robots: A tool for international stability. *15th Triennial World Congress IFAC, 2002*. (pp. 1–5). Barcelona, Spain.

Kumar, S., & Berl, T. (1999). Chapter 1: Diseases of Water Metabolism. *Atlas of Diseases of the Kidney, 1,* 1–22. Philadelphia, PA: Current Medicine, Inc.

Kuo, P. C., Schroeder, R. A., Mahaffey, S., & Bollinger, R. R. (2003, December). Optimization of operating room allocation using linear programming techniques. *Journal of the American College of Surgeons, 197*(6), 889–895. doi:10.1016/j.jamcollsurg.2003.07.006

Kuwabara, K., Ishida, T., & Osato, N. (1995). AgenTalk: Describing Multiagent Coordination Protocols with Inheritance. *Proc. 7th IEEE International Conference on Tools with Artificial Intelligence (ICTAI '95)* (pp. 460-465).

Laing, W., & Buisson, C. (2001). *Private Medical Insurance: UK market sector report 2001.* London: Laing & Buisson.

Lanner Group, Inc. (2008). Retrieved Nov. 20, 2008, From www.lanner.com.

Lanzola, G., Gatti, L., Falasconi, S., & Stefanelli, M. (1999). A Framework for Building Cooperative Software Agents in medical applications. [Elsevier]. *Artificial Intelligence in Medicine, 16*(3), 223–249. doi:10.1016/S0933-3657(99)00008-1

Law, A. M. (2007). *Simulation modeling and analysis* (4th Edition) McGraw-Hill.

Lenz, R., Blaser, R., Beyer, M., Heger, O., Biber, C., & Bäumlein, M. (2007). IT support for clinical pathways - Lessons learned. *International Journal of Medical Informatics, 76*(S3), 397–402. doi:10.1016/j.ijmedinf.2007.04.012

Leonard, M. (1983). Elicitation of Honest Preferences for the Assignment of Individuals to Positions. *The Journal of Political Economy, 91*(3), 461–479. doi:10.1086/261158

Leong, T.-Y., Kaiser, K., & Miksch, S. (2007). Free and Open Source Enabling Technologies for Patient-Centric, Guideline-Based Clinical Decision Support: A Survey. *IMIA Yearbook of Medical Informatics . Methods of Information in Medicine, 46*(Suppl. 1), 74–86.

Lesser, V., Decker, K., Wagner, T., Carver, N., Garvey, A., Horling, B., Neiman, D., & Podorozhny, R., NagendraPrasad, M., Raja, A., Vincent, R., Xuan, P., & Zhang, X.Q. (2004). Evolution of t he GPGP/TAEMS Domain- Independent Coordination Framework. *Au-*

tonomous Agents and Multi-Agent Systems, 9(1), 87–143. doi:10.1023/B:AGNT.0000019690.28073.04

Levin, S., Aronsky, D., Hemphill, R., Han, J., Slagle, J., & France, D. (2007). Shifting toward balance: Measuring the distribution of workload among emergency physician teams. *Annals of Emergency Medicine, 50*(4), 419–423. doi:10.1016/j.annemergmed.2007.04.007

Lewis, S., & Donaldson, C. (2001). The future of healthcare in Canada. *BMJ (Clinical Research Ed.), 323,* 926–929. doi:10.1136/bmj.323.7318.926

Li, M., & Istepanian, R. S. H. (2003). 3G Network Oriented Mobile Agents for Intelligent Diabetes Management: A conceptual Model. *Information Technology Applications in Biomedicine* (pp. 31-34).

Li, Y. C., Liu, L., Chiu, W. T., & Jian, W. S. (2000). Neural Network modeling for surgical decisions on traumatic brain injury patients. *International Journal of Medical Informatics,* (57): 1–9. doi:10.1016/S1386-5056(99)00054-4

Liu, J., Juo, S. H., Dewan, A., Grunn, A., Tong, X., & Brito, M. (2003). Evidence for a putative bipolar disorder locus on 2p13-16 and other potential loci on 4q31, 7q34, 8q13, 9q31, 10q21-24, 13q32, 14q21 and 17q11-12. *Molecular Psychiatry, 8*(3), 333–342. doi:10.1038/sj.mp.4001254

Liu, Q. (2002). *Master Degree Thesis: A Mobile Agent System for Distributed Mammography Image Retrieval.* Regina, Saskatchewan, Canada: University of Regina.

Lopez, A. D., & Murray, C. C. J. L. (1998). The Global Burden of Disease, 1990-2020. *Nature Medicine, 4,* 1241–1243. doi:10.1038/3218

Lowery, J. C., Hakes, B., Lilegdon, W. R., Keller, L., Mabrouk, K., & McGuire, F. (1994). Barriers to Implementing Simulation in Health Care. *Proceedings of Winter Simulation Conference* (pp. 868-875).

Luck, M., & d'Inverno, M. (1995). A Formal Framework for Agency and Autonomy. *Proceedings of the First International Conference on Multi-Agent Systems (ICMAS-95)* (pp. 254-260). AAAI Press/ MIT Press.

Maedche, A. D. (2003). *Ontology Learning for the Semantic Web.* Norwell, Massachusetts, Kluwer Academic Publishers.

Mago, V. K., & Devi, M. S. (2007). A Multi-Agent Medical System for Indian Rural Infant and Child Care. In

M.M. Veloso (Ed.), *IJCAI -07, The 20th International Joint Conference on Artificial Intelligence*. Menlo Park, California, USA: AAAI press

Mago, V. K., Devi, M. S., & Mehta, R. (2007). Decision Making System Based on Bayesian Network for an Agent Diagnosing Child Care Diseases. In D. Riaño (Ed.), *Knowledge Management for Health Care Procedures, From Knowledge to Global Care, AIME 2007 Workshop K4CARE 2007*, (pp. 127-136) *Lecture Notes in Computer Science*. Berlin Heidelberg: Springer-Verlag.

Mahapatra, S., Koelling, C. P., Patvivatsiri, L., Fraticelli, B., Eitel, D., & Grove, L. (2003). Pairing Emergency Severity Index 5-level Triage Data with Computer aided System Design to Improve Emergency Department Access and Throughput. *Proceedings of the 2003 Winter Simulation Conference* (pp. 1917-1925).

Makroglou, A., Li, J., & Kuang, Y. (2005). Mathematical Models and Software Tools for the Glucose-Insulin Regulatory System and Diabetes: An Overview. [Elsevier.]. *Applied Numerical Mathematics, 56*, 559–573. doi:10.1016/j.apnum.2005.04.023

Mao, K. Z., Tan, K. C., & Ser, W. (2000). Probabilistic Neural-Network Structure Determination for Pattern Classification. *IEEE Transactions on Neural Networks, 11*(4), 1009–1016. doi:10.1109/72.857781

Maria, D. B. A., Silva, V. T., & Lucena, C. J. P. (2005). Developing Multi-Agent Systems Based on MDA. *Proceedings of the 17th Conference on Advanced Information Systems Engineering (CAiSE'05)*. Porto, Portugal.

Marshall, A., Vasilakis, C., & El-Darzi, E. (2005). Length of Stay-Based Patient Flow Models: Recent Developments and Future Directions. [Springer Science+Business Media, Inc.]. *Health Care Management Science, 8*, 213–220. doi:10.1007/s10729-005-2012-z

Martens, R., Hu, W., Liu, A., Mahovsky, J., Saenchai, K., Schauenberg, T., et al. (2001). *TEEMA TRLabs Execution Environment for Mobile Agents*. Regina: Telecommunication Research and Laboratories (TRLabs) Regina.

Martin, R. M., & Sterne, J. A. C. (2003). NHS waiting lists and evidence of national or local failure: analysis of health service data. *BMJ (Clinical Research Ed.), 326*, 188–192. doi:10.1136/bmj.326.7382.188

Martin, R., Sterne, J. A. C., & Gunnel, D. (2003, January). NHS waiting lists and evidence of national or local failure: analysis of health service data. *BMJ (Clinical Research Ed.), 326*, 188. doi:10.1136/bmj.326.7382.188

McGuinness, D., & van Harmelen, F. (2004). *OWL Web Ontology Language*. Retrieved August 24, 2008, from http://www.w3.org/TR/owl-features/.

Merelli, E., Culmone, R., & Mariani, L. (2002). BioAgent - A mobile agent system for bioscientists. *Proceedings of the Network Tools and Applications in Biology Workshop Agents in Bioinformatics*, Italy.

Mersmann, S., & Dojat, M. (2004). SmartCareTM - Automated Clinical Guidelines in Critical Care. In R. L. de Mántaras & L. Saitta (Eds.), *Proc. of the 16th European Conference on Artificial Intelligence, ECAI 2004* (pp. 745-749). València, Spain.

Mes, M., Heijden, M., & Harten, A. (2007). Comparison of agent-based scheduling to look-ahead heuristics for real-time transportation problems. *European Journal of Operational Research, 181*, 59–75. doi:10.1016/j.ejor.2006.02.051

Michie, S., & Johnston, M. (2004). Changing clinical behaviour by making guidelines specific. *British Medical Journal, 328*, 343–345. doi:10.1136/bmj.328.7435.343

Miksch, S., Shahar, Y., & Johnson, P. (1997). Asbru: A Task-Specific, Intention-Based, and Time-Oriented Language for Representing Skeletal Plans. In E. Motta, F. V. Harmelen, C. Pierret-Golbreich, I. Filby & N. Wijngaards (Eds.), *Proc. of the 7th Workshop on Knowledge Engineering: Methods & Languages, KEML-97* (pp. 1-20). Milton Keynes, UK.

Milgrom, P. (1985). The Economics of Competitive Bidding: a Selective Survey. In L. Hurwicz, D. Schmeidler, & H. Sonnenschein (Eds.), *Social Goals and Social Organization: Essays in Memory of Elisha Panzer*.

Milgrom, P., & Roberts, J. (n.d.). *Economics, Organization and Management*. Englewood Cliffs, NJ: Prentice Hall.

Miller, M. J., Ferrin, D. M., & Messer, M. G. (2004). Fixing the Emergency Department: A Transformational Journey with EDSIM. *Proceedings of Winter Simulation Conference* (pp. 1988-1993).

Milne, F., Redman, C., Walker, J., Baker, P., Bradley, J., & Cooper, C. (2005). The pre-eclampsia community guideline (PRECOG): how to screen for and detect onset of pre-eclampsia in the community. *British Medical Journal, 330*, 576–580. doi:10.1136/bmj.330.7491.576

Mirkin, B. (2005). *Clustering for Data Mining: A Data Recovery Approach* (1ˢᵗ ed.). London: Chapman & Hall/ CRC. *Monitoring asthma symptoms*. Retrieved July 4, 2007, from http://chealth.canoe.ca/channel_section_details.asp?text_id=3405&channel_id=2014&relation_id=18605

Miró, O., Sánchez, M., & Millá, J. (2004). Hospital mortality and staff workload. *Lancet, 356*(9238), 1356–1357. doi:10.1016/S0140-6736(05)74269-0

Mohan, R., Mirmirani, S. (2008, December). *An assessment of OECD health care system using panel data analysis*. OECD Health Data (2001). *A comparative analysis of 30 countries CD-ROM*. Paris: OECD and CREDES.

Mok, W. Y., Palvia, P., & Paper, D. (2006). On the computability of agent-based workflows. *Decision Support Systems, 42*, 1239–1253. doi:10.1016/j.dss.2005.10.010

Moreno, A., & Garbay, C. (2003). Editorial: Software agents in health care. [Amsterdam, The Netherlands: Elsevier.]. *Artificial Intelligence in Medicine, 27*, 229–232. doi:10.1016/S0933-3657(03)00004-6

Moreno, A., & Isern, D. (2002). A first step towards providing health-care agent-based services to mobile users. *Proceedings of the First International Joint Conference on Autonomous Agents and Multi-agent Systems* (pp. 589-590).

Moreno, A., Isern, D., & Sanchez, D. (2001). Provision of Agent-Based Healthcare Services. *Proc. of AIME 2001*.

Moreno, A., Sánchez, D., & Isern, D. (2003). Security Measures in a Medical Multi-Agent System. In I. Aguiló, L. Valverde & M. T. Escrig (Eds.), *Proc. of the Artificial Intelligence Research and Development. Proceedings of 6th Catalan Conference in Artificial Intelligence, CCIA 2003* (pp. 244-255). Palma de Mallorca, Spain.

Moreno, A., Valls, A., Isern, D., & Sanchez, D. (2006). Applying Agent Technology to Healthcare: The GruSMA Experience. [New York, NY: IEEE Press]. *IEEE Intelligent Systems, 26*(6), 63–67. doi:10.1109/MIS.2006.108

Morris, M. (2004). Overview of network survey designs. In M. Morris (Ed.), *Network epidemiology: A handbook for survey design and data collection* (pp. 8-24). London: Oxford University Press.

Morrison, B. P., & Bird, B. C. (2003). A Methodology for Modeling Front Office and Patient Care Processes in Ambulatory Health Care. *Proceedings of Winter Simulation Conference* (pp.1882-1886).

Mouratidis, H., Giorgini, P., & Manson, G. A. (2003). Modelling secure multi-agent systems, *Proceedings of the Second International Joint Conference on Autonomous Agents and Multiagent Systems* (pp. 859-866).

Muller, G., Grébaut, P., & Gouteux, J. P. (2004, January). An agent-based model of sleeping sickness: simulation trials of a forest focus in southern Cameroon. *Comptes Rendus Biologies, 327*(1), 1–11. doi:10.1016/j.crvi.2003.12.002

Mulyar, N., van der Aalst, W. M. P., & Peleg, M. (2007). A Pattern-based Analysis of Clinical Computer-interpretable Guideline Modeling Languages. *Journal of the American Medical Informatics Association, 14*(6), 781–787. doi:10.1197/jamia.M2389

Munro, B. H. (2005). *Statistical Methods for Health Care Research* (5ᵗʰ ed.). Philadelphia: Lippincott Williams & Wilkins.

NASA. (2008). *The Remote Agent Project*. Retrieved August 28, 2008, from http://ti.arc.nasa.gov/projects/remote-agent/.

NationMaster. (2009). Retrieved March 2, 2009, from http://www.nationmaster.com/encyclopedia/Pathophysiology

Nealon, J. L., & Moreno, A. (2003). Agent-Based Applications in Health Care. In J. L. Nealon & A. Moreno (Eds.), *Applications of Software Agent Technology in the Health Care Domain* (pp. 3-18). Basel, Switzerland: Birkhäuser Verlag.

Newman, M. E. J. (2002). The spread of epidemic disease on networks . *Physical Review E: Statistical, Nonlinear, and Soft Matter Physics, 66*, 016128. doi:10.1103/PhysRevE.66.016128

Nicholls, A. G., & Young, F. R. (2007). Innovative Hospital Bed Management Using Spatial Technology. *Spatial Science Queensland* (pp. 26-30)

Nielsen, J., & Landauer, T. K. (1993). A mathematical model of the finding of usability problems. *Proceedings of the INTERACT '93 and CHI '93 Conference on Human Factors in Computing Systems* (pp. 206-213). New York, NY: ACM Press.

Nutrition Data. (2006). *Glycemic Index.* Retrieved December 12, 2006 from http://www.nutritiondata.com/glycemic¬index.html

Odell, J., Van Dyke, H. P., & Bauer, B. (2001). Representing Agent Interaction Protocols in UML. In P. Ciancarini, & M. Wooldridge (Ed.), *Agent-Oriented Software Engineering* (pp. 121-140). Springer-Verlag.

Omron, H. *J-720ITC Pocket Pedometer with Advanced Omron Health Management Software.* Retrieved December 20, 2007, from http://www.amazon.com/Omron-HJ-720ITC-Pedometer-Advanced-Management/dp/B000MN92WM/ref=pd_sbs_sg_title_3

Orr, R. K. (1997). Use of a Probabilistic Neural Network to Estimate the Risk of Mortality after Cardiac Surgery. *Medical Decision Making*, (17): 178–185. doi:10.1177/0272989X9701700208

Osidach, V. Z., & Fu, M. C. (2003). Computer Simulation of a Mobile Examination Centre. *Proceedings of Winter Simulation Conference* (pp. 1868-1875).

Pacher, P., & Kecskemeti, V. (2004). Cardiovascular Side Effects of New Antidepressants and Antipsychotics: New Drugs, old Concerns? *Current Pharmaceutical Design*, *10*(20), 2463–2475. doi:10.2174/1381612043383872

Padgham, L., & Winikoff, M. (2004). *Developing Intelligent Agent Systems: A Practical Guide*: John Wiley and Sons.

Pan, J., Yung, C., Liang, C., & Lai, L. (2007). An Intelligent Homecare Emergency Service System for Elder Falling. *IFMBE Proceedings*, 424–428. doi:10.1007/978-3-540-36841-0_114

Paranjape, R. (2006, May 9-12). Macroscopic Modeling of Information Flow in an Agent-Based Electronic Health Record System. *Fifth International Workshop on Agents and Peer-to-Peer Computing(AP2PC 2006)Fifth International Joint Conference on Autonomous Agents and Multi Agent Systems (AAMAS06)*, Hakodate, Japan.

Paranjape, R., Ogrady, M., & Ghoreshi-Nejad, S. (2008, August 18–20). A neuro-surgery ward bed-allocation modeling system using software agents. *Internet and Multimedia Systems and Applications*, Kailu-Kona, Hawaii, USA.

Parzen, E. (1962). On estimation of a probability density function and mode . *Annals of Mathematical Statistics*, *33*, 1065–1076. doi:10.1214/aoms/1177704472

Patel, D., Patel, S., & Hanley, D. (1995). Object Oriented Artificial Neural Network in Decision Support Systems for Dermatological Research. *Health Informatics Journal*, (1): 56–68. doi:10.1177/146045829500100206

Pavón, J., Gómez-Sanz, J. J., & Fuentes, R. (2005). The INGENIAS Methodology and Tools. In B. Henderson-Sellers & P. Giorgini (Eds.), *Agent-Oriented Methodologies* (pp. 236-276). Idea Group.

Peleg, M., Keren, S., & Denekamp, Y. (2008). Mapping computerized clinical guidelines to electronic medical records: Knowledge-data ontological mapper (KDOM). *Journal of Biomedical Informatics*, *41*(1), 180–201. doi:10.1016/j.jbi.2007.05.003

Peleg, M., Tu, S. W., Bury, J., Ciccarese, P., Fox, J., & Greenes, R. A. (2003). Comparing Computer-Interpretable Guideline Models: A Case-Study Approach. *Journal of the American Medical Informatics Association*, *10*(1), 52–68. doi:10.1197/jamia.M1135

Piatetsky-Shapiro, G., & Tamayo, P. (2003). Microarray data mining: Facing the challenges. *SIGKDD Explorations*, *5*(2), 1–6. doi:10.1145/980972.980974

Poulopoulos, V., Gortizis, L., Bakettas, I., & Nikiforidis, G. (2006). *In Proceedings of the International Conference on Information Technology: Research and Education* (pp. 253-257). New York, NY and Piscataway, NJ: IEEE Press.

Prado, M., Roa, L., Reina-Tosina, J., Palma, A., & Milan, J. A. (2001). Virtual Center for Renal Support: Definition of a Novel Knowledge-Based Telemedicine System. *Proceedings of the 23 Annual IEEE Engineering and Medicine in Biology Society Conference* (pp. 3878-3881). New York, NY and Piscataway, NJ: IEEE Press.

Priori, S. G., Klein, W., & Bassand, J.-P. (2003). Medical Practice Guidelines: Separating science from economics. *European Heart Journal*, *24*(21), 1962–1964. doi:10.1016/S0195-668X(03)00438-X

Province of Alberta. (1994). *Regional health authorities act.* Edmonton: Queen's Printer for Alberta.

Python software foundation. (2008). Retrieved Nov. 20, 2008, From http://www.python.org/

Quaglini, S., Stefanelli, M., Cavallini, A., Micieli, G., Fassino, C., & Mossa, C. (2000). Guideline-based Careflow Systems. *Artificial Intelligence in Medicine, 20*(1), 5–22. doi:10.1016/S0933-3657(00)00050-6

Rahmandad, H., & Sterman, J. (2008). Heterogeneity and network structure in the dynamics of diffusion: Comparing agent-based and system dynamics models. *Management Science, 54*(5), 998–1014. doi:10.1287/mnsc.1070.0787

Raymond, S. A., Gordon, G. E., & Singer, D. B. (1998, July 14, 1998). *US Patent 5778882 - Health monitoring system*. Retrieved July 4, 2007, from http://www.patentstorm.us/patents/5778882/fulltext.html

Reeves, W. T. (1983). Particle systems - a technique for modeling a class of fuzzy objects. *In SIGGRAPH '83: Proceedings of the 10th annual conference on computer graphics and interactive techniques* (pp. 359–375). New York, NY: ACM Press.

Riaño, D. (2004). Time-Independent Rule-Based Guideline Execution. In R. L. de Mántaras & L. Saitta (Eds.), *Proc. of the 16th European Conference on Artificial Intelligence, ECAI 2004* (pp. 535-538). Valencia, Spain.

Riaño, D. (2007). The SDA* Model: A Set Theory Approach In P. Kokol, V. Podgorelec, M. Dušanka, M. Zorman, & M. Verlic (Eds.), *Proc. of the 20th IEEE International Symposium on Computer-Based Medical Systems, CBMS 2007* (pp. 563-568). Maribor, Slovenia.

Ricci, S., Celani, M. G., & Righetti, E. (2006). Development of clinical guidelines: methodological and practical issues. *Neurological Sciences, 27*(S3), 228–230. doi:10.1007/s10072-006-0623-x

Riley, S. (2007). Large-scale spatial-transmission models of infectious diseases . *Science, 316*, 1298–1301. doi:10.1126/science.1134695

Roberts, M. S. (1992). Markov process-based Monte Carlo simulation: a tool for modeling complex disease and its application to the timing of liver transplantation. *In WSC '92: Proceedings of the 24th conference on winter simulation* (pp. 1034–1040). New York, NY: ACM Press.

Robocup (2008). *Robocup Federation homepage*. Retrieved August 22, 2008, from http://www.robocup.org/

Robocup-rescue. (2008). *Robocup Rescue homepage*. Retrieved August 7, 2008, from http://www.rescuesystem.org/robocuprescue/

Rodríguez, M. D., Favela, J., Preciado, A., & Vizcaíno, A. (2005). Agent-based ambient intelligence for healthcare. *AI Communications, 18*, 201–216.

Roth, A. (2003). The Origins, History and Design of the Resident Match. *Journal of the American Medical Association, 289*(7), 909–912. doi:10.1001/jama.289.7.909

Rvachev, L. A., & Longini, I. M. (1985). A mathematical model for the global spread of influenza. *Mathematical Biosciences, 75*, 3–22. doi:10.1016/0025-5564(85)90064-1

Saenchai, K., Benedicenti, L., & Paranjape, R. (2004, May). The design of an architecture for software agents on mobile platforms. *Canadian Conference on Electrical and Computer Engineering* (CCECE04), *3*, 1389-92. Niagara Falls, Canada.

Saenchai, K., Benedicenti, L., & Paranjape, R. (2005, May 1-4). A Dynamic Extension of the Asynchronous Weak-Commitment Search Algorithm. *Canadian Conference on Electrical and Computer Engineering* (CCECE05), Saskatoon, Canada (pp. 1112-1115).

Saenchai, K., Benedicenti, L., & Paranjape, R. (2006). Solving Dynamic Distributed Constraint Satisfaction Problems with a Modified Weak-Commitment Search Algorithm. *Lecture Notes in Computer Science, 3910*, 130–137. doi:10.1007/11734697_10

Sakane, A., Tsuji, T., Yoshiyuki Tanaka, Y., Shiba, K., Saeki, N., & Masashi Kawamoto, M. (2004). Realtime Monitoring of Vascular Conditions Using a Probabilistic Neural Network. *Lecture Notes in Computer Science*, 488–493.

Sandholm, T. (1996). Limitations of the Vickrey Auction in Computational MultiagenSystems. *Proceedings of the International Joint Conference on Artificial Intelligence(IJCAI)*.

Sandholm, T., & Lesser, V. (1997). Coalitions among Computationally Bounded Agents. [Special issue on Economic Principles of Multiagent Systems.]. *Artificial Intelligence, 94*(1), 99–137. doi:10.1016/S0004-3702(97)00030-1

Santana, P., Barata, J., Cruz, H., Mestre, A., Lisboa, J., & Flores, L. (2005, September). A Multi-Robot System for Landmine Detection. *Emerging Technologies and Factory Automation, 2005. ETFA 2005. 10th IEEE Conference on, 1*, 721-728.

Scalem, M., Bandyopadhyay, S., & Sircar, A. (2004, October). An approach towards a decentralised Disaster Management Information Network. *Lecture Notes on Computer Science, Springer Publications, 3285, AACC2004.*

Schaerf, A. (1999). A Survey of Automated Timetabling. *Artificial Intelligence Review*, 87–127. doi:10.1023/A:1006576209967

Schmickl, T., Thenius, R., & Crailsheim, K. (2005). Simulating swarm intelligence in honey bees: foraging in differently fluctuating environments. *In GECCO '05: Proceedings of the 2005 conference on genetic and evolutionary computation* (pp. 273–274). New York, NY: ACM Press.

Schumaker, J. F. (1992). *Religion and Mental Health.* Oxford University Press.

Sestito, S., & Dillon, T. S. (1994). *Automated knowledge acquisition.* Sydney: Prentice Hall of Australia.

Seyfang, A., Miksch, S., Marcos, M., Wittenberg, J., Polo-Conde, C., & Rosenbrand, K. (2006). Bridging the Gap between Informal and Formal Guideline Representations. In G. Brewka, S. Coradeschi, A. Perini & P. Traverso (Eds.), *Proc. of the 17th European Conference on Artificial Intelligence* (pp. 447–451). Riva del Garda, Italy.

Shaalana, K., ElBadryb, M., & Rafea, A. (2004). A multiagent approach for diagnostic expert systems via the internet. *Expert Systems with Applications, 27*, 1–10. doi:10.1016/j.eswa.2003.12.018

Shahar, Y., Young, O., Shalom, E., Galperin, M., Mayaffit, A., & Moskovitch, R. (2004). A Framework for a Distributed, Hybrid, Multiple-Ontology Clinical-Guideline Library and Automated Guideline-Support Tools. *Journal of Biomedical Informatics, 37*(5), 325–344. doi:10.1016/j.jbi.2004.07.001

Shahar, Y., Young, O., Shalon, E., Mayaffit, A., Moskovitch, R., Hessing, A., et al. (2003). DEGEL: A Hybrid, Multiple-Ontology Framework for Specification and Retrieval of Clinical Guidelines. In M. Dojat, E. Ker-

avnou & P. Barahona (Eds.), *Proc. of the 9th Conference on Artificial Intelligence in Medicine in Europe, AIME 2003* (pp. 122-131). Protaras, Cyprus.

Sibbel, R., & Christoph, U. (2001). *Agent-Based Modeling and Simulation for Hospital Management.* Retrieved Nov. 20, 2008, From http://cuong.tgs.vn/ebook/Agent-Based. Modeling.and.Simulation.for. Hospital.Management. pdf.

Siciliani, L., & Hurst, J. (2003). *Explaining waiting times variations for elective surgery across OECD countries.*

Sidhu, A. S., Dillon, T. S., & Chang, E. (2006). Integration of Protein Data Sources through PO. *Proceedings of the 17th International Conference on Database and Expert Systems Applications* (DEXA 2006) (pp. 519-527).

Sinreich, D., & Marmor, Y. N. (2004). A Simple and Intuitive Simulation Tool for Analyzing Emergency Department Operations. *Proceedings of Winter Simulation Conference* (pp.1994-2002).

Sklar, E., Davies, M., & Co, M. S. T. (2004). SimEd: Simulating Education as a Multi Agent System. *In AAMAS '04: Proceedings of the Third International Joint Conference on Autonomous Agents and Multiagent Systems* (pp. 998-1005). New York, NY: ACM Press.

Smith, B. (2006). From concepts to clinical reality: An essay on the benchmarking of biomedical terminologies. *Journal of Biomedical Informatics, 39*, 288–298. doi:10.1016/j.jbi.2005.09.005

Smith, D. G., Ebrahim, S., Lewis, S., Hansell, A. L., Palmer, L. J., & Burton, P. R. (2005). Genetic epidemiology and public health: hope, hype, and future prospects. *Lancet, 366*(9495), 1484–1498. doi:10.1016/S0140-6736(05)67601-5

Snijders, T. A. B., Steglich, C. E. G., & Schweinberger, M. (2007). Modeling the co-evolution of networks and behavior. In K. van Montfort, H. Oud, & A. Satorra (Eds.), *Longitudinal models in the behavioral and related sciences* (pp. 41-71). Mahwah, NJ: Lawrence Erlbaum.

Song, T., Jamshidi, M. M., Lee Roland, R., & Mingxiong, H. (2007). A Modified Probabilistic Neural Network for Partial Volume Segmentation in Brain MR Image. *IEEE Transactions on Neural Networks, 18*(5). doi:10.1109/TNN.2007.891635

Soto, J. P., Vizcaino, A., Portillo, J., & Piattini, M. (2006). Modelling a Knowledge Management System Architecture with INGENIAS Methodology*of the 15th International Conference on Computing (CIC 2006)* (pp. 167-173). Mexico City, Mexico.

Specht[1], D.F. (1990). *Probabilistic* neural networks Source. *Neural Networks, 3*(1), 109-118.

Specht[2], D.F. (1990). Probabilistic neural networks and the polynomial Adaline ascomplementary techniques for classification. *Neural Networks, IEEE Transactions on Neural Networks, 1*(1). 111-121.

Srinivasan, P., Mitchell, J., Bodenreider, O., Pant, G., & Menczer, F. (2002). Web Crawling Agents for Retrieving Biomedical Information. *Proceedings of International Workshop on Agents in Bioinformatics,* Italy.

Statistics Canada, Estimates of Population, Canada, the Provinces and Territories (Persons), CANSIM Table No. 051-0001, Ottawa.

Sterman, J. (2000). Business Dynamics. Systems Thinking and Modeling for a Complex World. Irwin/McGraw-Hill, New York.

Sulaiman, R., Sharma, D., Ma, W., & Tran, D. (2007). A Multi-Agent Security Framework for e-Health Services. *Knowledge-Based Intelligent Information and Engineering Systems and the XVII Italian Workshop on Neural Networks on Proceedings of the 11th International Conference, 4693,* 547-554. Berlin/Heidelberg: Springer.

Sutton, D. R., & Fox, J. (2003). The syntax and semantics of the PROforma guideline modeling language. *Journal of the American Medical Informatics Association, 10*(5), 433–443. doi:10.1197/jamia.M1264

Takakuwa, S., & Shiozaki, H. (2004). Functional Analysis for Operating Emergency Department of a General Hospital. *Proceedings of Winter Simulation Conference* (pp. 2003-2011).

Tang, Z., Johnson, T., Tindall, D., & J. Zhang (2006). Applying heuristic evaluation to improve the usability of a telemedicine system. *Telemedicine and e-Health, 12*(1), 24-34.

Tarapornsin, V., Ray, P., & Chowdhury, A. (2006). Mobile Software Agents for the Support of Chronic Illness: A Case Study in Diabetes Management for Rural Areas. *e-Health Networking, Applications and Services; 2006 HealthCom 2008. 10th International Conference* (17-19, 72-77)

ten Teije, A., Marcos, M., Balser, M., van Croonenborg, J., Duelli, C., & van Harmelen, F. (2006). Improving medical protocols by formal methods. *Artificial Intelligence in Medicine, 36*(3), 193–272. doi:10.1016/j.artmed.2005.10.006

Terenziani, P., Montani, S., Bottrighi, A., Molino, G., & Torchio, M. (2005). Clinical Guidelines Adaptation: Managing Authoring and Versioning Issues. In S. Miksch, J. Hunter, & E. Keravnou (Eds.), *Proc. of the 10th Conference on Artificial Intelligence in Medicine, AIME 2005* (pp. 151-155). Aberdeen, Scotland.

Terenziani, P., Montani, S., Bottrighi, A., Torchio, M., Molino, G., & Correndo, G. (2004). The GLARE Approach to Clinical Guidelines: Main Features. In K. Kaiser, S. Miksch, & S. W. Tu (Eds.), *Proc. of the Symposium on Computerized Guidelines and Protocols, CGP 2004* (pp. 162-166). Viena, AU.

Teweldemedhin, E., Marwala, T., & Mueller, C. (2004). Agent based modelling: A case study in HIV epidemic. *Proceedings of the 4th International Conference on Hybrid Intelligent Systems (HIS'04)* (pp. 154–159). Washington, DC, USA: IEEE Computer Society.

The six dimensional wellness model. Retrieved May 29, 2007, from http://www.nationalwellness.org/index.php?id=391&id_tier=381

Thomas, S. R., Layton, A. T., Layton, H. E., & Moore, L. C. (2006). Kidney Modeling: Status and Perspectives. *Proceedings of the IEEE, 94*(4), 740–752. doi:10.1109/JPROC.2006.871770

Tian, B., Azimi-Sadjadi, M. R., & Haar, T.H.V., B., & Reinke, D. (2000). Temporal Updating Scheme for Probabilistic Neural Network with Application to Satellite Cloud Classification. *IEEE Transactions on Neural Networks, 11*(4), 903–920. doi:10.1109/72.857771

Tian, J., & Tianfield, H. (2003). A Multi-agent Approach to the Design of an E-medicine System, *Multiagent system technologies, 2831,* 85-94. Berlin/Heidelberg: Springer.

Tse, B., & Paranjape, R. (2005, May 1-4). Mathematical Analysis of Agent Swarm Behavior in an Agent-Based Electronic Health Record System. *Canadian Conference on Electrical and Computer Engineering*, Saskatoon, (CCECE05) (pp. 996–1001), Saskatoon, Canada.

Tse, B., & Paranjape, R. (2007). Macroscopic Modeling of Information Flow in an Agent-Based Electronic Health Record System. In H. Lin (Ed), *Architectural Design of Multi-Agent Systems: Technologies and Techniques* (pp. 305-334). Information Science Reference.

Tse, B., Paranjape, R., & Joseph, S. (2008). Information Flow Analysis in Autonomous Agent and Peer-to-Peer Systems for Self-Organizing Electronic Health Records. In J.S.R.H., Despotovic, G. Moro, & S. Bergamaschi (Eds.), *Agents and Peer to Peer Computing, Lecture Notes in Artificial Intelligence, 4461*, 1-20.

Tu, S. W., & Glasgow, J. (2006). *The SAGE Guideline Model Technical Specification* (Research report No. SMI-2006-1243). Stanford, CA: Stanford Medical Informatics.

Tu, S. W., & Musen, M. A. (2001). Modeling Data and Knowledge in the EON Guideline Architecture. In V. Patel, R. Rogers & R. Haux (Eds.), *Proc. of the 10th Triennial Congress of the International Medical Informatics Association, MEDINFO 2001* (pp. 280-284). London, UK.

Tu, S. W., Campbell, J. R., & Musen, M. A. (2004). SAGE Guideline Modeling: Motivation and Methodology. In K. Kaiser, S. Miksch & S. W. Tu (Eds.), *Proc. of the Symposium on Computerized Guidelines and Protocols, CGP 2004* (pp. 167-171). Prague, Czech Republic.

Tu, S. W., Campbell, J. R., Glasgow, J., Nyman, M. A., McClure, R., & McClay, J. (2007). The SAGE Guideline Model: Achievements and Overview. *Journal of the American Medical Informatics Association, 14*(5), 589–598. doi:10.1197/jamia.M2399

Turner, K. M. E., Adams, E. J., Gay, N., Ghani, A. C., Mercer, C., & Edmunds, W. J. (2006). Developing a realistic sexual network model of chlamydia transmission in Britain. *Theoretical Biology & Medical Modelling, 3*(3), 1–11.

Ulieru, M. (2003). Internet-enabled soft computing holarchies for e-Health applications. *New Directions in Enhancing the Power of the Internet* (pp. 131-166).

University of Virginia Health System. (2006). *Diabetes and High Blood Pressure*. Retrieved December 12, 2006 from http://www.healthsystem.virginia.edu/uvahealth/ adult_diabetes/hbp.cfm

Vahabzadeh, M., Jia-Ling, L., Epstein, D. H., Mezghanni, M., Schmittner, J., & Preston, K. L. (2007). Computerized contingency management for motivating behavior change: automated tracking and dynamic reward reinforcement management computer-based medical systems. CBMS '07. Twentieth IEEE International Symposium on June 20–22. Pages: 85-90. Digital Object Identifier 10.1109/CBMS.2007.35

Vartziotis, F., Fotiadis, D. I., Likas, A., & Lagaris, I. E. (2003). A Portable Decision making tool for Health Professionals based on neural networks. *Health Informatics Journal*, (9): 273–282. doi:10.1177/1460458203094005

Vicari, R. M., Flores, C. D., Silvestre, A. M., Seixas, L. J., Ladeira, M., & Coelho, H. (2003). A multi-agent intelligent environment for medical knowledge. *Artificial Intelligence in Medicine, 27*(3), 335–366. doi:10.1016/S0933-3657(03)00009-5

Vincent, R., Horling, B., & Lesser, V. (2001). An Agent Infrastructure to Build and Evaluate Multi-Agent Systems: The Java Agent Framework and Multi-Agent System Simulator. *Lecture Notes in Artificial Intelligence: Infrastructure for Agents, Multi-Agent Systems and Scalable Multi-Agent Systems, 1887*.

Vivian, A., Venky, S., & Zhu, Y. Y. (2001). A Multi-agent Healthcare System-An Example for Diabetes Management. [Aquila, Italy.]. *Proceedings of IEEE Healthcom, 2001*, L.

Wagner, T., & Lesser, V. (2002). Evolving Real-Time Local Agent Control for Large-Scale MAS. In J.J. Meyer & M. Tambe (Eds.), *Intelligent Agents VIII (Proceedings of ATAL-01), Lecture Notes in Artificial Intelligence*. Springer-Verlag, Berlin.

Wagner, T., Garvey, A., & Lesser, V. R. (1997). Complex Goal Criteria and its Application in Design-to-Criteria Scheduling. *Proceedings of the Fourteenth National Conference on Artificial Intelligence*.

Walker, G. A. (2002). *Common Statistical Methods for Clinical Research with SAS® Examples* (2nd ed.). Cary, North Carolina, USA: Institute Inc.

Wang, D., & Shortliffe, E. H. (2002). GLEE – A Model-Driven Execution System for Computer-Based Implementation of Clinical Practice Guidelines. In AMIA (Ed.), *Proc. of the American Medical Informatics Association*

Annual Symposium, AMIA 2002 (pp. 855-859). San Antonio, TX, USA.

Wang, D., Nagalingam, S. V., & Lin, G. C. I. (2007). Development of an agent-based Virtual CIM architecture for small to medium manufacturers. *Robotics and Computer-integrated Manufacturing, 23*, 1–16. doi:10.1016/j.rcim.2005.09.001

Wang, D., Peleg, M., Tu, S. W., Boxwala, A. A., Ogunyemi, O., & Zeng, Q. (2004). Design and Implementation of the GLIF3 Guideline Execution Engine. *Journal of Biomedical Informatics, 37*(5), 305–318. doi:10.1016/j.jbi.2004.06.002

Wang, D., Peleg, M., Tu, S. W., Shortliffe, E., & Greenes, R. A. (2001). Representation of Clinical Practice Guidelines for Computer-Based Implementations. In V. Patel, R. Rogers & R. Haux (Eds.), *Proc. of the 10th Triennial Congress of the International Medical Informatics Association, MEDINFO 2001* (pp. 285-289). London, UK.

Wang, S., Xi, L., & Zhou, B. (2008). FBS-enhanced agent-based dynamic scheduling in FMS. *Engineering Applications of Artificial Intelligence, 21*, 644–657. doi:10.1016/j.engappai.2007.05.012

Watts, D. (1999). *Small worlds*. Princeton, NJ: Princeton University Press.

Web, M. D. (2006). *Heart Disease Health Center*. Retrieved December 12, 2006 from http://www.webmd.com/hw/heart_disease/hw233473.asp

Webopedia (2009). Retrieved February 10, 2009, from http://www.webopedia.com/DidYouKnow/Computer_Science/2005/rfid.asp

Weiss, G. (1999). *Multiagent Systems: A Modern Approach to Distributed Artificial Intelligence*. The MIT Press.

Weng, M. X., Wu, Z., Qi, G., & Zheng, L. (2008). Multiagent-based workload control for make-to-order manufacturing. *International Journal of Production Research, 46*(8), 2197–2213. doi:10.1080/00207540600969758

Wenner, M. (2008). Infected with Insanity: Could Microbes Cause Mental Illness? *Scientific American*. Retrieved from http://www.sciam.com/article.cfm?id=infected-with-insanity.

Werneke, U., Northey, S., & Bhugra, D. (2006). Antidepressants and sexual dysfunction. *Acta Psychiatrica Scandinavica, 114*(6), 384–397. doi:10.1111/j.1600-0447.2006.00890.x

What is wellness. Retrieved June 12, 2007, from http://www.hooah4health.com/overview/wellness.htm

Wheaton, W. D., Allpress, J. L., Chasteen, B. M., Cajka, J. C., Wagener, D. K., Cooley, P. C., & Roberts, D. J. (2006). *Nationwide geographically-explicit synthetic populations using public use microdata*. Presented at Congress of Epidemiology, Seattle, WA, June 21–24, 2006.

WHO. (2008). Core Health Indicators the latest data from multiple WHO sources. *WHO Statistical Information System (WHOSIS)*. Retrieved September 8, 2008, from http://www.who.int/whosis/database/core/core_select_process.cfm?country=cai&indicators=healthpersonnel

WHO. (2008). Primary Health Care – Now More Than Ever. The *World Health Report* (p. 82). Retrieved Nov. 20, 2008, from http://www.who.int/whr/2008/en/index.html

Wilczynski, N. L., Haynes, R. B., & Hedges, T. (2006). Optimal search strategies for identifying mental health content in MEDLINE: an analytic survey. *Annals of General Psychiatry, 5*.

Williamson, M., Decker, K. S., & Sycara, K. (1996). Unified information and control flow in hierarchical task networks. *Proceeding of the AAAI-96 workshop on Theories of Planning, Action and Control*.

Wooldridge, M. (2002). *An Introduction to Multiagent Systems*. Chichester, England: John Wiley & Sons

Wooldridge, M., & Jennings, N. (1995). Intelligent agents: theory and practice. *The Knowledge Engineering Review, 10*(2), 115–152. doi:10.1017/S0269888900008122

Wooldridge, M., Jennings, N., & Kinny, D. (2000). The Gaia Methodology for Agent-Oriented Analysis and Design. *Journal of Autonomous Agents and Multi-Agent Systems, 3*, 285–312. doi:10.1023/A:1010071910869

Wu, Hsin-I. (2005). *A Case Study of Type 2 Diabetes Self-Management*. Retrieved January 22, 2005 from http://www.biomedical-engineering-online.com/

Wyatt, J. C., & Sullivan, F. (2007). eHealth and the future: promise or peril? *British Medical Journal, 331*, 1391–1393. doi:10.1136/bmj.331.7529.1391

Xiang, W., & Lee, H. P. (2008). Ant colony intelligence in multi-agent dynamic manufacturing scheduling. *Engineering Applications of Artificial Intelligence, 21*, 73–85. doi:10.1016/j.engappai.2007.03.008

Xu, H., & Zhang, X. (2005). A Methodology for Role-Based Modeling of Open Multi-Agent Software Systems. *ICEIS, (3),* 246–253.

Xu, H., Zhang, X., & Patel, R. J. (2007). Developing Role-Based Open Multi-Agent Software Systems. [IJCITP]. *International Journal of Computational Intelligence Theory and Practice, 2*(1), 39–56.

Yang, Y. Paranjape, R., & Benedicenti, L. (2004). An Examination of Mobile Agents System Evolution in the Course-Scheduling Problem. *Proceedings of the 2004 IEEE Canadian Conference on Electrical and Computer Engineering* (pp 5782-5785)

Yang, Y., Paranjape, R., & Benedicenti, L. (2006). A Hierarchical Multi Agent Architecture For The University Course Timetabling Problem. *Autonomous Agents and Multi-Agent Systems (AAMAS05),* Hokodate, Japan.

Yang, Y., Paranjape, R., Benedicenti, L., & Reed, N. (2005, December). A Mobile Agent System for University Course Timetabling. *Proceedings of the Second Indian International Conference on Artificial Intelligence* (IICAI 2005) (pp. 2926-2937), Pune, India.

Yang, Y., Paranjape, R., Benedicenti, L., & Reed, N. (2006). A System Model for University Course Scheduling using Mobile Agents. *Multiagent and Grid Systems -. International Journal (Toronto, Ont.), 2*(3), 267–275.

Yergens, D., Hiner, J., Denzinger, J., & Noseworthy, T. (2006a). IDESS - A Multi Agent Based Simulation System for Rapid Development of Infectious Disease Models. [ITSSA]. *International Transactions on Systems Science and Applications, 1*(1), 51–58.

Yergens, D., Noseworthy, T., Hamilton, D., & Denzinger, J. (2006b, May). Agent Based Simulation combined with Real-Time Remote Surveillance for Disaster Response Management. *5th International Joint Conference on Autonomous Agents and Multi-Agent Systems, (Workshop on Agent Technology for Disaster Management),* Hakodate, Japan.

Yoon, J. S., & Maher, M. L. (2005). A swarm algorithm for wayfinding in dynamic virtual worlds. *In VRST '05: Proceedings of the ACM symposium on virtual reality software and technology* (pp. 113–116). New York, NY: ACM Press.

Young, O., & Shahar, Y. (2005). The Spock System: Developing a Runtime Application Engine for Hybrid-Asbru Guidelines. In S. Miksch, J. Hunter, & E. Keravnou (Eds.), *Proc. of the 10th Conference on Artificial Intelligence in Medicine, AIME 2005* (pp. 166-170). Aberdeen, Scotland.

Young, O., Shahar, Y., Liel, Y., Lunenfeld, E., Bar, G., & Shalom, E. (2007). Runtime application of Hybrid-Asbru clinical guidelines. *Journal of Biomedical Informatics, 40*, 507–526. doi:10.1016/j.jbi.2006.12.004

Yu, S. N., & Chou, K. T. (2008). Integration of independent component analysis and neural networks for ECG beat classification. *Expert Systems with Applications, (34)*: 2841–2846. doi:10.1016/j.eswa.2007.05.006

Zafar, K., Qazi, S. B., & Baig, A. R. (2006). Mine detection and route planning in military warfare using multi agent system. *In COMPSAC '06: Proceedings 30th annual international computer software and applications conference* (pp. 327-332). Los Alamitos, CA: IEEE Computer Society Press.

Zambonelli, F., Jennings, N. R., & Wooldridge, M. (2003). Developing Multiagent Systems: The Gaia Methodology. *ACM Transactions on Software Engineering and Methodology, 12*(3), 317–370. doi:10.1145/958961.958963

Zhang, D. Z., Anosike, A., & Lim, M. K. (2007). Dynamically Integrated Manufacturing Systems (DIMS) - A Multiagent Approach. *IEEE Transactions on Systems, Man, and Cybernetics. Part A, Systems and Humans, 37*(5), 824–850. doi:10.1109/TSMCA.2007.897710

Zhang, W. J., & Xie, S. Q. (2007). Agent technology for collaborative process planning: a review. *International Journal of Advanced Manufacturing Technology, 32*, 315–325. doi:10.1007/s00170-005-0345-x

Zhang, X., & Xu, H. (2006) Towards Automated Development of Multi-Agent Systems Using RADE. *Proceedings of the 2006 International Conference on Artificial Intelligence (ICAI'06)* (pp. 44-50). Las Vegas, Nevada.

Zhang, X., Xu, H., & Shrestha, B. (2007). An Integrated Role-Based Approach for Modeling, Designing and Implementing Multi-Agent Systems. *Journal of the Brazilian Computer Society (JCBS) . Special Issue on*

Software Engineering for Multi-Agent Systems, 13(2), 45–60.

Zule, W. A., & Bobashev, G. V. (in press, 2008). High dead-space syringes and the risk of HIV and HCV infection among injecting drug users. *Drug and Alcohol Dependence.*

About the Contributors

Raman B. Paranjape completed the B.Sc. (1981), M.Sc. (1984), and Ph.D (1989) degrees at the University of Alberta. His research interests are in both physical and software agent systems. Research in physical systems has focused on the development of sensor systems and new technologies in image and signal processing for real world application in robotics and automated systems for team formation using both passive and active sonar arrays. Research in software agents is focused on analysis and retrieval of medical data from distributed databases and modeling of agent and human societies. Dr. Paranjape has worked as Research Scientist, Software Engineer, Project Leader, and Project Manager in Canadian Industry. He joined the University of Regina in 1997, and is currently the Professor of Electronic Systems Engineering and Director of the Centre for Sustainable Communities.

Asha B. Sadanand completed a BSc Honors in Mathematics at the University of Alberta, Canada. She then completed an MA in Economics at the University of Alberta, Canada. She went on to do a PhD in Microeconomics at the California Institute of Technology, U.S.A. While she was at the California Institute of Technology she worked on designing market mechanisms for resource allocation and property rights. She is currently a professor of Economics at the University of Guelph. She specializes in microeconomic theory, information economics and game theory. In addition she has interested in industrial organization, experimental economics and law and economics.

* * *

Luigi Benedicenti received his Laurea in Electrical Engineering and Ph.D. in Electrical and Computer Engineering from the University of Genoa, Italy. Benedicenti is a professor in the Faculty of Engineering at the University of Regina, where he performs his research. He is the Associate Dean of Engineering in charge of Special Projects. He has served on several advisory boards and is currently a member of the Board of Directors of SpringBoard West Innovation. Benedicenti's current research is in three areas: Software Agents, Software Metrics, and New Media Technology. Research in Software Agents involves the characterization of software agents and the best applications for the agent model. Research in Software Metrics aims at characterizing agile development methods with a corresponding lightweight metrics program. Research in New Media Technology is directed towards harnessing distributed computing and advanced visualization techniques like augmented reality for appropriate creation and delivery of media content.

Ajay Bhatia received the B.Sc. in information technology and the Masters in Computer Application from Guru Nanak Dev University and ICFAI University in 2004 and 2007 respectively. He is serving as a lecturer in the department of computer science at CTIM&IT, India. His research interests include intelligent agents, Web 2.0 and mathematical computing languages.

Georgiy Bobashev is a Senior Research Statistician at RTI International with almost 20 years of experience in complex systems analysis, mathematical modeling, and statistical methods. He has received his Master's degree in Mechanics and Control Processes from St-Petersburg Technical University in 1989, Ph.D. in Biomathematics from the North Carolina State University in 1997, and Postdoctoral training from the School of Public Health at Johns Hopkins University in 1998. At RTI Georgiy leads a modeling domain team, and his research interests are focused on the application of mathematical and simulation methods to health and behavior, as well as on mathematical foundations of agent-based modeling. Georgiy is a non-resident Fellow at the Brookings Institution and an Adjunct Faculty at North Carolina State University

Andrei Borshchev, Co-founder and CEO, XJ Technologies. Andrei received his MSc in 1989 from Technical University of St.-Petersburg, Russia in Computer Science & Complex Systems Modeling. In early 1990s he worked for Hewlett-Packard Labs applying verification and simulation techniques to a number of HP products. Co-founded XJ Technologies in 1992. Completed PhD in Simulation Modeling in the Technical University of St.-Petersburg in 1995. From 1998 he led the design and development of an innovative multi-method simulation tool AnyLogic, and then its launch in the commercial simulation tool market. Andrei is a member of the System Dynamics Society and a constant contributor to the International System Dynamics Conference, the Winter Simulation Conference and other major events in the worldwide simulation community. Andrei has published over 50 papers and conducted numerous lectures, workshops, and training sessions on simulation modeling and AnyLogic.

Jörg Denzinger is an Associate Professor of Computer Science at the University of Calgary and his main areas of interest are Artificial Intelligence and Multi-Agent Systems. He has a PhD from the University of Kaiserslautern (1993), where he also did his Habilitation (2000). His students and he have done projects ranging from AI-based software and policy testing over distributed heterogeneous data mining and learning of cooperative behavior of agents to cooperative / competitive multi-agent search. He is a member of the Centre for Information Security and Cryptography and a fellow of the Institute of Advanced Policy Research, both at the University of Calgary.

Syamala Devi was born in Vizianagaram, India in 1958. She received her M.Sc. degree in Applied Mathematics from Andhra University, M.E. degree in Computer Science & Engineering from Allahabad University and Ph.D. degree in Computer Science from Andhra University in 1980, 1994 and 2004 respectively. Presently she is a Professor in the Department of Computer Science and Applications, Panjab University, Chandigarh. She is a senior member of Computer Society of India. Her main research interests include distributed artificial intelligence, educational computing, and simulation of computer based laboratory experiments.

Darshan Dillon is a Masters by Research student at the Digital Ecosystems and Business Intelligence Institute of the Curtin University of Technology. His major area of research is the use of multi-agent ontology's to detect financial statement fraud. He has special interest in the use of UML to do conceptual modeling of Multi-Agent Systems. He has also co-authored papers a large number of papers on these and related topics.

Tarek Y. ElMekkawy received his BSc and an MSc from the Department of Mechanical Design and Production, Cairo University, Egypt in 1990 and 1994, respectively. He received his PhD from the Department of Industrial and Manufacturing Engineering, University of Windsor, Canada, in 2001. He joined the University of Manitoba (UM) in 2003 after working for two years in automotive industry, Ontario, Canada. His research interest is in the areas of scheduling optimization, and applications of operational research and industrial engineering techniques to improve healthcare delivery. He has published many papers in international journals, such as *IJPR, IJPE, IJCIM, IJAMT, IJOR,* and *CIRP Annals*.

Simerjit Gill is M.A.Sc. student in the Department of Electronic Systems Engineering at the University of Regina, Regina, Canada. Simerjit received his Master in Information Technology (M.I.T.) degree from De La Salle University Manila, Philippines in 2007. He completed his Bachelor's degree in Computer Engineering from AMA Computer College Makati, Philippines in 2006. His research interests are in software agents, e-health, healthcare simulation and modeling, information security and web development. He is presently doing a research on agent-based healthcare simulation and modeling, funded by TRLabs Canada.

Maja Hadzic holds PhD in Health Information Systems and is currently a Research Fellow at the Digital Ecosystems and Business Intelligence Institute of the Curtin University of Technology. She has a multi-disciplinary background and her current research interests include Ontologies, Multi-agent Systems, Data Mining, Mental Health and Total Wellbeing. She has a large number of publications on these topics, including 1 book, 5 book chapters, 5 journals and more than 10 conference papers.

Julie Hiner is currently a model architect for military communication systems at General Dynamics Canada. She received both her BSc and MSc in Computer Science with a specialty in network simulation from the University of Calgary. Julie has applied research and industry experience in network simulation of telecommunication and military systems. She also has experience in model driven systems engineering of military communication systems. Her research interests include architecture modeling, model driven system engineering, simulation, health informatics, multi agent system and global health.

David Isern is a researcher of the University Rovira i Virgili's Department of Computer Science and Mathematics. He is also associate professor of the Open University of Catalonia. He received his PhD in Artificial Intelligence (2009) and an MSc (2005) from the Technical University of Catalonia. His research interests are intelligent software agents, distributed systems, user's preferences management, and ontologies, especially applied in healthcare and information retrieval systems. He has been involved in several research projects (National and European), and published several papers and conference contributions.

Vijay Kumar Mago received the B.A. degree in Mathematics and the Masters degree in Computer Application in 1998 and 2001 respectively from Guru Nanak Dev University, India. Currently he is pursuing Ph.D degree in Computer Science from Panjab University, India. His research interests include decision making in multi-agent environment, probabilistic networks, neural networks and fuzzy based expert systems. He has served on the program committees of many international conferences and workshops, including the International Conference on Artificial Intelligence and Pattern Recognition (AIPR-08), International Conference on Enterprise Information Systems and Web Technologies (EISWT-08) and Indian International Conference on Artificial Intelligence (IICAI-09).

Ravinder Mehta received his M.B.B.S. degree from Medical College, Patiala (Punjabi University, Patiala) and the M.D. degree from L.L.R.M. Medical College, Meerut (C.C.S. University, Meerut) in 1998 and 2002 respectively. He was Senior Resident (Pediatric) at U.C.M.S. & G.T.B. Hospital, Delhi in 2002. He has spent 3 years as Consultant Pediatrics at Vijayanand Diagnostic Center at Ludhiana. Currently, he is working as pediatric consultant at Community Health Center, Punjab, India. His main research interests include Neonatal Sepsis and application of soft computing techniques in medical decision making.

Antonio Moreno is a Lecturer at the University Rovira i Virgili's Computer Science and Mathematics Department. He is the founder and head of the ITAKA research group (Intelligent Techniques for Advanced Knowledge Acquisition). His main research interests are the application of agent technology to problems in diverse domains (health care, Tourism) and ontology learning from the Web. He was the coordinator of the Spanish network on agents and multi-agent technology. He has organised several workshops on agents applied in healthcare in the most prestigious international scientific conferences. He has acted as invited editor of special issues in AI Communications, Artificial Intelligence in Medicine and IEEE Intelligent Systems, and he has also edited several books.

Qing Niu is a Master student of the Department of Mechanical and Manufacturing Engineering, University of Manitoba, Canada. She received her Bachelor's Degree from Southwest Jiaotong University, Chengdu, China. Her research is simulation modeling and optimization for healthcare systems.

Qingjin Peng is an Associate Professor of the Department of Mechanical and Manufacturing Engineering at the University of Manitoba, Canada. He received his Doctorate at the University of Birmingham, UK in 1998. His research areas cover virtual manufacturing, system modeling and simulation. He has published over 80 refereed papers in international journals and conferences. He is a registered professional engineer and a member of ASME.

Nancy E. Reed received the Bachelor of Science degree in Biology, and the Masters and Ph.D. degrees in Computer Science from the University of Minnesota, Minneapolis. She is an Assistant Professor in the Information and Computer Sciences Department at the University of Hawai'i at Mānoa. Before coming to Hawai'i, Dr. Reed was an Associate Professor in the Computer and Information Sciences Department at Linköping University in Sweden. Earlier, she was an Adjunct Assistant Professor in the Computer Science Department at the University of California, Davis. Dr. Reed's primary research interests are in artificial intelligence, specifically autonomous agents, knowledge-based systems, and medical informatics. Recent research activities include the design of autonomous agent systems and developing computational diagnostic models for medical applications. Dr. Reed is a member of the AAAI, ACM, AHA, AMIA, and IEEE, including the IEEE Computer and Bioinformatics Societies.

Venkatraman Sadanand is currently an Associate Professor of Neurosurgery and Pediatrics in the Division of Neurosurgery, Department of Surgery in the University of Saskatchewan. He is also the Director of Research and Graduate Studies in the Department of Surgery and the Surgical Director of the Saskatchewan Epilepsy Program. He completed his undergraduate degree in Electrical Engineering at the Indian Institute of Technology and a M.S and Ph.D from the California Institute of Technology. He earned an MD from the University of Toronto, trained in Neurosurgery at the University of Saskatchewan and completed a research fellowship at the University of Toronto and a Pediatric neurosurgery fellowship at the Children's Memorial Hospital, Northwestern University in the United States. His current clinical interests are in pediatric neurosurgery and epilepsy surgery and research interests are in health economics and epidemiology.

Bhavesh Shrestha received B.E degree(2003) in Computer Engineering from Kathmandu University, Nepal, the M.S. degree (2007) in Computer Science from University of Massachusetts, Dartmouth, MA. During his study at University of Massachusetts, he worked as a research assistant under the supervision of Dr. Xiaoqin(Shelly) Zhang. Beginning March 2008, he has been working as a Software Engineer for Vecna Technologies at Cambridge. His research interests include multi-agent systems and web services.

Chitsutha Soomlek is a Ph.D. student in the Department of Electronic Systems Engineering at the University of Regina, Regina, Canada. Soomlek received her MA.Sc. in Electronic Systems Engineering from the University of Regina, Regina, Canada in 2007. She received her B.E. in Computer Engineering from King Mongkut's Institute of Technology Ladkrabang, Bangkok, Thailand in 2004. Soomlek has been a Thai scholar since 2004. Her research interests are in the areas of mobile agents and their applications, software engineering, computer network, visualization, distributed computing, computer and network security, and database system. Soomlek's current research involves software agents, visualization systems, and clinical decision-support systems.

Dale Vincent is a graduate of the United States Military Academy at West Point, and received his M.D. degree from the University of Texas Southwestern Medical School at Dallas. He completed a fellowship in General Internal Medicine at Walter Reed Army Medical Center, and holds a Masters Degree in Public Health. Board Certified in Internal Medicine and Geriatrics, and a Fellow of the American College of Physicians, Dr. Vincent is an Adjunct Associate Professor at the Telehealth Research Institute, and an Assistant Clinical Professor of Medicine at the University of Hawai'i John A. Burns School of Medicine. Dr. Vincent has extensive experience in using advanced distributed learning methods and human patient simulators for medical education. He and his colleagues recently demonstrated the efficacy of a 3D immersive virtual reality application developed at the Telehealth Research Institute to teach mass casualty triage skills to first responders.

Kin Lik Wang received his Bachelor of Science and Master of Science degrees in Computer Science from the University of Hawai'i at Mānoa in 2003 and 2006, respectively. For his M.S., he developed "A Multi-agent Simulation of Kidney Function". In 2004, he was a research assistant and became a software developer in 2007 at the Telehealth Research Institute, John A. Burns School of Medicine at the University of Hawai'i. His projects include the Virtual Nephron and Virtual Reality Triage simulations. His fields of interest are artificial intelligence, autonomous agents, computer graphics, virtual reality, simulation, and web programming. Recent research activities include a simulator and trainer for extracorporeal membrane oxygenation (ECMO) and a web-based patient monitoring system.

Yikun Xie is a Master student of the Department of Mechanical and Manufacturing Engineering, University of Manitoba, Canada. He received his Bachelor's Degree from Anhui University of Science & Technology. He served for Siemens Ltd., China, Industry Sector, Industry Automation & Drive Technologies (SLC I IA&DT) for 5 years and GEA Group, Division of Process Engineering for 4 years. His current research includes agent- based systems and applications in simulation with value stream mapping for healthcare systems

Haiping Xu received the B.S. degree (1989) in Electrical Engineering from Zhejiang University, Hangzhou, China, the M.S. degree (1998) in Computer Science from Wright State University, Dayton, Ohio, and the Ph.D. degree (2003) in Computer Science from the University of Illinois at Chicago. Prior to 1996, he successively worked with Shen-Yan Systems Technology, Inc. and Hewlett-Packard Co., as a software engineer, in Beijing, China. Since 2003, he has been with the University of Massachusetts Dartmouth, where he is currently an Assistant Professor at the Computer and Information Science Department, and a Co-Director of the Concurrent Software Engineering Laboratory (CSEL). His research interests include distributed software engineering, formal methods, Internet security, multi-agent systems, and service-oriented architecture (SOA). His research has been supported by the National Science Foundation (NSF) and the U.S. Marine Corps. He is a senior member of the IEEE Computer Society and a professional member of the ACM.

Dean Yergens is Manager, Medical Informatics at the University of Manitoba, Faculty of Medicine and Director, Medical Informatics in the Department of Research at the Health Sciences Centre in Winnipeg, Canada. He received his BSc in Computer Science from the University of Calgary and has worked in the area of Medical Informatics for over 10 years in various positions at the Calgary Health Region, Alberta Research Council, University of Calgary and the University of Manitoba. He also lived in Malawi, Africa and continues to be in involved in international medical informatics projects in Malawi, Zambia, Kenya and the Philippines. His primary research agenda is deriving secondary information from primary data sources utilizing simulation, multi-agent systems, machine learning, geographical information systems and real-time data management systems.

Xiaoqin Zhang received her B.S. degree in computer science from University Of Science & Technology Of China in 1995, and the M.S. and Ph.D degree in computer science from University of Massachusetts at Amherst in 1998 and 2002, respectively. She is an Associate Professor of CIS Department at the University of Massachusetts on the Dartmouth campus, she joined this campus since 2002. Her major research focus is on multi-agent systems and intelligent agents. She has done research work in the following areas: sophisticated negotiation and cooperation in multi-agent systems, intelligent agent architecture designing, agent control and reasoning under uncertainty, and information gathering.

Index